THE GYNECOLOGIST AND THE OLDER PATIENT

Edited by
James L. Breen, MD

Chairman, Department of Obstetrics and Gynecology
Saint Barnabas Medical Center
Livingston, New Jersey

Clinical Professor of Obstetrics and Gynecology
Jefferson Medical College
Philadelphia, Pennsylvania

AN ASPEN PUBLICATION®
Aspen Publishers, Inc.
1988
Rockville, Maryland
Royal Tunbridge Wells

Library of Congress Cataloging-in-Publication Data

The Gynecologist and the older patient/[edited by] James L. Breen.
p. cm.
"An Aspen publication."
Includes bibliographies and index.
ISBN: 0-87189-773-3
1. Geriatric gynecology. 2. Aged women--Diseases. I. Breen, James L., 1926- .
[DNLM: 1. Geriatric Diseases, Female--in old age. 2. Geriatrics.
WP 140 G99714]
RG103.G97   1988   618.97'81--dc19   DNLM/DLC
for Library of Congress
88-6328
CIP

Copyright © 1988 by Aspen Publishers, Inc.
All rights reserved.

Aspen Publishers, Inc., grants permission for photocopying for personal or internal use, or for the personal or internal use of specific clients registered with the Copyright Clearance Center (CCC). This consent is given on the condition that the copier pay a $1.00 fee plus $.12 per page for each photocopy through the CCC for photocopying beyond that permitted by the U.S. Copyright Law. The fee should be paid directly to the CCC, 21 Congress St., Salem, Massachusetts 01970.
0-87189-773-3/88 $1.00 + .12.

This consent does not extend to other kinds of copying, such as copying for general distribution, for advertising or promotional purposes, for creating new collective works, or for resale. For information, address Aspen Publishers, Inc., 1600 Research Boulevard, Rockville, Maryland 20850.

The author's have made every effort to ensure the accuracy of the information herein, particularly with regard to drug selection and dose. However, appropriate information sources should be consulted, especially for new or unfamiliar drugs or procedures. It is the responsibility of every practitioner to evaluate the appropriateness of a particular opinion in the context of actual clinical situations and with due consideration to new developments. Authors, editors, and the publisher cannot be held responsible for any typographical or other errors found in this book.

Editorial Services: Mary Beth Roesser

Library of Congress Catalog Card Number: 88-6328
ISBN: 0-87189-773-3

Printed in the United States of America

1 2 3 4 5

Table of Contents

List of Contributors xv

Preface xi

PART I—INTRODUCTION 1

Chapter 1—**A Look at Older Americans** 3
        Morton A. Lebow

        Proportion of Men/Women 4
        The Aged Aged 7
        Women and Morbidity 7
        Use of Health Services 9
        Where They Live 10
        Attitudes Toward Health Care 11
        Conclusion 12

PART II—MEDICAL PROBLEMS OF THE OLDER WOMAN ... 15

Chapter 2—**Geriatric Endocrinology** 17
        Robert S. Modlinger

        Pituitary 17
        Thyroid 18
        Parathyroid 23
        Adrenal Gland 27
        Ovary 29
        Diabetes Mellitus 30

Chapter 3—Mammography in the 1980s: The Detection of
          Minimal Breast Cancer 39
          Robert J. DiBenedetto

Chapter 4—Dermatologic Lesions in the Elderly
          Gynecologic Patient 75
          Roger Harrison Brodkin and Cynthia E. Saporito

     Dermatitis 75
     Papulosquamous Dermatoses 77
     Infections and Infestations 78
     Nonsymptomatic Conditions 80
     Conditions That Affect the Vulva 81
     Tumors 84
     Alopecia 90
     Pruritus Vulvae 92

Chapter 5—Hypertension and Renal Diseases in Elderly Women .. 93
          Michael Gutkin and Lawrence H. Byrd

     Introduction 93
     Determinants of High Blood Pressure 94
     Changes in Circulation with Aging 94
     Changes in Renal Function with Aging 95
     Definitions of Hypertension 95
     Rise of Systolic Blood Pressure with Age 96
     Wasted Cardiac Work 96
     Cardiovascular Disease in Hypertensive Women 96
     Risk Factors for Heart Disease in Elderly Women 98
     Risk Factors for Stroke in Elderly Women 100
     High-Risk Patients 102
     The Principle of Multiple Risk Factors 102
     The Benefit of Antihypertensive Therapy:
        Randomized Prospective Trials 104
     Trials That Compared Drug with Placebo Treatment 106
     Trials That Compared One Type of Treatment
        with Another 108
     Implications of Findings for Mild Hypertensives 109
     Blood Pressure Treatment in the Very Old 110
     Measurement of Blood Pressure 111
     Ambulatory Blood Pressure Monitoring 113

	Recommendations for Treating the Elderly	
	Hypertensive Woman	114
	Drug Therapy	116
	Pseudohypertension	121
	Renal Disease in the Aged	121
Chapter 6—	**Gastroenterology and the Aging Gastrointestinal Tract**	**131**
	William C. Sloan	
	Introduction	131
	Dysphagia	131
	Jaundice	133
	Gastrointestinal Endoscopy	134
	Ulcers	136
Chapter 7—	**Constipation and Rectal Bleeding in the Elderly**	**139**
	Glen Mogan	
	Introduction	139
	Constipation	139
	Rectal Bleeding	141
	Nutrition	146
Chapter 8—	**Infectious Diseases of the Aged**	**151**
	Leon G. Smith, Leon G. Smith, Jr., and Paul R. Summers	
	Introduction	151
	Host Defense	151
	Vaginal Flora	152
	Gardnerella Vaginalis, Trichomonas, and	
	Other Vaginitis	152
	Gonococcal Infection	153
	Bacteriologic Sepsis from Inapparent Atrophied	
	Gynecologic Site	153
	Postmenopausal Tubo-Ovarian Abscess	154
	Pyomyoma	155
	Pessary Infection	155
	Unusual Infections of the Female Genital Tract	155
	Genital Elephantiasis (Lymphedema)	156
	Postmenopausal Pelvic Tuberculosis	156

Pressure Ulcers 157
Genital Fistuals 157
Myiasis in the Genital Tract 158
Pyoderma Gangrenosum of the Genitalia 158
Interstitial Cystitis with Vaginitis 158
Actinomycosis of the Pelvic Organs 159
Pinworms 159
Virus of the Genital Tract 160
Toxic Shock Syndrome 160
Acquired Immunodeficiency Syndrome 160
Antibiotics 161

Chapter 9—Psychiatric Aspects of Aging **169**
Hilda B. Templeton and Donald D. Scalea

Introduction 169
Sexuality 172
Menopause 173
Diagnostic Categories 175

Chapter 10—Musculoskeletal Problems **197**
Sheldon D. Solomon

Introduction 197
Classification of Musculoskeletal Problems 197
Differential Diagnosis 197
Specific Rheumatic Diseases of the Elderly Woman 200
Management of the Elderly Female with
  Pharmacologic Therapy 211
Case Discussions 215
Summary 217

**PART III—SELECTED SURGICAL AND GYNECOLOGICAL
PROBLEMS OF THE OLDER WOMAN** **219**

**Chapter 11—Urinary Incontinence in the Elderly:
A Clinician's Viewpoint** **221**
George L. Sexton, Jr.

Introduction 221
Classifications of Incontinence 221

Factors That Predispose to Types of
  Geriatric Incontinence 222
Diagnostic Evaluation of Geriatric Incontinence 226
Treatment Modalities for Geriatric Incontinence 231
Conclusion 243

Chapter 12—Urology for the Elderly Female 247
Eugene A. Stulberger and Stanley Bloom

Introduction 247
Urinary Tract Infection 247
Renal Calculi 261
Urinary Vaginal Fistula 267
Tumors 269

Chapter 13—Vulvar Changes with Aging 283
James A. Wilson II

Introduction 283
The Normal Aging Process 283
Age-Associated Vulvar Pathology 285
Vulvar Dystrophy 292

Chapter 14—Vaginal Changes with Aging 299
Paul A. Bergh

Introduction 299
Atrophic Vaginitis 299
Anatomy 299
Physiology 300
Ecology 303
Vaginal Infections 304
Noninfectious Vaginitis 308

Chapter 15—Anesthesia for the Aging Gynecologic Patient 313
Norman J. Zeig

Introduction 313
Aging and Anesthetic Risk 313
Anesthetic Risk 315

Ambulatory Care of the Aged Surgical
   Gynecological Patient 318
Monitoring 319
Temperature Control 322
Preoperative Medication 323
Recovery Room 326
Hypotension 329
Hypertension 329
Pain Control 329

Chapter 16—A Radiologist Looks at the Aging Patient 333
Alan G. Dembner

PART IV—OTHER ASPECTS OF AGING 337

Chapter 17—The Cost-Effectiveness of the Geriatric Patient 339
Richard Caruana, Alex MacDonald, and John D. Phillips

Educational Programs for the Elderly 340
Transportation for the Elderly 341
Discharge Planning and Placement 342
Geriatric Evaluation Unit 343
Additional Opportunities for Hospitals to Help
   the Elderly 344
Conclusion 345

Chapter 18—Medicolegal Issues in the Care of the Aged 347
Albert L. Strunk

Introduction 347
Preliminary Considerations 347
Competency 348
Informed Consent 349
No-Code Orders 350
Withdrawal of Life-Sustaining Treatment 351
Prognosis or Ethics Committees 351
The Role of the Courts 352
Abuse of the Elderly Patient 353
Conclusion 354

PART V—AN OVERVIEW OF GERONTOLOGY 357

Chapter 19—Assessment of the Older Woman 359
Maria A. Fiatarone and Laurence Z. Rubenstein

    Introduction 359
    Components of Assessment 361
    Principles of History Taking 377
    Physical Examination 381
    Specialized Geriatric Assessment Programs and
        Their Effectiveness 387
    Conclusions 391

Index 399

Editor

JAMES L. BREEN, M.D.
Chairman, Department of Obstetrics
  and Gynecology
St. Barnabas Medical Center
Livingston, New Jersey
Clinical Professor of Obstetrics and
  Gynecology
Jefferson Medical College
Philadelphia, Pennsylvania

Contributing Authors

PAUL A. BERGH, M.D.
Third Year Resident
Department of Obstetrics and
  Gynecology
St. Barnabas Medical Center
Livingston, New Jersey

STANLEY BLOOM, M.D.
Senior Attending Urologist
St. Barnabas Medical Center
Livingston, New Jersey
Clinical Instructor of Urology
The University of Medicine and
  Dentistry of New Jersey
Newark, New Jersey

ROGER HARRISON BRODKIN,
  M.D.
Clinical Professor of Medicine
Division of Dermatology
University of Medicine and Dentistry
  of New Jersey
Newark, New Jersey

LAWRENCE H. BYRD, M.D.
Attending Physician, Hypertension
  Section
St. Barnabas Medical Center
Livingston, New Jersey

RICHARD CARUANA, M.P.A.
Administrative Assistant for DRG
  Management
St. Barnabas Medical Center
Livingston, New Jersey

ALAN G. DEMBNER, M.D.
Attending Radiologist
St. Barnabas Medical Center
Livingston, New Jersey

ROBERT J. DiBENEDETTO, M.D.
Attending Physician, Department of
  Obstetrics/Gynecology
St. Barnabas Medical Center
Livingston, New Jersey

MARIA A. FIATARONE, M.D.
Instructor in Medicine
Division on Aging
Harvard Medical School
Boston, Massachusetts
Scientist III
Human Nutrition Research Center on
  Aging
Tufts New England Medical Center
Boston, Massachusetts

MICHAEL GUTKIN, M.D.
Chief, Hypertension Section
St. Barnabas Medical Center
Livingston, New Jersey

MORTON A. LEBOW, B.S.S.,
M.A.
Associate Director for Public
 Information
The American College of
 Obstetricians and Gynecologists
Washington, D.C.

ALEX MacDONALD, B.S., R.R.A.
Administrative Assistant
DRG Management
St. Barnabas Medical Center
Livingston, New Jersey

ROBERT S. MODLINGER, M.D.
Chief of Hypertension
Veteran's Administration Medical
 Center
East Orange, New Jersey
Chief of Endrocrinology
Mountainside Hospital
Mountclair, New Jersey

GLEN MOGAN, M.D.
Attending in Medicine and
 Gastroenterology
St. Barnabas Medical Center
Livingston, New Jersey

JOHN D. PHILLIPS, M.H.A.
Executive Vice-President
St. Barnabas Medical Center
Livingston, New Jersey

LAURENCE Z. RUBENSTEIN,
M.D.
Clinical Director of Geriatric
 Research Education and Clinical
 Center
Veteran's Administration Medical
 Center
Sepulveda, California

CYNTHIA E. SAPORITO, M.D.
Attending Physician
Department of Medicine
Cleveland Clinic
Cleveland, Ohio

DONALD D. SCALEA, M.D.
Associate Clinical Chief, Department
 of Psychiatry
St. Barnabas Medical Center
Livingston, New Jersey

GEORGE L. SEXTON JR., M.D.
Past Chairperson, Section of
 Gynecology
The Reading Hospital and Medical
 Center
Reading, Pennsylvania

WILLIAM C. SLOAN, M.D.
Attending in Medicine and
 Gastroenterology
St. Barnabas Medical Center
Livingston, New Jersey
Assistant Clinical Professor of
 Medicine
NJCMD
Newark, New Jersey

LEON G. SMITH, M.D.
Director of Medicine
Chief of Infectious Diseases
St. Michael's Medical Center
Professor of Medicine and Preventive
 Medicine
New Jersey Medical School
Newark, New Jersey

LEON G. SMITH JR., M.D.
Resident in Obstetrics and
 Gynecology

Tulane University Medical School
New Orleans, Louisiana

SHELDON D. SOLOMON, M.D.
Codirector, Arthritis Unit
Garden State Community Hospital
West Jersey Health Systems
Clinical Associate in Medicine
Department of Medicine
School of Medicine
University of Pennsylvania
Philadelphia, Pennsylvania

ALBERT L. STRUNK, J.D., M.D.
Attending Staff
Department of Obstetrics and
    Gynecology
St. Barnabas Medical Center
Livingston, New Jersey
Attending Staff
Department of Obstetrics and
    Gynecology
Muhlenberg Regional Medical Center
Plainfield, New Jersey

EUGENE A. STULBERGER
Senior Attending Urologist
St. Barnabas Medical Center
Livingston, New Jersey

Clinical Instructor of Urology
The University of Medicine and
    Dentistry of New Jersey
Newark, New Jersey

PAUL R. SUMMERS, M.D.
Assistant Professor
Department of Obstetrics and
    Gynecology
Tulane University School of Medicine
New Orleans, Louisiana

HILDA B. TEMPLETON, M.D.
Clinical Chief, Department of
    Psychiatry
St. Barnabas Medical Center
Livingston, New Jersey

JAMES A. WILSON II, M.D.
Attending Physician
Department of Obstetrics and
    Gynecology
Shore Memorial Hospital
Somers Point, New Jersey

NORMAN J. ZEIG, M.D.
Chairman, Department of
    Anesthesiology
St. Barnabas Medical Center
Livingston, New Jersey

Preface

As futurists speak of reassessment, reevaluation, and reinvention, little attention is given to one of our major health problems: the medical and social responsibility of properly caring for the elderly. We hear about the aging of America, but how large a problem is it? Statistics indicate that it is rapidly becoming a national crisis. Americans over age 65 represent the fastest-growing age group in the United States. Between 1900 and 1980 the population as a whole tripled, while the subgroup of those over 65 increased eightfold. By the year 2030, when our current younger generation will be into its seventh decade, the number of people over age 65 is expected to reach 55 million, constituting nearly one sixth of the US population.

A woman born today can look forward to a life span of 78.3 years, 7.5 years longer than that of a man. By the middle of the next century, her great granddaughter can expect to live for 83.6 years; and she, too, will outlive a man by 8.5 years.

The US population will increase from its current 230 million to an all-time high of 309 million by the year 2050, but the annual rate of growth will shrink from the current 0.9% to virtually zero. As we live through this decline, the trend toward an aging population will accelerate and become accentuated. Our attention, which is now focused on debates over social security, will be drawn more and more to that part of our population.

Pathological entities encountered in the elderly will become more and more prevalent as the 28 million women who are today aged 55 or older will grow to 68 million by the middle of the next century. As more women live longer, these population trends will have a profound effect on their health care. With increasing age comes an increase in the incidence of chronic conditions. Women have higher rates of all major chronic conditions, with the specific exceptions of coronary heart disease, emphysema, and gastrointestinal disorders.

Sources: Obstetrics and Gynecology (1983;62:403), Copyright © 1983, The American College of Obstetricians and Gynecologists; *Clinical Therapeutics* (1986;8:462), Copyright © 1986, Excerpta-Medica. Used with permission of Elsevier Science Publishing Company Inc.

As our patients age, we as physicians will be dealing with a clientele who will have looked for years on their gynecologist-obstetrician as their principal health care physician. These individuals will be coming to us with a variety of disorders that we are not used to seeing. We must, through one mechanism or another, train ourselves both mentally and medically to deal with an aging population who will continue to look on us as their principal health care source. We must also realize that we will no longer exist in a seller's but rather a buyer's market; therefore, with increasing competition, we must project that we will be obligated to continue caring for our patients in their waning years.

Is it not reasonable to assume that if pediatricians are extending care of their patients to age 21, thus becoming a new breed of physician—part psychiatrist, part gynecologist, part internist, part dermatologist, as well as pediatrician—that other specialists will do the same? Is it not reasonable to assume that specialties will begin to impinge on other specialties, whenever it becomes reasonable to do so, in the forthcoming geriatric era of medicine?

Of nearly 400,000 current members of the American Medical Association, only 720 identify themselves as having a major practice commitment to geriatrics. Many physicians feel uncomfortable and are not prepared to deal with the elderly. Recommendations for the elderly are mostly extrapolations from studies done on middle-aged adults; therefore, health care professionals are often ill-equipped to care for elderly patients.

Estimates indicate that by 1990, the United States will need 8,000 to 10,000 geriatric physicians to care for the growing elderly population. There is now no such category of individual with specific certification, and there probably never will be. It is predicted that each specialty will eventually develop a subset of criteria and training that relates specifically to geriatrics.

We gynecologists can give much more to our elderly patients than we are currently giving. Unfortunately, during our training years, we may have had minimal patient contact with elderly women. Residents and students are more likely to think of the elderly patient in terms of the 70-year-old whom they saw with terminal cancer rather than as the 70-year-old widow who is planning to remarry and is requesting sexual counseling. There is little literature on gerontology, and most practicing gynecologists are not well prepared to treat the aged. Yet women in this population will become the patients who will constitute a significant portion of our future practice.

As gynecologists, we must increase our skills in those areas that apply to the aged, a few of which are as follows:

1. *Oncology.* Elderly women are still at high risk for development of malignancies of the reproductive system.
2. *Treatable nonmalignant disorders that affect the quality of life.* Stress incontinence, vulvar dystrophy, uterine procidentia, and vaginal vault prolapse are examples.

3. *Sexuality*. With greatly increased longevity, sexuality has become an important concern of older women.
4. *Screening and preventive care*. Periodic screening, appropriate evaluation for high-risk patients, and early diagnosis for symptomatic women are important in this age group.
5. *Health maintenance counseling*. Osteoporosis can be prevented by appropriate diet, exercise, and estrogen therapy.
6. *Medical health maintenance*. Elderly patients need care for their noninsulin-dependent diabetes, hypertension, emotional disorders, and other medical problems. They may also need advice about organ replacement.
7. *Physician input into legislation concerning the elderly*. Such areas include Social Security, Medicare, and control of physician and hospital costs.

These seven entities, as they apply to any age category, fall within the area of expertise for the practicing gynecologist. The one area in which we are lacking, and in which we will be called on to serve, relates to the medical specialties that increasingly will impact on our aging population. It is not unreasonable to assume that when we anticipate that 1 out of every 4 of our patients will be age 65 or older, and that we will be treating many of their medical problems while caring for their gynecologic problems, in essence gynecology will take on certain medical overtones.

This text addresses the expanding spectrum of clinical patient care that may be managed by the gynecologist. A major portion of the book is directed toward the medical aspect of our specialty. That is, within what areas, and how far, may we go in treating our gynecologic patients (e.g., their arthritis or endocrinopathies, etc.).

It is not the purpose of this text to encompass all the problems facing our gerontologic patients. For example, because the literature is already so profuse with regard to upper genital tract abnormalities as seen in the elderly, cancer of the ovary, uterus, and cervix is not covered.

It is the intent of the authors that all chapters be written in a manner to cover those areas that we, as obstetricians and gynecologists, should feel professionally competent about when it comes to taking care of the gynecologic infirmities of the aging patient as relating to medicine and, selectively, several surgical areas that may present problems.

There will be limitations, however, to how much we should do, and therefore we will still maintain the concept of triage for problems that exceed our knowledge and capabilities.

James L. Breen
June 1988

Part I
Introduction

Chapter 1

A Look at Older Americans

Morton A. Lebow

On July 1, 1983, for the first time in history, there were more elderly people living in the United States than there were teenagers.[1] Never again will teenagers outnumber senior citizens. A trend that has been going on, like the aging processes, inexorably and unnoticed, has now captured national attention.

Since 1960 the over-65 age group has grown more than twice as fast as the younger population. In 1960 there were 16.7 million elderly in the United States; by 1985 there were 28.7 million, an increase of 72%. This compares with an increase of less than 25% for the rest of the population. During the same period—1960 to 1985—in addition to increasing in numbers, the elderly increased as a proportion of the population. In 1960 those who were 65 or over accounted for 9.1% of the population (fewer than 1 in 10). By 1985 the elderly had become 12% of the population.[1] The number and the rapidly rising proportion have caused us as a nation to take a searching look at our national policies.

As more and more people join the ranks of the elderly, we have reexamined our national employment and retirement policies and have taken a searching look at the entire range of social and political issues. The graying of America has provoked congressional debate over the future of Social Security, Medicare, and Medicaid and has caused the government, industry, the medical establishment, and almost all segments of society to undertake careful and, in some cases, frantic consideration of the effect a growing, aging population will have on our institutions.

Today's aged population of 28.7 million is just the forerunner of a wave of the future. By the turn of the century the elderly population will grow to 35 million, or 13.1% of the population; and by the year 2050—the midpoint of the next century—the elderly will number 67 million and make up almost 22% of the population—more than 1 out of every 5 (Figure 1-1).[1]

The increasing life expectancies will mean an older age structure than we have now. The median age will increase from 1981's 30.3 years to 36.3 in the year

4   THE GYNECOLOGIST AND THE OLDER PATIENT

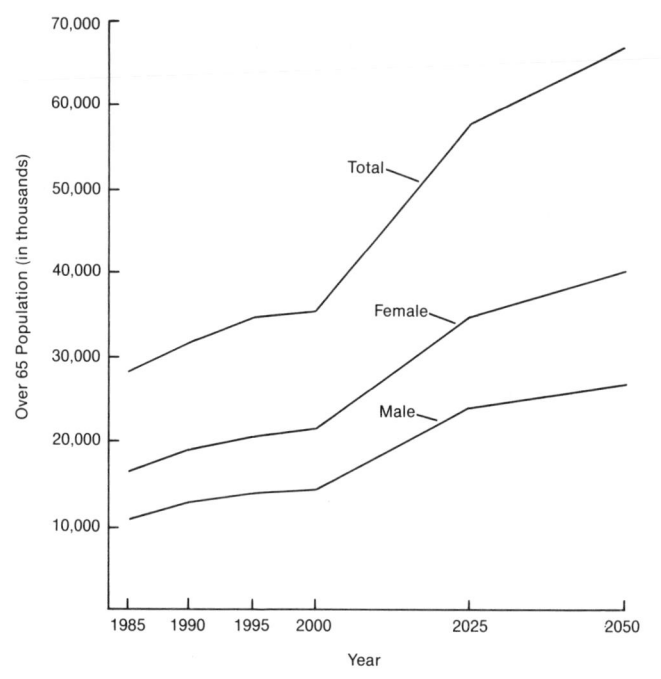

Figure 1-1 Population over age 65, by sex. *Source: Projection of Population of the United States: 1982 to 2050,* Series P-25, No 922, Bureau of the Census, October 1982.

2000 and 41.6 in 2050. As more people live longer, chronic diseases become the major causes of death and disability—quite different from the infectious disease causes we saw in the first half of the 20th century. Our success in reducing death rates from heart disease, influenza, cerebrovascular disease, and other frequent causes of death has contributed greatly to the growth of the elderly population.[2] As this population continues to grow, we will witness an increase in the total number of deaths. It will grow from its current 2 million annually to more than 3.7 million in 2035, when, for the first time, deaths will outnumber births in the United States. Immigration will keep the US population growing until about the year 2050. After that, the population will begin to decline. By then the number of deaths will reach 3.9 million annually (Figure 1-2).[1]

PROPORTION OF MEN/WOMEN

In the United States, as in practically all industrialized countries, women live longer than men. This was not always so. In 1920, in the aftermath of the great influenza epidemics, the traditional advantage that men had over women in average life expectancy had all but vanished, especially for those people age 65 or

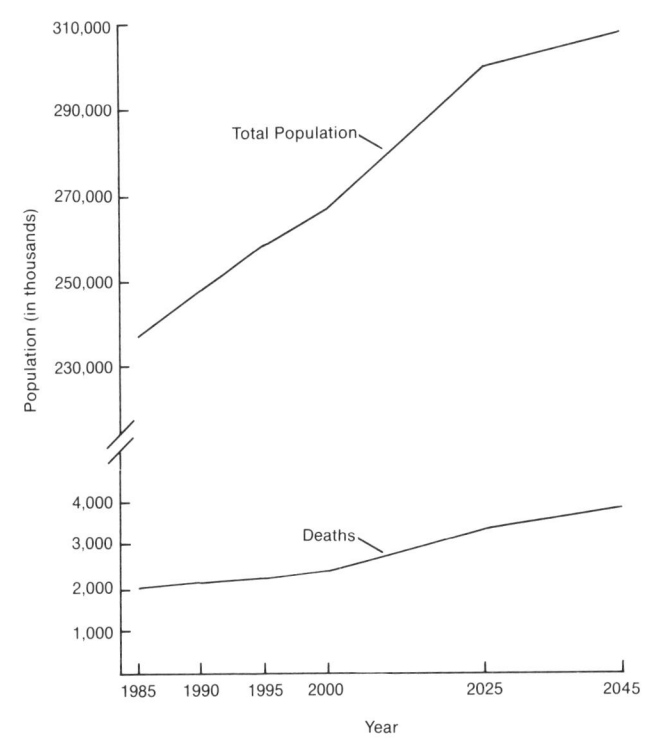

Figure 1-2 Population and deaths. *Source: Projection of Population of the United States: 1982 to 2050,* Series P-25, No 922, Bureau of the Census, October 1982.

---

older. Since 1920 the gap in life expectancy has steadily increased. A girl born today can look forward to a life expectancy of 78.3 years. This is 7.3 years longer than her twin brother.

Since 1970 there has been some stabilization in the difference between the life expectancy of men and women. Although the gap has widened by 1 year or more in each decade since 1920, it has not increased in the 15 years since 1970 (Figure 1-3).[3]

Our great granddaughters who will be born in the year 2050 may expect to live for 83.6 years, more than 5 years having been added to their life expectancies. By then women may be outliving men by 8.5 years.

Much of this increase in life expectancy has taken place at the beginning of life, where we have been so successful in reducing infant mortality to its current impressively low levels. We have also been successful in adding years at the end of life. Today a woman who reaches age 65 can expect to live for another 18.8 years, compared with a man's expectations of 14.5 years.[1] This represents an increase of almost 4 years for women since 1950, compared with less than a 2-year increase

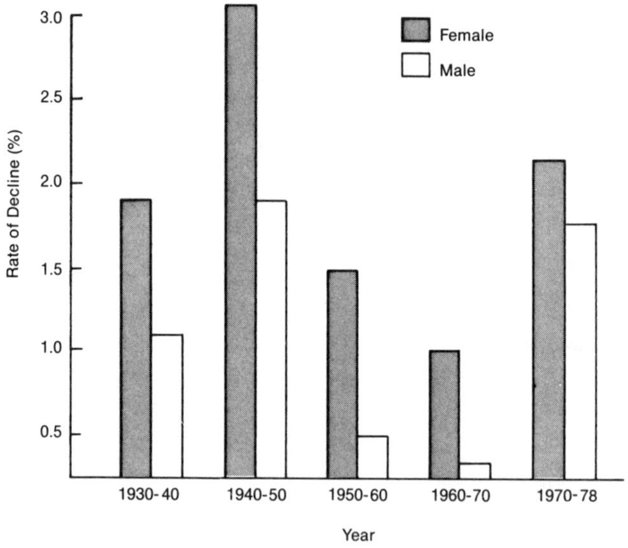

6   THE GYNECOLOGIST AND THE OLDER PATIENT

Figure 1-3 Anuual rates of decline in age-adjusted death rates. *Source: Vital and Health Statistics,* Series 13, Number 51, DHHS Pub No 81-1,712, National Center for Health Statistics, US Government Printing Office, April 1981.

---

for men. The advantage that women have is growing more slowly than in the past. This slowing does not indicate any deterioration in the health of women, but a great improvement, especially in the past decade, in the death rates of men.[2]

The age-adjusted death rate for males exceeds that for females. In 1930 it was 1.2 times the rate for females, by 1960 it was 1.6 times, and in 1978 it had reached 1.8. The age-adjusted rate for males was 80% higher than that for females.[3]

Women in the age group of 65 or over are the fastest growing segment of this nation's population. Today's 17.2 million women who are 65 or over will grow to 21.3 million by the year 2000. At that time there will be 21.3 million elderly women and 13.7 million elderly men. By the year 2050 America's 40 million elderly women will continue to outnumber the country's 27 million elderly men.[1]

The increased survivorship of women is an important accomplishment. Looking back just 100 years we get the picture of many women dying in childbirth. As recently as 1940, 376 out of every 100,000 women died as a result of childbirth. Today maternal mortality is the rare exception, and more and more women reach a healthy and active old age.[4]

Since the latter part of the 1960s there has been a decline in mortality rates for all groups in the population. The declining mortality rates for the over-65 group of both men and women have been more persistent and striking. This has led to a much higher rate of growth in the number and proportion of elderly in the population. Despite the fact that both men and women are living longer, the numerical advantage held by women continues to increase with time, especially in the elderly population. The expected leveling off of this advantage as more and more women entered the job market and competed for jobs along with men has failed to materialize. Women continue to hold their lead in life expectancy at all ages and are expected to slowly add to that lead well into the next century.

THE AGED AGED

The percentage of the population that reaches age 85 and beyond is growing at a faster rate than the population aged 65 to 84. As this phenomenon accelerates, the advantage in female survivorship will become more pronounced. This has led Dr Robert Butler, former Director of the National Institute on Aging, to call the next century "the Century of the Older Woman."

Today there are 2.8 million persons over age 85: 2 million women and 800,000 men—a 5-to-2 advantage. By the year 2000 this population group will grow by 82% to 5.1 million, made up of 3.7 million women—an increase of 85%—and 1.4 million men—an increase of 75%. By the midpoint of the next century the number of people age 85 or over will reach more than 16 million, an increase of more than 57%. In the year 2050 we can expect to see 11.4 million women and 4.6 million men who have reached their 85th birthday (Figure 1-4).[1]

One dramatic indication of this trend is the number who reach their 100th birthday. In the past decade we could see this trend develop clearly and suddenly. In 1970, according to the Social Security Administration, 4,574 persons reached this landmark; by 1985 more than 25,000 Americans had become centenarians, and more than two thirds of these were women.[5]

WOMEN AND MORBIDITY

Women's advantage in mortality and life expectancy figures does not extend to morbidity. Women have more illnesses and disabilities than do men; they visit doctors more often and are hospitalized at higher rates.

In looking at the data we can agree with Dr Robert Butler, who says that "the problems of old age in America are largely the problems of women." Women have a higher incidence of respiratory conditions than do men (pneumonia excepted). They also have a higher incidence of digestive system conditions and infectious diseases, but they do have significantly fewer injuries from accidents. Once women reach age 65 they die at much lower rates than men from diseases of the heart, malignant neoplasms, and influenza and pneumonia, but they have a slightly higher death rate from cerebrovascular diseases and arteriosclerosis.

8   THE GYNECOLOGIST AND THE OLDER PATIENT

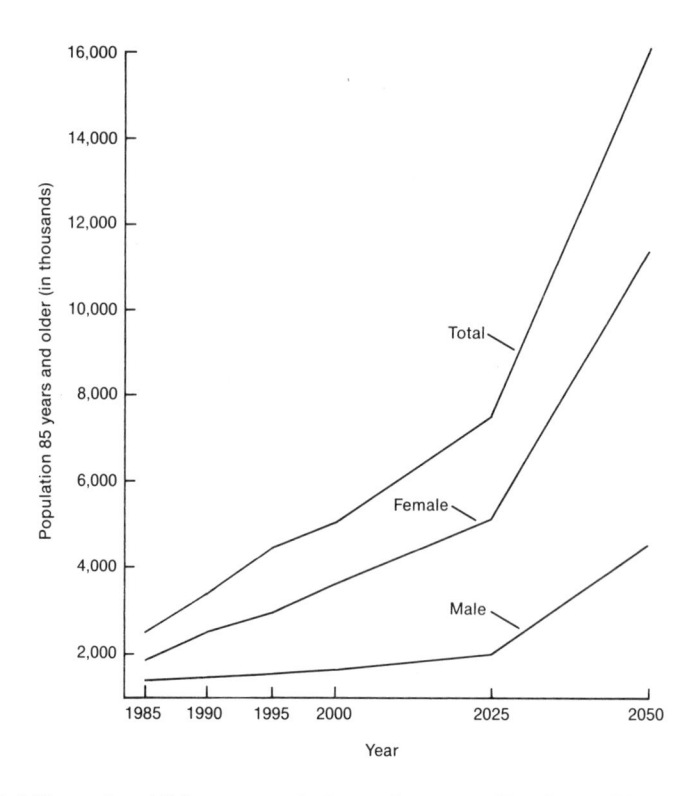

Figure 1-4 The aged aged (85 years or over). *Source: Projection of Population of the United States: 1982 to 2050,* Series P-25, No 922, Bureau of the Census, October 1982.

Women also have a tremendously higher incidence of such chronic conditions as varicose veins, poor circulation, constipation, gallbladder condition, enteritis and colitis, and intestinal conditions. They are five times more likely than men to have thyroid and anemia disorders and about three times more likely to suffer migraine and diseases of the urinary system. But they suffer significantly lower rates of visual, hearing, and speech impairments.

Improvement in survival to advanced ages gives some indication that many people who survive to advanced ages will do so in good health. Studies of this phenomenon are in progress.[6]

Looking at the major causes of death today for people over age 65, the data show that women die at a much lower rate than men at all age groupings. Today the rate of death for all causes for the 65-to-69 age group is twice as high for men as for women. In the future there will be a steady drop in the death rate, but the rate for women will hold at one half that for men well into the next century.

USE OF HEALTH SERVICES

Women's use of health services and facilities is quite different from that of men. In 1979 the average American woman visited her physician's office more than three times; the average man went twice. Older people visit doctors more often than young people. The number of physician visits by Americans of all ages will increase in the future as a larger percentage of the population becomes older. The 1.1 billion physician visits in 1980 will grow to 1.6 billion in the year 2040, an increase of 47% largely because of the greater number of visits by the aged.[7]

There will be a different effect on hospitals and nursing homes—different and more intense. Short-stay hospital days will almost double from 264 million in 1980 to 508 million in 2040, with more than half of this increase owing to the aging factor. The very old, 85 years or older, will account for 56% of the days of care in 2040, compared with 37% in 1980.[7]

Over the past 20 years the number of people in nursing homes substantially increased, and indications are that the number will continue to grow at a considerable rate. One prominent reason is the large increase in the population 85 or older. In 1980 nearly $21 billion was spent on nursing home care, with Medicaid providing a major share. By 2040 there will be a projected 5.2 million nursing home residents, compared with 1.5 million in 1980—a 350% increase. About 87% of the residents will be aged 75 or over.

The vast majority of elderly people in the United States, however, live in the community. About 95% of all people 65 or older are *not* in nursing homes; however, women 65 or older are twice as likely as men to be living in nursing homes. In 1977 that ratio was 59.7 women for each 1,000, compared with 30.7 for men.[3]

Adult women visited physicians' offices approximately 350 million times in 1978, an average of 3.2 visits for each woman in the civilian population. Although women over age 65 made only 16% of these visits, they averaged 4.2 visits a year. This rate was higher than for all other groups in the population.

Visits to the gynecologist, not surprisingly, did not loom large. Only 2.3% of all visits by women between the ages of 65 and 74 were to the gynecologist. For the female population age 75 or older, this percentage dropped to 0.9%. Visits to general and family practitioners and internists accounted for 61.2% of the 65-to-74 age group and 63.5% of the 75 or older group.[8]

For each 1,000 women age 65 or older, 8.2 would see their physicians for female troubles other than breast disease. More than 600,000 (1.1%) visited doctors' offices for malignant neoplasm of the breast.

In 1978, 17.9% of women between ages 65 and 74 had general, and 64.6% had limited, medical examinations. Only 4.8% had Pap tests. In the group age 75 or over, 66.5% had limited examinations, 18.6% had general examinations, and 2.2% had Pap tests.

Malignant neoplasms of the breast, uterus, and other female genital organs accounted for 1.2% of all office visits and 2.8% of all hospital discharges for the 65-or-over group. Fractures accounted for 1.0% of office visits and 5.3% of hospital discharges.

An estimated 4.8 million women 65 years of age or older were discharged from short-stay hospitals in 1978. Of these 31.2% were married, 59.0% were widowed, 3.2% were divorced or separated, and 6.6% were never married.

Heart disease was the most common diagnosis for all hospitalized women 45 years of age or over; this diagnosis becomes more common as age increases. It ranges from 3% for the 45-to-64 age group to 11% for those 85 years or over. The incidence of surgery for breast and gynecologic reasons drops with advancing age. The rate for each 10,000 population drops from 54 in the 45-to-64 group for breast surgery to 47 for the 65-to-74 group, and to 46 for those 75 years or older. For gynecologic surgery the rate drops from 366 to 166 to 102, respectively.

Gynecologic operations such as dilation and curettage and hysterectomy, which accounted for 20% of the operations performed on women of middle age, dropped in frequency and were not in the top 62% of operations for women age 85 or over.

The average length of stay in hospitals varied according to the severity of the condition and the living arrangements once out of the hospital. The average length of stay for a single elderly woman was 13.2 days, compared with 10.4 days for a married woman. Because it is likely that more older women will live alone, they may use the hospital for a longer period after an illness.[8]

In 1977 about 1.3 million persons in the United States lived in nursing homes. Some 86% of these were 65 or over; 70% were 75 or over; and 35% were 85 or over. Fewer than 1 out of 20 persons over age 65 was in a nursing home, but nearly 1 out of every 4 over age 85 resided there.[9]

Of special interest to us is the fact that 7 out of every 10 residents in nursing homes are female. Three out of 4 of those over 65 and 4 out of 5 of those over 85 are female. The number and proportion of females have been rising since the 1960s.

If we compare the population in institutions with the population that is not, we see that females are the larger proportion in both groups, but they make up a much greater proportion in the nursing home population. In 1977 the elderly population outside of institutions was 59% female and 41% male; in nursing homes the ratio was 74% female to 26% male.

Marital status was significantly different between the two groups. Outside the nursing home 54% of the elderly were married. Inside, only 12% were.

WHERE THEY LIVE

The greatest proportion of elderly people live in the largest states. California, with 2.4 million, and New York, with 2.16 million, lead all states in elderly population. Five states have more than 1 million persons over age 65 each: Florida (1,685,000), Pennsylvania (1,530,000), Texas (1,370,000), Illinois (1,260,000), and Ohio (1,170,000). These seven states have about 45% of all the elderly people in the United States, which is about the same proportion of total population in those states.

Between 1970 and 1980 the population of people over age 65 shifted. The most rapid growth of aged population occurred in seven states; none except Florida were among the largest states described above. As a section of the country, the South increased its share of elderly people by 41.1% between 1970 and 1980; the West followed closely with an increase of 39.5%. By state Nevada increased its older population by 113.7%, Arizona by 90.8%, Hawaii by 73.3%, Florida by 71.0%, Alaska by 69.6%, New Mexico by 64.8%, and South Carolina by 51.1%. These states experienced these large jumps while the nation as a whole added 27.9% to its elderly population.

These states were the pacesetters, while the number of elderly in seven states—Massachusetts, New York, Iowa, Missouri, South Dakota, Nebraska, and Kansas—and the District of Columbia grew at rates of less than 15%.

Counties show a much greater swing in proportions of elderly than do states. More than one quarter of the counties in Kansas and more than one fifth of the counties in Missouri and Texas had more than 20% of elderly people in 1980. The national average was about 11%. People over age 65 move relatively little. In the years 1975 to 1979 the rate of interstate migration for this group was 3.6%, which was only two fifths that of the general population. Approximately 82% of this group lived in the same house during this period, compared with about 58% for the general population.

The elderly population also tends to cluster in neighborhoods. For example, in the District of Columbia, elderly people ranged from 0.3% in one census tract and 60% in another compared with a citywide average of 11.6% in the 1980 census. Some of the reasons for this clustering include low income, movement into cities when families break up because of the death of one of the partners, and choices because of convenience of shopping, transportation, and other facilities.[4]

ATTITUDES TOWARD HEALTH CARE

Generally the elderly are more apt to be satisfied with their health care than any other segment of the adult population. Asked how satisfied they were with their last visit to the physician, in a 1984 American Medical Association survey, 69% were very satisfied with the treatment by the doctor's staff compared with 47% of the 18-to-34-year-old age group. Some 68% were very satisfied with the doctor's explanations and 75% were very satisfied with the medical care they received. This was about 20% higher than the opinion of the young age group.[10]

The over-65 age group was much more satisfied with key patient comfort issues, such as waiting time in the office and waiting times for appointments. Some 55% were very satisfied with office waiting time and 65% felt the same way about the waiting time to get an appointment. This compared with the 34% very satisfied rating for the 18-to-34-year-old group for office waiting time and 50% for appointment waiting time.

Generally 64% of the elderly population thought that the elderly are able to get needed medical care, compared with only 48% of the younger age group who agreed with this statement.

Strangely enough, the elderly were even more content than the younger age groups with the funds being spent on health care and financial support for the elderly. Some 44% of the elderly, compared with 58% of the younger group, felt that not enough was being spent on health care. When asked whether enough was being spent for financial support of the elderly, 53% of the elderly and 80% of the younger group felt that the amount was insufficient.

Even on highly personal cost matters such as their own doctors' fees, the elderly, by a larger margin, felt that the fees are usually reasonable. Some 79% of the elderly and 69% of the younger group agreed with this premise.

CONCLUSION

In the past 100 years our society has moved from the point at which our major health concerns were the death of women in childbirth and childhood deaths from infectious diseases to our current viewpoint that we have to concern ourselves with the health care of the aged. For in the past 100 years we have largely eliminated maternal death and death in infancy resulting from infectious diseases. As a greater percentage of our population live past infancy and experience a longevity that was unthought of even 50 years ago, our medical problems have turned into advances and opportunities to provide even better health care in the next century. The face of medicine will change, and our methods of dealing with gynecologic problems will, in many instances, be the difference between a fulfilling and active old age and one of institutionalization.

REFERENCES

1. *Projection of Population of the United States: 1982 to 2050,* Series P-25, No 922, Bureau of the Census, October 1982, Table 2.

2. Rice DP, Hing E, Kovar MG, et al: Sex differences in disease risks. Presentation at Johns Hopkins School of Public Health, Baltimore, Md, October 22, 1981.

3. Huig E: Characteristics of nursing home residents, health status and care received. *Vital and Health Statistics,* Series 13, No 51, DHHS Pub No (PHS) 81-1,712, National Center for Health Statistics, Government Printing Office, April 1981.

4. *Statistical Abstract of the United States, 1986,* ed 106, Bureau of the Census, 1986, p 72, Table 112.

5. Metropolitan Life Insurance Company: *Statistical Bulletin* 1987;68(January-March).

6. Manton KG, Soldo BJ: Dynamics of health changes in the oldest old: New perspectives and evidence. *Milbank Mem Fund Q* 1985;63(Spring):206–285.

7. Rice DP, Feldman JJ: *Demographic Changes and the Health Needs of the Elderly.* National Center for Health Statistics. Presentation at Institute of Medicine Annual Meeting, Washington, DC, October 20, 1982.

8. Huig E, Cypress BK: Use of health services by women 65 years of age and over in the United States. *Vital and Health Statistics,* Series 13, No 59, DHHS Pub No (PHS) 81-1,720, National Center for Health Statistics, Government Printing Office, August 1981.

9. Demographic and socioeconomic aspects of aging in the United States. *Current Population Reports,* Series P-23, No 138, Bureau of the Census, Government Printing Office, 1984.

10. American Medical Association: The elderly and medical care in America: Their own evaluation of quality, access and cost. *Survey and Opinion Briefs* 1984;3(April).

Part II

Medical Problems of the Older Woman

Chapter 2

Geriatric Endocrinology

Robert S. Modlinger

Although it was once popular to consider endocrine organ senescence as the basis for all aging, it is no longer possible to support this broad hypothesis. Indeed, current data indicate that many of the endocrine changes noted during the aging process develop as compensation for alterations in hormone degradation and end-organ sensitivity. This is not to imply that there are no primary age-related endocrine changes or that alterations in endocrine function do not cause at least some of the physical changes that accompany aging, but merely to indicate that blanket statements regarding geriatric endocrinology and the genesis of aging are inappropriate. In the sections that follow, the pathophysiology of each endocrine organ's response to growing older is briefly discussed. True endocrine pathology is considered when appropriate. It is to be anticipated that rapid expansion of research into the subject of aging will soon change the "facts" as we now see them.

PITUITARY

Autopsy surveys suggest that the weight of the pituitary gland diminishes by as much as 20% in old age. Mitoses become less frequent, vascularity decreases, and connective tissue increases. Stores of follicle-stimulating hormone (FSH) increase in postmenopausal women but are unchanged in elderly men. Growth hormone continues to be produced, but growth hormone release to various stimuli is reduced as aging progresses, so that 20% of subjects over 65 years of age would be classified as nonresponsive if youthful criteria were used. The majority of patients over 50 years of age also fail to demonstrate nocturnal growth hormone surges. At least some of the normal metabolic responses to exogenous growth hormone fail to occur in elderly subjects. Prolactin is probably unchanged in the elderly, but there may be some reduction in drug-induced stimulation.[1]

Most pituitary tumors of clinical significance present before age 60, but the actual incidence rate may continue to rise as age increases.[2] Unsuspected tumors are frequently found at autopsy. Magnetic resonance imaging with thin sections (2.5 mm or less), using transverse, sagittal, and coronal views, is superior to computed tomography in studying pituitary pathology by better defining relationships between abnormalities and perisellar anatomical structures. The two techniques may be equivalent in depicting suprasellar lesions.[3]

Elderly patients normally maintain plasma osmolality within the same range as younger individuals, indicating no change in the normal "set point." They do, however, have diminished sensitivity to blood volume and pressure changes, in that hypotension and hypovolemia are not met with the same increases in plasma vasopressin concentration as in youth. Vasopressin-secreting neurons themselves are unaffected, as indicated by the observation that vasopressin release in response to osmotic stress is actually increased twofold. The failure of older subjects to fully concentrate their urine is therefore a manifestation of the aging kidney rather than of the aging hypothalamic-pituitary unit. However, the tendency of elderly diabetics treated with chlorpropamide to develop hypo-osmolality (hyponatremia) does suggest some possible hypothalamic abnormality in the form of an inability to diminish vasopressin release when faced with the chlorpropamide-induced increased potency of this hormone.

THYROID

With advancing age the thyroid gland undergoes variable degrees of atrophy, fibrosis, and cellular infiltration, with the development of micronodules and, occasionally, macronodules. Virtually all studies have demonstrated a reduction in thyroid gland size with aging in patients without multinodular goiters, which, however, commonly occur in the elderly. Antithyroglobulin and antimicrosomal antibodies appear in low titer with increasing frequency, the former being detectable in almost 20% of normal subjects by the eighth decade.

The metabolic clearance rate of thyroxine (T_4) declines progressively to values approximately 50% of those of young subjects by the ninth decade, perhaps as a result of reduced hepatic metabolism. This decline is accompanied by a matching reduction in T_4 synthesis, resulting in preservation of normal serum total and free T_4 levels into the geriatric age group, although some investigators have reported a 15% to 20% reduction after age 60 to 65. There is more agreement that plasma triiodothyronine measured by radioimmunoassay (T_3 RIA) decreases 10% to 15% with aging, perhaps because of diminished conversion from T_4 in the periphery, but even this is not uniformly accepted.[4]

Thyrotropin (thyroid-stimulating hormone [TSH]) is unchanged by aging, and old reports suggesting increased levels probably reflected a high incidence of subclinical hypothyroidism occurring secondary to autoimmune thyroiditis. TSH response to the administration of thyrotropin-releasing hormone (TRH) has been variously reported as normal and subnormal—an uncertainty that may hamper the diagnosis of hyperthyroidism, since the TRH test is frequently used to determine the presence of hyperthyroidism in equivocal cases involving middle-aged adults and children. Release of T_3 RIA but not T_4 by TRH may be reduced in the elderly.[5]

Although absolute thyroid iodine uptake is reduced with aging, the 24-hour radioactive iodine uptake determination is within normal limits owing to reduced renal iodine clearance, which also occurs. The 6-hour uptake may be slightly low, however.

The assessment of thyroid function among the elderly is frequently complicated by medication and by coexisting caloric restriction or chronic illness (even unrecognized) that so alters the values of thyroid function tests as to give the false impression of hypothyroidism. This "euthyroid sick" syndrome can occur with almost any debilitating illness or cancer and may present with several patterns of thyroid function tests.[6,7] Most commonly the T_3 RIA is reduced, with the total T_4 and free thyroxine index falling as the illness becomes severer. The TSH is low and its response to TRH administration is blunted, but the TSH may be elevated when recovery occurs and the other indexes return to normal. In contrast to true hypothyroidism, the free T_4 determined by dialysis is either normal or high, reflecting the impairment of thyroxine binding caused by serious illness and the failure of the T_3 resin uptake test to adequately identify this abnormality. The substance, reverse triiodothyronine, is normal instead of low. Some investigators have suggested that the euthyroid sick syndrome reflects attempted adaptation to illness and impaired nutrition. Prognosis for recovery appears to be directly related to the magnitude of decrease in T_4, there being a 68% to 84% mortality in critically ill patients with T_4 under 3 µg/dL.[8,9]

Hypothyroidism

Although hypothyroidism most commonly presents at 30 to 60 years of age, many cases are first found among geriatric patients. Determination of serum TSH is the most sensitive screening test, and Sawin and colleagues[10] found clearly elevated values in 4.4% of the original Framingham cohort over age 60. Thyroid deficiency was more prevalent in women than in men (5.9% versus 2.3%). An additional 5.9% had slightly elevated TSH levels, suggesting the need for close monitoring. Only 39% of those with definitely elevated TSH had low serum T_4 values, thus establishing the inferiority of this latter test (when used alone), despite its low cost. It may, however, be a fine first step, with a TSH obtained in those patients whose T_4 falls within the lower 30% of the normal range. Symptoms are the same among the elderly as among younger subjects but are frequently overlooked because lethargy, constipation, cold intolerance, dry skin, cardiomegaly, and diminished mental acuity are also signs of aging.[11] Indeed, a substantial number of patients who develop myxedema coma do so after admission to the hospital when the unsuspecting physician administers anesthetics or sedatives to patients with undetected severe hypothyroidism. Most such patients have underlying Hashimoto's thyroiditis, idiopathic myxedema (with elevated antibody titers), or a history of Graves' disease treated long before with surgery or radioactive iodine. Pituitary hypofunction is seldom the cause but should be investigated before therapy, lest the patient suffer hypoadrenalism (adrenocortical crisis) after replacement with thyroid hormone. In contrast to the more common primary hypothyroidism, TSH is normal or low if pituitary or hypothalamic dysfunction is responsible.

Replacement with thyroid hormone begins with 0.025 mg/day of the thyroxine (or equivalent) and proceeds slowly with at least 2- to 3-week intervals (preferably longer) between dose increments of 0.025 mg. Occasionally angina supervenes before full replacement is reached, and the dosage must be cut back. In most cases, however, further attempts to increase the dose in even smaller increments at longer intervals are successful. Beta blockers may be added to the regimen. Replacement may be considered adequate when the TSH concentration is within normal limits, even if the T_4 is not within the upper or midnormal range. It may require 6 weeks for blood tests to fully reflect the effect of the thyroid replacement. Elderly patients may need smaller replacement doses of thyroid than younger patients, occasionally only 0.05 mg/day. Myxedema coma is treated with intravenous L-thyroxine (0.5 mg) as a single injection followed by oral replacement (as indicated above) when the patient regains consciousness. Respiratory therapy and other supportive measures are usually required, and concomitant early therapy with glucocorticoids (100 to 300 mg of hydrocortisone or equivalent every 24 hours) is advised.

Hyperthyroidism

Some 10% to 20% of patients with hyperthyroidism (mainly women) are over age 60 at presentation. Enlarged glands are palpable in only 35% to 85% of these patients, in contrast to almost 100% of younger patients. Patients with normal-sized glands almost always have Graves' disease. Among patients with thyromegaly, Graves' disease accounts for 30% to 50% with most of the remainder caused by multinodular goiter and approximately 20% to 30% by a single toxic nodule.[12,13] Severe Graves' ophthalmopathy is infrequent, but stare, lid lag, and a widened palpebral fissure commonly occur. Blepharoptosis is occasionally seen in the ''apathetic'' form of hyperthyroidism, which occurs in some 15% of elderly patients. These patients appear chronically ill, depressed, and wasted. Appetite is usually poor. Other cases present as single-system disorders in which cardiovascular (usually) or gastrointestinal complaints so overshadow the other features of hyperthyroidism that the underlying thyroid disorder is overlooked. Indeed, 10% of unexplained atrial fibrillation results from unsuspected hyperthyroidism.[14] Dyspnea and palpitations are present in more than 40% to 60% of patients. In contrast to younger patients, the elderly often present with only minimal hyperkinetic adrenergic symptomatology. Tachycardia is absent in more than 30%, and fewer than 50% report nervousness. Hyperactive reflexes occur in only 25%. The incidence of tremors appears to diminish even as patients over age 75 are compared with those aged 60 to 75.[13] Hyperthyroidism is suspected on a clinical basis alone in fewer than 75% of elderly patients found to have it. Periodic screening for hyperthyroidism, therefore, appears wise.

The serum T_4, free T_4 index, and free T_4 by dialysis are probably the most reliable tests for diagnosing hyperthyroidism in the elderly. Triiodothyronine is normal in 34% to 50%, perhaps as a reflection of the failure to "correct" the normal range for age. T_3 toxicosis occurs but is decidedly uncommon. It is to be suspected most strongly in patients with single "hot" nodules. The 24-hour radioactive iodine uptake was normal in 5/18 patients studied,[13] and is nonspecific. The new highly sensitive immunoradiometric assays for TSH can diagnose hyperthyroidism at younger ages: Values are suppressed below the normal range. However, such low values occasionally occur among the normal elderly. The TRH test is similarly flawed. Patients who respond to TRH administration with a normal TSH rise are not hyperthyroid, but failure to respond cannot be taken as evidence of hyperthyroidism in view of the debate centering about the frequency of nonresponse in normal aged subjects.

Radioactive iodine is the therapeutic modality of choice for this age group unless a very enlarged multinodular goiter is producing respiratory embarrassment, in which case surgery is used after first controlling hypermetabolism with antithyroid agents and inorganic iodine. Because radiation thyroiditis with leakage of performed thyroid hormone occasionally occurs after radioactive iodine administration, and because this may result in exacerbation of the thyrotoxicosis in a patient with a compromised cardiovascular system, this author prefers to pretreat elderly toxic patients with antithyroid drugs for 2 to 4 months (until they are completely euthyroid) before administering the radioactive iodine. The oral agents are stopped for a few days to permit iodine 131 administration and are then restarted 5 to 7 days later and continued for 6 to 10 weeks while awaiting destruction of the gland by the radioactive iodine. Fairly large doses of radioactive iodine are often needed in elderly patients with nodular disease. Patients who present as thyrotoxic emergencies are treated by the same modalities as young patients and eventually receive radioactive iodine.

Goiters and Cancer

With advancing age an increasing percentage of patients are found to have multinodular goiters. Unless the goiter is threatening to compress surrounding structures, there appears little point in attempting to suppress the gland with thyroid hormone. In fact, such an attempt may be hazardous, since many of the nodules may be autonomous and therefore unsuppressible. In such cases, administration of thyroid hormone causes hypermetabolism at an unexpectedly low dosage. Each nodule within such a goiter must be carefully assessed for hardness, recent growth, and attachment to surrounding structures. Similarly, solitary nodules must be evaluated by these classic criteria and functional activity determined by scanning techniques. Ultrasound may be of value in further evaluating "cold" nodules. Fine-needle aspiration biopsy continues to look promising and is probably the favored technique in the evaluation of single cold nodules at institutions where pathologists have experience in interpreting such specimens.

Papillary carcinoma accounts for 35% to 50% of thyroid cancers among geriatric patients.[15] The 10-year survival exceeds 80% among all patients affected, but prognosis is somewhat poorer among older patients, in whom the disease is notably more aggressive. Follicular cancer, which most commonly presents in the fifth or sixth decade, accounts for 15% to 30% of geriatric thyroid cancer. The 5-year survival is approximately 65%. Giant cell (spindle cell) anaplastic cancer is found almost exclusively among patients over 60 years of age. It grows quite large and spreads rapidly, causing respiratory tract obstruction and the superior vena cava syndrome. It may become manifest as metastatic disease several years after incomplete therapy for a differentiated thyroid cancer. The average survival is 6 months, with almost no survival beyond 3 years. Small-cell anaplastic thyroid carcinoma spreads more slowly, with a 5-year survival of 20% to 25%. Together these two tumors account for approximately 25% of geriatric thyroid cancer. Medullary thyroid carcinoma accounts for 10% of thyroid malignancies in patients over 60 years of age. Almost all patients have elevated titers of serum calcitonin, either in the basal state or after stimulation with calcium or pentagastrin. Some 20% of these tumors occur in the setting of familial multiple endocrine neoplasia, while the rest are spontaneous. Whereas the familial tumors may occur at any age, the spontaneous variety usually presents at 40 years of age. The virulence of this tumor is quite variable, with a mean 5-year survival of 50%. Because medullary carcinoma is frequently multicentric, total thyroidectomy is almost always indicated, even if surgical findings suggest that more limited surgery may be curative. Pentagastrin testing may be used postoperatively to assess the presence of metastatic disease or tumor recurrence.

Calcitonin is normally secreted by the C cells of the thyroid. Incompletely understood control mechanisms maintain levels under 80 to 100 pg/mL. Basal levels decline with advancing age but are always higher in men than in women. Men also respond to calcium challenge with greater rises in plasma levels of calcitonin than do women. Because calcitonin protects the skeleton from resorption by vitamin D and parathormone, it is possible that progressive calcitonin deficiency contributes to the increased bone loss that accompanies aging, especially in women. Estrogen therapy raises calcitonin levels.

PARATHYROID

It is now generally agreed that parathormone levels rise with age, at least when measured with assays directed at the C-terminal fragment of the hormone. Although the mechanism for this change is subject to debate, it seems likely that it is at least partly due to reduced renal function with aging.[16] Because commercially available assays may offer no correction for age when describing their normal range, the physician must be wary in the interpretation of elevated parathormone values that are less than twice the upper limit of normal.

Although a review in 1974 indicated that most cases of primary hyperparathyroidism occurred in patients 40 to 60 years of age (somewhat earlier in men and somewhat later and more commonly in women), with only approximately 20% of cases appearing in patients over age 60,[17] a study in 1980, after introduction of routine serum calcium measurement, reported a sharply increased incidence in women over age 40, with an annual incidence of hypercalcemia rising from 8.0 per 100,000 below age 39 to 103.6 per 100,000 for ages 40 to 59, to 188.5 per 100,000 for women over age 60.[18] Renal lithiasis, the most common presenting symptom among younger patients, is infrequent in the geriatric population, while bone pain is much more common. Surprisingly common, too, is the occurrence of elevated sedimentation rates, significant anemia, and profound weight loss so that their existence with hypercalcemia does not automatically indicate the presence of malignancy.[17] Another form of hyperparathyroidism, although uncommon, also appears in the geriatric age group, with almost 50% of patients suffering from "acute" primary hyperparathyroidism being over 60 years of age.[19] This disorder is marked by severe hypercalcemia (17.5 ±2.1 mg/dL), anorexia, polyuria, dehydration, reduced renal function, and central nervous system dysfunction. Nonetheless, almost 50% of elderly patients with hyperparathyroidism are asymptomatic, and their disorder is disclosed only through routine serum testing.

The hypercalcemia of primary hyperparathyroidism is most commonly accompanied by a serum chloride greater than 102 mEq/L (often greater than 107 mEq/L) and a serum phosphorus less than 3.0 mg/dL (often less than 2.5 mg/dL). Urine testing demonstrates phosphaturia and a diminished tubular reabsorption of phosphorus in most patients. Serum parathormone levels provide significant assistance in arriving at the diagnosis of hyperparathyroidism, but they are not uniformly helpful—often returning at the upper limit of normal or just beyond and leaving the physician with the question as to whether they should be judged "elevated" in view of the coexisting hypercalcemia. In most laboratories the C-terminal parathormone assay is preferred in making the diagnosis of primary hyperparathyroidism in the absence of renal disease, but some laboratories use N-terminal assays more effectively.[17,20]

Surgical removal of the involved parathyroid gland(s) is the treatment of choice. The procedure is well tolerated even among patients in their 70s, indicating that age alone should not exclude patients from being considered as surgical candidates. Naturally, careful postoperative management of hypocalcemia and hypomagnesemia is mandatory. Patients who are not surgical candidates usually respond well to oral phosphorus, and their serum calcium concentrations can almost always be lowered to less than 12.0 mg/dL by slowly increasing phosphorus load. Failure of calcium to fall despite increasing phosphorus indicates the necessity of stopping this form of therapy. Long-term therapy may adversely affect kidney function. Estrogen and/or progestogen administration is also helpful in postmenopausal women.[21]

Given the high frequency of asymptomatic patients suffering from hyperparathyroidism, one is often faced with the need to decide on the necessity of operative intervention. There is significant debate on this issue.[22] At Massachusetts General Hospital criteria for surgery include (a) calcium levels persistently within the range of 11 to 12 mg/dL or steadily increasing; (b) parathormone levels 1 or 2 times above normal; (c) urine calcium levels greater than 250 mg/24 hours; and (d) overt evidence of loss of bone mass, or impaired renal function.[23]

Malignancy is the most common cause of hypercalcemia among geriatric patients. Breast and lung cancer and multiple myeloma are the most frequent. A large proportion of patients with malignancy-related hypercalcemia—perhaps the majority—do not have evidence of bone metastases to account for the calcium elevation. Rather, their malignancies appear to secrete one of a large number of "hormonal" substances capable of increasing bone breakdown. These include parathormone-like substances, prostaglandin E–like material, vitamin D–like sterols, and osteoclast-activating factor (OAF). Hypercalcemia secondary to OAF or sterol production responds well to glucocorticoid administration, whereas that owing to prostaglandin synthesis responds to a variety of prostaglandin synthetase inhibitors, including indomethacin and aspirin. Ectopic hyperparathyroidism has been studied best. Serum phosphorus is often depressed, while chloride tends to be less than 102 mEq/L (unlike true hyperparathyroidism). Assays designed to detect the C-terminal end of the molecule frequently reveal levels that, although not suppressed, are lower than usually found in primary hyperparathyroidism (for the simultaneously determined serum calcium), but assays vary greatly in their sensitivity to ectopic parathyroid hormone and the physician must have familiarity with the assay used by his or her laboratory.[20] Oral phosphate therapy is often of value in treating these patients when therapy directed at the malignancy is unavailable or ineffective. Calcitonin can be used in all forms of hypercalcemia, even in the presence of renal or hepatic disease or heart failure, but it is not a powerful agent. Mithramycin is almost always effective in the hypercalcemia of malignancy. Adequate hydration is basic to the treatment of hypercalcemia. The use of furosemide in mild hypercalcemia is well established.

Vitamin D intoxication, usually occurring in patients treated with vitamin D and calcium for osteoporosis, is not uncommon, and responds to hydration and glucocorticoid administration. Adrenal insufficiency, usually occurring when the physician withdraws steroid therapy after long-term administration and before the pituitary-adrenal axis has had time to recover, also may present with hypercalcemia that responds to glucocorticoid adminstration, but here only physiological replacement, rather than pharmacologic doses, is needed. Thiazide administration, especially when coupled with dehydration, is a common cause of hypercalcemia, and it is wise to see the effect of drug withdrawal before engaging in a long and costly investigation.

Osteoporosis

Osteoporosis is the disorder of having abnormally porous bones. There is an absolute decrease in bone mass with a normal ratio of mineralized to unmineralized bone matrix. Remaining bone is morphologically normal. It is to be distinguished from osteomalacia, which represents a failure of normal mineralization owing to diminished availability of calcium and phosphorus, usually secondary to vitamin D deficiency. The ratio of bone mineral to bone protein matrix is decreased.

Osteoporosis presents most commonly in women after the menopause, in whom it is at least 5 to 10 times more common than in age-matched men. Slender women of north European or Oriental extraction are most at risk. It is uncommon in blacks. Predisposing factors include premature or surgical menopause or prolonged estrogen deficiency of any cause (eg, exercise-induced amenorrhea, hyperprolactinemia); sedentary life style; excess caffeine, smoking, alcohol, protein, and phosphate intake; low calcium intake; family history of osteoporosis; and use of certain drugs, such as steroids, anticonvulsants, and excess thyroid hormone. As many as 15 to 20 million Americans may have this disorder that accounts for at least 1.2 million fractures per year.[24,25] The vertebrae, hip, and distal forearm (in this order) are the most frequently involved sites. Hip fractures are fatal in 12% to 20% of cases and often lead to long-term nursing home care. Vertebral compression fractures most commonly involve T-12 to L-3, with fractures above T-6 being rare: they should be viewed with suspicion.

Peak bone mass is normally obtained by ages 30 to 35 years. Bone is not quiescent thereafter, but continues to undergo remodeling, with bone resorption being coupled to bone formation in order to respond to changing stress patterns while preserving bone mass. With aging, however, for reasons that are unclear, bone is lost during this process, and osteoporosis develops. It has been proposed that at least two distinct syndromes exist. According to Riggs and Melton,[24] type I osteoporosis ("postmenopausal") primarily involves trabecular bone with relative sparing of cortical bone, and therefore mainly affects the vertebrae, the ultradistal radius, and the mandible (tooth loss). Crush injury and acute collapse of the vertebrae occur. Type I osteoporosis is triggered by estrogen deficiency, which (perhaps mediated by reduced calcitonin production) increases bone susceptibility to parathormone action, resulting in accelerated bone loss, increased calcium mobilization, and diminished parathormone production by way of the normal serum calcium–parathormone feedback loop. With reduced parathyroid hormone production, renal conversion of 25-hydroxyvitamin D to 1,25-dihydroxyvitamin D decreases and intestinal calcium absorption (strongly controlled by the latter vitamin D metabolite) diminishes, further aggravating bone loss. It remains unclear why osteoporosis varies so greatly among patients despite similar degrees of estrogen deficiency among menopausal women.

In contrast to type I osteoporosis, with its disproportionate frequency among women (6:1 versus men), type II ("senile") osteoporosis is more evenly distributed (2:1). Bone turnover is slower and involves both cortical and trabecular bone, causing multiple wedge fractures of the vertebrae as well as hip fractures in the elderly (over age 70 as opposed to type I, which is more common at ages 51 to 75). Impaired production of 1,25-dihydroxyvitamin D (with consequent impaired intestinal calcium absorption) and decreased osteoblast (bone-forming) function appear to be the primary factors responsible with secondary *increase* in parathyroid function (versus *decrease* in type I).

The calcium intake of most American adults falls below the 1,000 mg/day recommended by public health agencies with the possible result that the maximum bone mass achieved may be suboptimal and that negative calcium balance may commence before its anticipated onset secondary to factors already noted. Calcium requirements among the elderly seem likely to be higher owing to decreased intestinal absorption, and most authorities recommend intake of 1,500 mg/day or more for postmenopausal women. It remains unclear whether provision of more than "required" amounts of calcium will result in normalization of bone calcium balance in estrogen-deficient patients who are not receiving estrogen or other therapy.[26] Although some studies, including that of Riggs and Melton,[24] demonstrated significant (50%) reduction in vertebral fracture rate produced by calcium supplementation alone, other studies[27,28] have found little effect of calcium supplementation on spinal mineral content. In the absence of hypercalcemia or nephrolithiasis, calcium supplementation is safe.

There is no question but that provision of estrogens at the menopause helps to preserve bone density for 5 to 10 years, with decreasing but still observable effects at 15 to 20 years. Such therapy is now widely recommended.[29,30] Together with calcium supplementation, vertebral fracture rate may be decreased by 78%.[31] It is possible that such combinations may also permit use of doses lower than the customarily prescribed 0.625 to 1.25 mg of conjugated estrogen.[28] Progestogen therapy must be added to at least those patients with intact uteri. Such agents themselves may have a protective effect on the skeleton.

Calcitonin is of uncertain use in the treatment of osteoporosis. It is expensive and has to be administered parenterally. As such, it certainly has no role in prophylaxis. It may have its primary use in patients with extremely high rates of bone turnover, but it cannot now be generally recommended.

Use of vitamin D and its metabolite, 1,25-dihydroxyvitamin D, is another therapy not fully evaluated at this time.[32] Its use is based on the observation of diminished calcium absorption in many elderly and low serum 1,25-dihydroxyvitamin D levels in some. Although it is clear that use of vitamin D can increase intestinal calcium absorption, studies have shown that it may stimulate rather than depress bone turnover and thus be detrimental. It may be that doses capable of increasing calcium absorption without ill effect can be found, but this has not been clearly demonstrated. Additional problems involve the development of vitamin D intoxication in many treated patients. Riggs and associates[31] found a 69% reduction of vertebral fractures when this drug was used. Serum 1,25-dihydroxyvitamin D levels can be obtained and may perhaps serve to select patients suitable for vitamin D therapy. Vitamin D in doses of 50,000 units once per week may be helpful in preventing osteoporosis in patients treated with high-dose glucocorticoids.

Sodium fluoride is the only well-studied agent known to stimulate bone formation rather than simply stabilize existing bone. It is not approved by the Food and Drug Administration for this purpose, and is not recommended for prophylaxis in the asymptomatic individual. When administered with calcium in doses of 40 to 80 mg/day, vertebral trabecular bone increases and the incidence of new fractures falls by 64%. When estrogens are added, fracture rate falls by 94%.[29] Although the bone formed seems less strong than normal, it appears likely that this is overcome by the large amount of new bone produced. Only about 75% of patients so treated respond, and a significant number complain of gastric irritation and joint pain. The author restricts use of this agent to patients who are already suffering from osteoporotic bone fractures at the time of presentation.

Weight-bearing exercise and emphasis on a life style with a low risk of falls (including avoidance of medication that causes orthostatic hypotension and unsteadiness) may be as important as drug prescriptions in the avoidance of osteoporotic fractures.[26]

ADRENAL GLAND

Adrenal Cortex

It is generally agreed that the cortisol secretory rate decreases with aging, falling by approximately 25% by the end of the seventh decade. This fall is accompanied by a diminished volume of distribution and rate of disposal so that plasma cortisol levels remain the same as those observed in younger subjects. Urinary free cortisol levels do not diminish with age, while the quantity of 17-hydroxycorticoids (17-

OHCS) excreted in the urine is reduced by 30% to 40% among patients 60 to 90 years of age. Interestingly, when expressed per milligram of excreted creatinine, urinary 17-OHCS levels show no fall with age. This observation is clinically useful.[32]

Although there is a tendency for serum adrenocorticotropic hormone (ACTH) levels to decline with age, almost all existing data confirm normal response of the entire hypothalamic-pituitary-adrenal axis to stress as tested by the insulin tolerance test and the intravenous (but not oral) metyrapone test. Cortisol release after ACTH administration is brisk. Normal adrenocorticotropin suppressibility has been documented by use of dexamethasone, and the periodicity of cortisol feedback mechanisms that control cortisol secretion is unaltered. This further supports the suppositions that the feedback mechanisms that control cortisol secretion are unaltered by aging and that the diminished synthesis of glucocorticoids in older patients represents a controlled response to slowed metabolic degradation.

In contrast, adrenal androgen synthesis seems to fall with aging by a greater degree than can be explained simply by altered disposal. This seems to be particularly so for dehydroepiandrosterone. Urinary ketosteroids fall to approximately 50% of youthful values. The potential significance of this androgen decline on the maintenance of nitrogen metabolism and bone integrity among the elderly has not been fully explored.

Plasma aldosterone concentrations and aldosterone excretion fall by 50% with aging. Although both aldosterone synthesis and metabolic clearance decline (the latter by 20%), there is at least the suggestion that these declines are not completely the result of altered degradation rates, since it has now been well documented that plasma renin activity also declines with aging. Basal renin levels may be fully one third lower at age 70 than at age 20, and stimulated levels appear to be at least equally blunted.

Diseases of the adrenal cortex continue to occur among geriatric patients but account for only a small percentage of all patients with these diseases. Attention is directed to the fact that urinary free cortisol determination, an important diagnostic test in the search for adrenal hyperfunction, has diminished utility in the presence of moderate to severe renal dysfunction. Also, cortisol replacement doses for patients with adrenal insufficiency tend to be lower in older than in younger patients: approximately 25 mg/g of excreted creatinine administered in divided doses—two thirds on arising and one third in the late afternoon or evening.

Adrenal Medulla

Pheochromocytomas most commonly present in the fourth through sixth decades and are rare in people over 60 years of age. Most cases are suspected because of sustained hypertension or a history of paroxysms, or both. Characteristically, paroxysms are marked by the sudden onset of headache, sweating, palpitations, tachycardia, and blanching or flushing. Headaches may be absent, and symptoms may be mistakenly attributed to the "menopausal syndrome." A metanephrine determination is the best screen in patients suspected of having this disorder, including patients first developing sustained hypertension after 40 years of age. In patients having paroxysms, urine collection should be started immediately after such an attack. Recent information has indicated the potential diagnostic use of plasma catecholamine determinations (despite occasional overlap with values observed in essential hypertension) and the localizing value of computed axial tomography (CAT) scans. It must be emphasized that initial therapy is by use of alpha-adrenergic blocking agents rather than beta blocking agents, which can cause severe hypertensive crises when used in the absence of adequate alpha blockade.[33]

OVARY

Until Costoff and Mahesh reported the presence of normal primordial follicles in menopausal ovaries[34] it was commonly accepted that ovarian ovum depletion triggered the menopause. Recent data suggest that alterations in follicular sensitivity to gonadotropins are responsible. According to this concept, those follicles most sensitive to FSH are stimulated early in a woman's reproductive life, whereas those most resistant are unstimulated and form a progressively higher percentage of the ovarian store of primordial follicles. By the time of menopause, remaining follicles cannot be stimulated by FSH levels 10 times those present in youth. This developing ovarian resistance is mirrored by rising FSH and luteinizing hormone (LH) levels even before cessation of menstruation, so that menopausal FSH and LH levels usually exceed 50 mIU/mL. Simultaneously the ovary becomes smaller and more fibrotic, and connective tissue increases. The ovarian stroma becomes unable to aromatize androgens to estrogens, and ovarian estrogen secretion (mainly estradiol) essentially ceases. Plasma estradiol falls by 90%. However, androgen secretion (androstenedione and testosterone) continues and may even increase. Maximum FSH and LH levels occur 3 to 5 years after the menopause, with subsequent decline toward "normal" levels.[35]

Accompanying these changes, postmenopausal women develop an increased capacity for peripheral conversion of androgens, produced by both the adrenal gland (95%) and the ovary (5%) into estrone, a relatively weak estrogen. Adipose tissue is particularly active in this conversion, and estrogen production is quite pronounced in obese women. This continued estrogen secretion in obese women may account for their higher incidence of endometrial carcinoma. Estrogen excretion falls from the time of menopause until 60 years of age, after which it remains stable at about 20% of youthful levels. Progesterone production falls about 60% soon after menopause. The mild hirsutism that commonly occurs in postmenopausal women is usually the result of a fall in estrogen production greater than the concomitant fall in androgen production.

Endocrinologically active ovarian tumors may appear for the first time in postmenopausal women. Most commonly they announce their presence by causing endometrial stimulation and subsequent uterine bleeding. Granulosa–theca cell tumors account for 70% of estrogen-secreting tumors (3% of all ovarian tumors), and 60% of cases occur postmenopausally. Pure theca cell tumors are less common and may cause feminization or virilization, although the former syndrome is more common. Arrhenoblastomas are the most common androgenic ovarian neoplasm, but they seldom occur in the age group under consideration.

DIABETES MELLITUS

With advancing age, glucose tolerance decreases to such an extent that more than 40% of geriatric patients in some groups have glucose tolerance test values that exceed those found in normal youthful subjects.[36] The Framingham Heart Study data indicate a prevalence rate of 10% to 15% in those over 60 years of age, with individuals overweight by more than 40% having twice the prevalence of those of normal weight. The annual incidence of noninsulin-dependent diabetes mellitus (NIDDM) exceeds 5 per 1,000 persons over age 60.[37]

According to criteria endorsed by the American Diabetes Association, diabetes mellitus should be diagnosed in any patient found to have fasting plasma glucose values of 140 mg/dL or higher on more than one occasion.[38] Other patients suspected of having diabetes should undergo a two-hour oral glucose tolerance test. Testing should be delayed at least 2 weeks after any stressful illness (eg, myocardial infarction, cerebrovascular accident, significant trauma) and until the patient has consumed a diet containing a minimum of 150 g of carbohydrate (more if previously malnourished) for at least three days. Drugs capable of interfering with glucose tolerance must also have been discontinued for at least 2 weeks. The test is performed in the morning after a 10- to 16-hour fast, using 75 g of glucose. Diabetes is diagnosed if the 2-hour value and either the 0.5-hour, 1-hour, or 1.5-hour plasma value equals or exceeds 200 mg/dL. These criteria are unaltered by advancing age. A diagnosis of impaired glucose tolerance (IGT) is made if the fasting plasma glucose is under 140 mg/dL, the 0.5-, 1-, or 1.5-hour plasma glucose is greater than or equal to 200 mg/dL, and the two-hour value is between 140 and 200 mg/dL. Many patients with IGT have return of normal glucose tolerance with time, while approximately 1% to 5% per year proceed to overt diabetes. Although short-term studies have indicated improvement of glucose tolerance with diet in such individuals, long-term improvement is unproved.

Patients with IGT do not develop the late microangiopathy of diabetes, but do show an increased prevalence of atherosclerotic complications.

Elderly diabetics are frequently asymptomatic, perhaps because of coexisting renal disease, which raises the glucose threshold and thereby lessens glycosuria, polyuria, and polydipsia, or because of the mildness of the insulin deficiency and/or resistance. Elderly diabetics, therefore, often present suffering from one of the long-term complications of diabetes rather than from the more acute metabolic disturbances of the disease.

Neuropathy is particularly common in patients with longstanding diabetes, and is usually manifest as a peripheral neuropathy with sensory loss. The feet may be painful. Ankle jerks are lost, along with vibration and position senses. Loss of perception of heat, cold, and touch may occur in severe cases, and such loss is accompanied by the risk of unrecognized injury to the feet. Patients must be warned about the dangers of using heating pads, soaking feet in excessively hot water, exposing the feet to excessive cold, and wearing poorly fitting shoes. Walking barefoot is prohibited, and the feet must be visually inspected daily lest minor skin breaks lead to large-scale infection, osteomyelitis, and amputation. Charcot joints of the foot and plantar ulcers result from impaired proprioception and pain sense. Routine care by a podiatrist is advisable for patients with peripheral neuropathy, visual impairment, or thickened, dystrophic nails.

Autonomic neuropathy may lead to orthostatic hypotension, gastroparesis, and diabetic enteropathy with malabsorption or diarrhea and subsequent nutritional deficiencies, anemia, and debility. Atonic bladder with large residual urine volumes predisposes to urinary tract infections and pyelonephritis and impairs monitoring of fractional urines.

Unusual syndromes of diabetic neuropathy include amyotrophy with its characteristic asymmetric weakness, muscle wasting, and pain in the pelvic and thigh muscles unaccompanied by sensory loss. A rare syndrome, diabetic neuropathic cachexia, has been reported. Patients present with profound weight loss, anorexia, cachexia, and depression and are usually felt to be suffering from malignancy until the true nature of the difficulty is found. Remission within 1.5 years is the rule. Patients with autonomic neuropathy that involves cardiac fibers are prone to sudden death. Extraocular muscle paresis, most commonly involving the third or sixth cranial nerve, occasionally occurs in diabetics. Characteristically, there is sparing of pupillary response.

Diabetes accelerates the development of atherosclerosis, leading to an increased incidence and severity of large vessel disease among elderly patients. Accordingly, intermittent claudication and peripheral vascular occlusion with skin and muscle atrophy and gangrene are more common among diabetics than among nondiabetics. The physician must search for early signs of cold feet, dependent rubor, and blanching of feet on elevation during physical examination. Diabetic patients respond well to replacement grafting of localized areas of vascular narrowing if such are found on arteriography.

Microangiopathy is unique to diabetes and seems to progress with increasing duration of diabetes. It is frequently manifest by patchy areas of gangrene and atrophic skin and nail changes in the feet, despite palpable pulses. Such areas may require minor amputations. Ulcerated areas may become infected, leading to larger areas of gangrene. Failure of the patient with sensory disturbances to note this occurrence and seek care not uncommonly results in the classic "diabetic foot" and extensive amputation. More than 80% of patients with diabetes of 20 years' duration have some form of vascular disease.

Diabetic nephropathy is of two types. Although nodular glomerulosclerosis (Kimmelstiel-Wilson lesion) is best known, diffuse glomerulosclerosis is undoubtedly more common. Clinically they are indistinguishable. Diabetic nephropathy usually appears at least 10 years after the onset of clinical diabetes and therefore is uncommon in patients first diagnosed as diabetic after 60 years of age. On the other hand, known diabetics often develop proteinuria for the first time at this age. As disease progresses, creatinine clearance begins to diminish and proteinuria becomes severer. The average duration of life after the appearance of sustained proteinuria is 7 to 10 years. Recent work has indicated that diabetic patients do not fare as well as nondiabetics when treated with hemodialysis. Renal transplantation offers a better chance for survival. Stress testing and cardiac catheterization may predict posttransplant mortality and help to select the best candidates.[39] Microangiopathy may develop in the transplanted kidneys. Diabetic patients may also be affected by nephrosclerosis, acute and chronic pyelonephritis, and gouty nephropathy. Papillary necrosis frequently precipitates terminal renal failure.

The risk of developing diabetic retinopathy increases with the duration of the diabetes. Background retinopathy is present in 65% of patients with diabetes of more than 15 years' duration and in more than 80% of patients with diabetes of more than 30 years' duration. Some 35% to 40% of patients over 60 years of age have mild disease. The lesions are not fixed, and the prognosis for vision is variable, depending on the degree and location of hard exudate formation and the state of the capillary bed. Severe maculopathy is more common in NIDDM than in IDDM (insulin-dependent diabetes mellitus).

A variable percentage of patients with background retinopathy progress to retinitis proliferans and advanced diabetic eye disease. Although the incidence of this complication also increases with the duration of diabetes (almost 50% of patients with diabetes of more than 20 years' duration), it is more common in IDDM than in NIDDM. It is present in 10% to 15% of patients first diagnosed as diabetic when over 60 years of age. Retinitis proliferans frequently, but not always, culminates in macular traction, retinal detachment, vitreous hemorrhage, and blindness. Recent advances in the use of photocoagulation and vitrectomy promise to preserve useful vision in large numbers of patients otherwise destined to become unemployable because of blindness. Blindness may also result from glaucoma, to which diabetics are prone, and cataract formation, which appears to occur at an earlier age and to progress more rapidly in diabetic patients than in normal subjects. Some 70% of diabetics over 70 years of age have this complication. The need for ophthalmologic consultation and follow-up in all diabetics cannot be overemphasized.

Skin complications that occur in diabetics include diabetic dermopathy (shiny spots), characterized by pigmented retracted scars of up to 1 cm (in the late stages); necrobiosis diabeticorum, characterized by papules or plaques that may ulcerate, leading to thinned areas surrounded by an erythematous border (usually on the anterior tibia); an increased incidence of Dupuytren's contracture; facial and plantar rubeosis; and a variety of xanthomas secondary to associated hyperlipidemias. There is no agreement as to whether or not generalized pruritus is more common among diabetics than among age-matched normals.

Elderly diabetics occasionally present with ketoacidosis. Management is the same as in younger patients, but the physician must be particularly wary of possible coexisting renal disease. Elevation of serum creatinine suggests extreme caution in administering fluids. Central venous pressure monitoring is advised in such cases. The author prefers use of intravenous insulin infusions (0.1 U/kg/h) as initial therapy, but has successfully used both large-dose and small-dose regimens. For hospitals in which continuous metered infusions cannot be used, intramuscular insulin works quite well. This author recommends a loading intravenous dose of 0.25 to 0.33 U/kg regular insulin, together with the first hourly intramuscular dose of 0.1 U/kg. Glucose should decline at 10% of baseline, or approximately 50 to 70 mg/dL/h. Failure to fall by 2 hours suggests a need for larger insulin doses.

Hyperglycemic hyperosmolar nonketotic coma tends to occur with unexpectedly high frequency among elderly diabetics. Most of these subjects have had longstanding mild disease managed by diet or oral agents. At the time of presentation, glucose is usually over 600 mg/dL, serum osmolality over 350 mosm/kg, and arterial pH only modestly depressed. In contrast to ketoacidosis, lipolysis is not severe, and ketones are produced in only moderate quantities. The patient, therefore, remains relatively well for long periods of time (average duration of symptoms before admission is 2 weeks), during which glucose continues to rise and osmotic diuresis causes profound dehydration. Neurologic deficits are common, and fever frequently is present. Treatment includes early use of normal saline until the blood pressure is stable with minimal orthostatic hypotension and urine output is established. At this time fluid may be changed to one half normal saline and this continued until glucose falls below 300 mg/dL, when dextrose in water or dextrose in one quarter or one third normal saline is begun. Most patients have a water deficit equal to 20% to 25% of total body water. This author recommends use of intravenous insulin infusions in this condition as well as in ketoacidosis, and has not been troubled by overly rapid falls in serum glucose. Such falls must be avoided because they are associated with the development of shock and central nervous system deterioration (brain edema?). Bolus insulin therapy, if used, must begin with smaller than usual doses because nonketotic patients may be more sensitive to insulin. Potassium is replaced as in ketoacidosis. Venous thrombosis and pulmonary embolism may be more frequent than in ketoacidosis. Mini-heparin therapy is controversial. The mortality of hyperosmolar coma approaches 70% in some studies. Particularly common is late nervous system deterioration.

Work completed since the late 1970s has significantly altered our understanding of insulin's role in the genesis of diabetes. Although it is still accepted that an absolute insulin deficiency is responsible for the metabolic derangements of juvenile type I or insulin-dependent diabetes, and that altered insulin secretion is present in most patients with type II (noninsulin-dependent) diabetes, many studies have suggested that insulin resistance (as indicated by coexisting hyperinsulinemia and hyperglycemia) is the causative factor in most adult patients.[40,41] Such resistance seems to exist not only in obese diabetics, in whom excess food intake or adipose tissue may account for it, but also in many nonobese diabetic patients with mild disease. Insulin antibodies are not present in excess titers in most of these patients, and coexisting diseases are absent. Rather, it appears that at least some of these patients have a diminished number of insulin receptors on insulin's target organs, accounting for insulin's diminished effect. Studies completed most recently have further indicated that patients with severe hyperinsulinemia may have both diminished insulin binding and undisclosed postreceptor abnormalities, accounting for their insulin resistance. Oral hypoglycemic agents increase insulin binding to circulating monocytes (and presumably other cells), which may account for at least part of their action in some adults. Glucagon, at one time considered an important factor in diabetes regulation, is no longer accorded so important a role by most investigators.

The majority of patients first diagnosed as diabetic after 60 years of age can be managed without insulin. Usually they are obese, and reduction of body weight to or toward normal by appropriate diet and exercise therapy eliminates glycosuria and reduces fasting plasma glucose to under 130 to 140 mg/dL and 2-hour postprandial glucose to under 160 to 180 mg/dL.

Diet therapy generally involves caloric restriction to 25 to 30 calories per kilogram of ideal body weight in nonobese, moderately active elderly women and 20 to 25 calories per kilogram of ideal weight in obese sedentary individuals. Carbohydrates (strongly favoring complex carbohydrates) constitute 50% to 60% of the total calories, with the protein content representing 15% to 20% and the fat content less than 30% of the total. Saturated fats should be less than one third to one half of the total fat intake. In some compliant patients these goals are not achieved despite progressive weight loss, and oral agents are suitable to control hyperglycemia until ideal body weight is achieved. Most authorities recommend these drugs for the nonobese 60-year-old with any degree of fasting hyperglycemia, as well as for the nonobese 80-year-old and all obese elderly with fasting glucoses over 140 mg/dL.[42] Although the second-generation oral agents glyburide and glipizide have not proved more efficacious than previously available drugs, their nonionic protein binding significantly reduces the likelihood of untoward hypoglycemia when patients are begun on sulfonamides, salicylates, phenylbutazone, and similar agents that can displace the older sulfonylureas from their ionic binding to plasma proteins. Given the poor eating habits of many elderly, the tendency to miss meals, and the progressive reduction in renal function and hepatic blood flow that occurs with aging, it seems best to avoid agents with prolonged action (chlorpropamide) and those only partially metabolized by the liver and requiring renal excretion for complete inactivation or clearance of active metabolic products (chlorpropamide, acetohexamide, and tolazamide to a lesser extent).

Oral agents are effective in 60% to 70%.[42] If one agent fails, as judged by fasting plasma glucose values exceeding 140 to 180 mg/dL or glycosylated hemoglobin values exceeding normal by 2%, a second agent may be tried. Patients who do not achieve control after two such trials are candidates for insulin therapy. So, too, are patients, originally controlled, who later fail to respond to their drug despite compliance with their diet. This phenomenon, termed secondary failure, occurs in 5% to 10% of patients per year.

Insulin is begun directly in patients with fasting glucoses of 300 mg/dL or more. If they are feeling well and are without metabolic complications such as dehydration and without renal insufficiency or complicating illness, such therapy can commence in the doctor's office, whereas a short period of hospitalization may be otherwise indicated. Human insulin is the agent of choice. It is associated with a lower incidence of allergic complications than earlier preparations that contained combined beef and pork, and there is no possibility that supply will be exhausted, as exists with the use of purified pork insulin. Patients must be motivated in this undertaking. They must be sufficiently flexible in their dietary habits to permit some alteration by the physician, at least in constancy of their carbohydrate load and division among meals. They must have the manual dexterity to self-administer insulin or have living or nursing care arrangements that permit assistance by others. Visual handicaps can be overcome with available insulin administration devices or the physician can prefill syringes for refrigerator storage.

Insulin prescriptions should be kept as simple as possible, since overly complicated regimens discourage compliance. It should be remembered that available insulin preparations include not only pure isophane insulin suspension (NPH) and regular, but also mixtures that contain 30% regular:70% NPH. In addition, the short-acting insulin promptinsulin zinc suspension (Semilente) and the long-acting insulin extended insulin zinc suspension (Ultralente) are stable in all ratios so that the physician can prepare a bottle with any ratio he or she feels is best and the patient draws up the preparation into the insulin syringe as simply as if it were a single substance. The widely prescribed insulin zinc suspension (Lente) insulin is itself a mixture of 30% Semilente:70% Ultralente.

The patient and physician must arrive at an understanding regarding the tightness of control desired. As a minimum, persistent glycosuria must be eliminated, since urinary tract infection and pyelonephritis are constant risks in patients whose urine provides food for bacterial proliferation. This is easily accomplished in most alert cooperative patients. Those who are unable to check urinary glucose at timely intervals can bring test tubes of their before-meal (ac) and at-bedtime (hs) urine (preceding day) to the physician's office. Negative urines, however, provide little information regarding blood glucose levels in the elderly with high renal thresholds for glucose and in patients with even mild renal disease. Moreover, they completely fail to provide information useful in avoiding hypoglycemia, a development associated with substantial risk in the elderly, particularly in patients with cardiovascular or cerebrovascular disease. The author has been gratified with the large number of aged patients who are willing and able to determine their fingerstick glucose values using strips interpreted visually or by a monitor. Most capable individuals are willing to check their capillary blood glucose once each 1 or 2 days. By having them check at different times, the physician obtains an accurate picture of the high and low values attained and can alter the diet and insulin prescription to achieve his or her aim: fasting capillary glucoses of approximately 100 to 140 mg/dL and premeal values of 110 to 160 mg/dL. These criteria provide an adequate margin against minor errors that cause unanticipated hypoglycemia in those who are relatively stable. Intermittent determinations of hemoglobin A_{1c} may represent an ideal method of assuring adequacy of treatment in patients with occasional spillage and inability to check fingerstick glucoses. It is otherwise a useful supplement to direct glucose measurements.

REFERENCES

1. Rolandi E, Magnani G, Sannia A, et al: Evaluation of prolactin secretion in elderly subjects. *Acta Endocrinol* 1982;100:351–357.

2. Annegers JF, Coulam CB, Laws ER Jr: Pituitary tumors: Epidemiology, in Givens JR (ed): *Hormone-secreting Pituitary Tumors*. Chicago, Year Book Medical Publishers, 1982, pp 393–403.

3. Karnaze MG, Sartor K, Winthrop JD, et al: Suprasellar lesions: Evaluation with MR imaging. *Radiology* 1986;161:77–82.

4. Gregerman RI: Intrinsic physiologic variables, in Ingbar SH (ed): *The Thyroid*. Philadelphia, JB Lippincott, 1986, pp 361–381.

5. Azizi F, Vagenakis AG, Portnay GI, et al: Pituitary-thyroid responsiveness to intramuscular thyrotropin-releasing hormone based on analysis of serum thyroxine, tri-iodothyronine and thyrotropin concentration. *N Engl J Med* 1975;292:273–277.

6. Kaplan MM, Larsen PR, Crantz FR, et al: Prevalence of abnormal thyroid function test results in patients with acute medical illness. *Am J Med* 1982;72:9–16.

7. Schussler GC: Nonthyroidal illness, in Ingbar SH (ed): *The Thyroid*. Philadelphia, JB Lippincott, 1986, pp 381–406.

8. Slag MF, Morley JE, Elson MK, et al: Hypothyroxinemia in critically ill patients as a predictor of high mortality. *JAMA* 1981;245:43–45.

9. Kaptein EM, Weiner JM, Robinson WJ, et al: Relationship of altered thyroid hormone indices to survival in nonthyroidal illnesses. *Clin Endocrinol* 1982;16:565–574.

10. Sawin CT, Castelli WP, Hershman JM, et al: The aging thyroid. Thyroid deficiency in the Framingham study. *Arch Intern Med* 1985;145:1386–1388.

11. Hurley JR: Thyroid disease in the elderly. *Med Clin North Am* 1983;67:497–516.

12. Felicetta JV, Sowers JR: The thyroid and aging, in Van Middlesworth L (ed): *The Thyroid Gland*. Chicago, Year Book Medical Publishers, 1986, pp 131–147.

13. Tibaldi JM, Barzel US, Albin J, et al: Thyrotoxicosis in the very old. *Am J Med* 1986;81:619–622.

14. Havard CWH: The thyroid and aging. *Clin Endocrinol Metab* 1981;10:163–178.

15. Ingbar SH: The thyroid gland, in Wilson JD, Foster DW (eds): *Williams' Textbook of Endocrinology*. Philadelphia, WB Saunders, 1985, pp 796–806.

16. Marcus R, Madvig P, Young G: Age-related changes in parathyroid hormone and parathyroid hormone action in normal humans. *J Clin Endocrinol Metab* 1984;58:223–230.

17. Mallettee LE, Bilezikian JP, Heath DA, et al: Primary hyperparathyroidism: Clinical and biochemical features. *Medicine* 1974;53:127–146.

18. Heath H III, Hodgson SF, Kennedy MA: Primary hyperparathyroidism. Incidence, morbidity, and potential economic impact in a community. *N Engl J Med* 1980;302:189–193.

19. Fitzpatrick LA, Bilezikian JP: Acute primary hyperparathyroidism. *Am J Med* 1987;82:275–282.

20. Aurbach GD, Marx SJ, Spiegel AM: Parathyroid hormone, calcitonin, and the calciferols, in Wilson JD, Foster DW (eds): *Williams' Textbook of Endocrinology*. Philadelphia, WB Saunders, 1985, pp 1170–1207.

21. Selby PL, Peacock M: Ethinyl estradiol and norethindrone in the treatment of primary hyperparathyroidism in postmenopausal women. *N Engl J Med* 1986;314:1481–1485.

22. Bilezikian JP: Surgery or no surgery for primary hyperparathyroidism. *N Engl J Med* 1985;102:402–403.

23. Wang C: Surgical management of primary hyperparathyroidism. *Curr Probl Surg* 1985;22:1–50.

24. Riggs BL, Melton LJ: Involutional osteoporosis. *N Engl J Med* 1986;314:1676–1686.

25. Silverberg SH, Lindsay R: Postmenopausal osteoporosis. *Med Clin North Am* 1987;71:41–57.

26. Santora AC: Role of nutrition and exercise in osteoporosis. *Am J Med* 1987;82 (suppl 1B):73–79.

27. Riis B, Thomsen K, Christiansen C: Does calcium supplementation prevent postmenopausal bone loss? A double blind, controlled clinical study. *N Engl J Med* 1987;316:173–177.

28. Ettinger B, Genant HK, Cann CE: Postmenopausal bone loss is prevented by treatment with low-dosage estrogen with calcium. *Ann Intern Med* 1987;106:40–45.

29. National Institutes of Health, Consensus conference: Osteoporosis. *JAMA* 1984;252:799–802.

30. Hall FM, Davis MA, Baran DT: Bone mineral screening for osteoporosis. *N Engl J Med* 1987;316:212–214.

31. Riggs BL, Seeman E, Hodgson SF, et al: Effect of the fluoride/calcium regimen on vertebral fracture occurrence in postmenopausal osteoporosis. Comparison with conventional therapy. *N Engl J Med* 1982;306:446–450.

32. Riggs BL: Osteoporosis, in Krieger DT, Bardin CW (eds): *Current Therapy in Endocrinology 1983-1984*. St Louis, CV Mosby, 1983, pp 259–263.

33. Modlinger RS, Ertel NH, Hauptman JB: Adrenergic blockade in pheochromocytoma. *Arch Intern Med* 1983;143:2245–2246.

34. Costoff A, Mahesh VB: Primordial follicles with normal oocytes in the ovaries of postmenopausal women. *J Am Geriatr Soc* 1975;23:193–196.

35. Asch RH, Greenblatt RB: The aging ovary: Morphological and endocrine correlations, in Greenblatt RB (ed): *Geriatric Endocrinology*. New York, Raven Press, 1978, pp 141–164.

36. Lipson LG: Diabetes in the elderly: Diagnosis, pathogenesis, and therapy. *Am J Med* 1986;80(suppl 5A):10–21.

37. Wilson PWF, Andersen KF, Kannel WB: Epidemiology of diabetes mellitus in the elderly. The Framingham study. *Am J Med* 1986;80(suppl 5A):3–9.

38. National Diabetes Data Group: Classification and diagnosis of diabetes mellitus and other categories of glucose intolerance. *Diabetes* 1979;28:1039–1057.

39. Philipson JB, Carpenter BJ, Itzkoff J, et al: Evaluation of cardiovascular risk for renal transplantation in diabetes patients. *Am J Med* 1986;81:630–634.

40. Halter JB, Ward WK, Porte D Jr, et al: Glucose regulation in non-insulin-dependent diabetes mellitus. *Am J Med* 1985;79(suppl 2B):6–12.

41. Truglia JA, Livingston JN, Lockwood DH: Insulin resistance: Receptor and post-binding defects in human obesity and noninsulin-dependent diabetes mellitus. *Am J Med* 1985;79 (suppl 2B):13–22.

42. The physician's guide to Type II diabetes (NIDDM): Diagnosis and management. New York, American Diabetes Association, 1984.

Chapter 3

Mammography in the 1980s: The Detection of Minimal Breast Cancer

Robert J. DiBenedetto

Before 1985 breast cancer had been the leading cause of death from malignancy in American women.[1] In that year it was surpassed by carcinoma of the lung.[2] In 1983 breast cancer resulted in the death of 37,900 women, followed by cancer of the lung, colon and rectum, ovary, and pancreas.[3] Although the mortality rates for several cancers, such as that of the uterus and stomach, have fallen significantly since the 1930s, the death rate for cancer of the breast remained virtually unchanged between 1930 and 1985.[3] With the exception of skin cancer, it is the most common site of cancer in American women.

The rate of incidence, however, presents a more accurate picture of the true frequency of breast carcinoma than mortality rate, because the latter does not take into account the proportion of women cured of the disease (Figure 3-3).[4] The Connecticut Cancer Registry, organized in 1935, is one of the most comprehensive in the United States and has provided breast carcinoma incidence data over a 40-year period. Between 1935 and 1976 the incidence of breast cancer in Connecticut rose from 50 per 100,000 to 87 per 100,000, an increase of 75%. The US mortality rates for breast cancer for this period, however, have changed very little.

The reasons for the constant mortality and rising incidence of breast carcinoma are complex and not totally understood. Improved surgical management resulting in cured patients and longer survival, with death from other disease, provides much of the explanation, as these patients do not appear in mortality rates.[4]

The most important factor affecting breast cancer survival is the presence or absence of axillary lymph node metastases at the time of surgery (Figure 3-4).[5] The 5-year survival is 83% if the nodes are free of disease and 55% if they are not. Mammography, which has dramatically improved in accuracy and reduced radiation absorption since its introduction by Salomon in 1913, outperformed physical examination in normal and abnormal nodal categories in the Breast Cancer Detection Demonstration Projects (BCDDP) sponsored by the National Cancer Institute and the American Cancer Society in 1973.

40 THE GYNECOLOGIST AND THE OLDER PATIENT

1988 ESTIMATED CANCER INCIDENCE BY SITE AND SEX[†]

Male			Female
SKIN	3%	3%	SKIN
ORAL	4%	2%	ORAL
LUNG	20%	28%	BREAST
PANCREAS	3%	11%	LUNG
COLON & RECTUM	14%	3%	PANCREAS
PROSTATE	20%	16%	COLON & RECTUM
URINARY	10%	4%	OVARY
LEUKEMIA & LYMPHOMAS	8%	10%	UTERUS
ALL OTHER	18%	4%	URINARY
		7%	LEUKEMIA & LYMPHOMAS
		12%	ALL OTHER

[†]Excluding nonmelanoma skin cancer and carcinoma in situ.

1988 ESTIMATED CANCER DEATHS BY SITE AND SEX

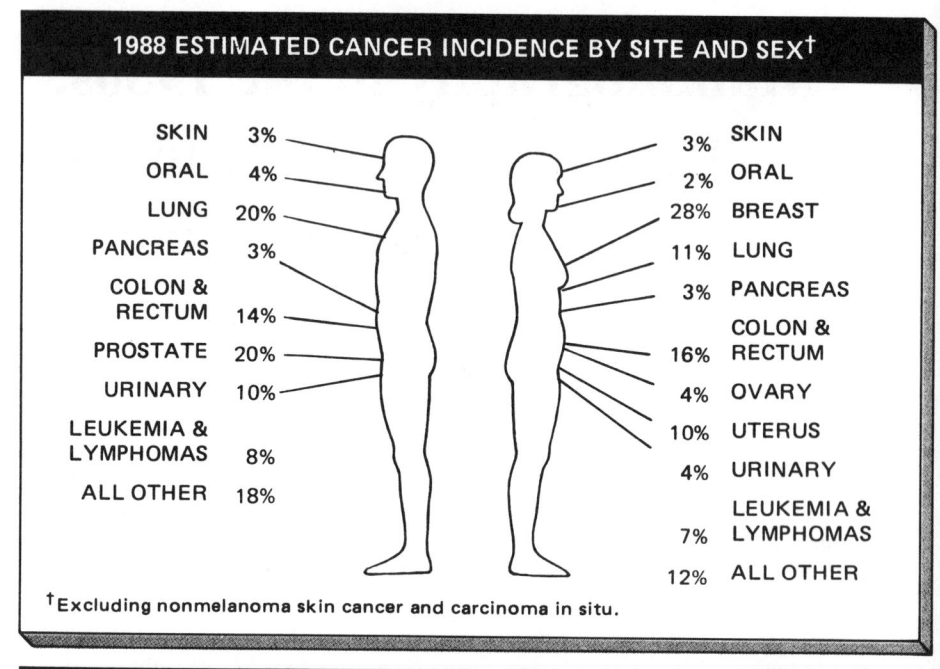

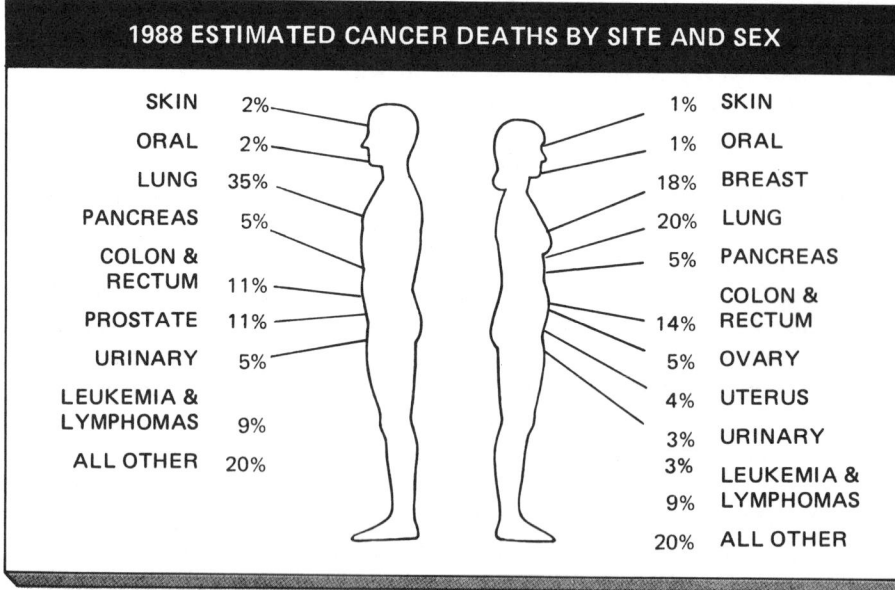

Male			Female
SKIN	2%	1%	SKIN
ORAL	2%	1%	ORAL
LUNG	35%	18%	BREAST
PANCREAS	5%	20%	LUNG
COLON & RECTUM	11%	5%	PANCREAS
PROSTATE	11%	14%	COLON & RECTUM
URINARY	5%	5%	OVARY
LEUKEMIA & LYMPHOMAS	9%	4%	UTERUS
ALL OTHER	20%	3%	URINARY
		9%	LEUKEMIA & LYMPHOMAS
		20%	ALL OTHER

Figure 3-1 1988 Estimated cancer incidence and death by site and sex. *Source:* Reprinted from *Cancer Statistics, 1988* (p 1) by E Silverberg and J Lubera with permission of American Cancer Society, © 1988.

Mammography in the 1980s 41

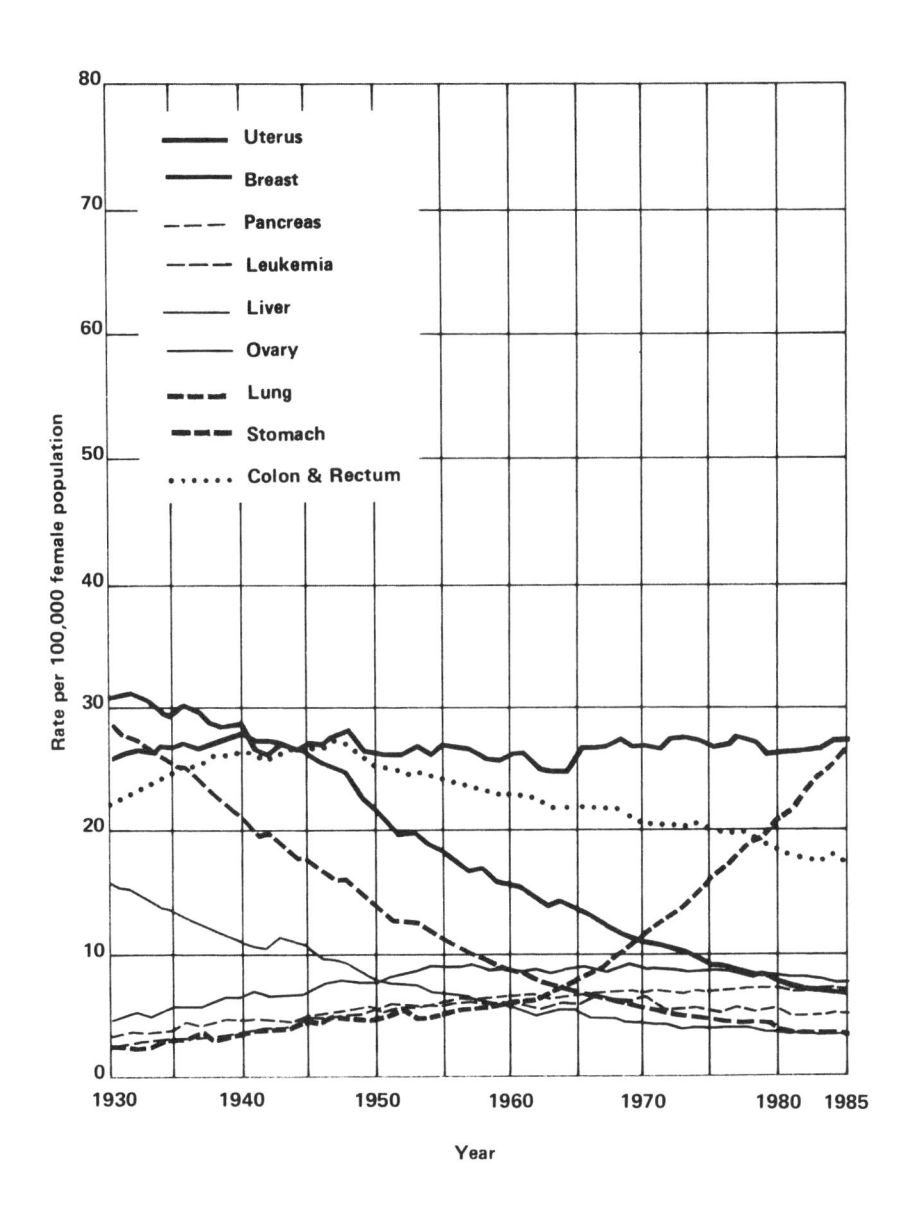

Sources of Data: US National Center for Health Statistics and US Bureau of the Census.

Figure 3-2 Age-adjusted cancer death rates for selected sites in US women, 1930-1983. Adjusted to the age distribution of the 1970 US Census Population. *Source:* Reprinted with permission from *CA: A Cancer Journal for Clinicians* (1986;36[1]:14), Copyright © 1986, American Cancer Society.

42   THE GYNECOLOGIST AND THE OLDER PATIENT

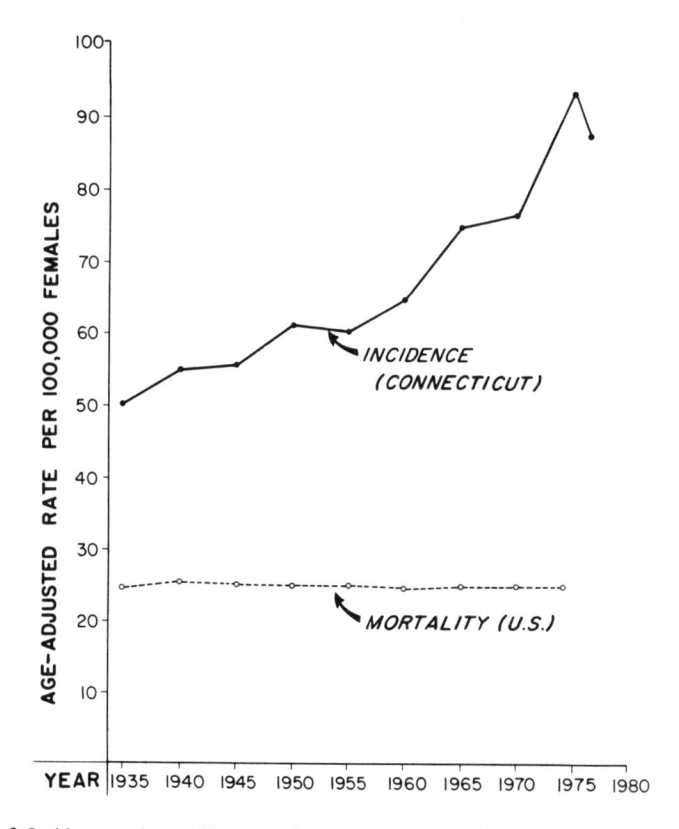

Figure 3-3 Incidence and mortality rates of data: for carcinoma of the breast—1935 to 1975, age-adjusted to the 1950 total US population. Sources: Cancer in Connecticut, Connecticut State Department of Health. Mortality Summary, Vital Statistics Special Reports (before 1945), US Department of Commerce, Bureau of the Census. Vital Statistics of the United States Vol I (1945–1959). US Public Health Service, National Office of Vital Statistics. Vital Statistics of the United States Vol II (1960 and subsequently), National Center for Health Statistics. *Source:* Reprinted from *Breast Carcinoma: Risk and Detection* (p 4) by CD Haagensen, C Bodian, and DE Haagensen Jr with permission of WB Saunders Company, © 1981.

In the BCDDP 50% of cancers with normal nodes were not detected on physical examination. If mammography had been omitted and breast palpation was the only mode of screening, half of the tumors in this favorable prognostic category might have been detected only after reaching a more advanced stage.

Low-dose mammography is by far the most effective means available to detect minimal breast cancer in asymptomatic women. Minimal carcinoma is defined by the BCDDP as a noninfiltrating (in situ) or infiltrating tumor less than 1 cm in diameter.[6] Cancer detection in asymptomatic women implies screening mam-

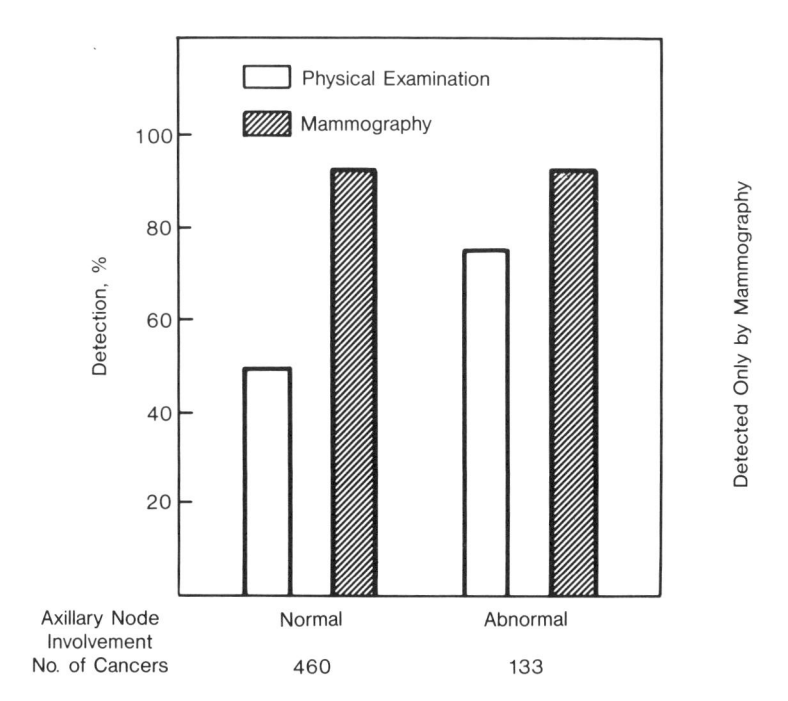

Figure 3-4 Detection of 593 cancers found on initial screening at Breast Cancer Detection Demonstration Projects by mammography and physical examination according to lymph node status. *Source:* Reprinted with permission from *Journal of the American Medical Association* (1979;242[19]:2108), Copyright © 1979, American Medical Association.

mography integrated into the patient's periodic health examination, as performed by her primary care physician in the office (Table 3-1).[7]

The human hand, regardless of how well trained, cannot reliably detect breast tumors less than 1 cm in size. To assume this capability often results in unjustified self-criticism on the part of the physician whose patient develops clinical breast cancer after a routine examination. In addition, this assumption produces unrealistic expectations in patients looking for a "clean bill of health" from an annual physical examination. Only the legal profession benefits from such misconception.

The incidence of deaths from cancer of the uterus and cervix has diminished dramatically since the 1930s, primarily because of the general acceptance of the Pap smear as a screening technique.[8] By means of the Pap smear the diagnosis of in situ and minimally invasive cervical cancer has led to the high cure rate of this disease. The test's popularity results from its diagnostic sensitivity and ease of performance in the office and from the absence of side effects. In contrast, screening asymptomatic women for nonpalpable breast lesions through the use of

Table 3-1 Periodic Health Examination Schedule for Women

Age	Complete Physical*	Screening Examinations	Screening Tests	Immunizations
20–39	Every 5 years	Blood pressure, annually Breast, every 1 to 3 years Pelvic, every 1 to 3 years	Papanicolaou smear, every 1 to 3 years† Serum cholesterol, every 5 years Rubella titer at age 20 Mammography at age 35	Diphtheria and tetanus, every 10 years Rubella, once if necessary
40–49	Every 3 years	Blood pressure, annually Breast, annually Pelvic, annually	Papanicolaou smear, every 1 to 3 years Mammography, every 2 years Occult blood, every 3 years Serum cholesterol, every 5 years Tonometry	Diphtheria and tetanus, every 10 years
50–69	Every 2 years	Blood pressure, annually Breast, annually Pelvic, annually Proctosigmoidoscopy, every 3 years†	Mammography, annually Occult blood, annually Papanicolaou smear, every 3 years Serum cholesterol, every 5 years Tonometry, every 2 years	Influenza, annually Pneumococcal vaccine, at age 65 Diphtheria and tetanus, every 10 years
70 and older	Annually	Proctosigmoidoscopy, every 3 years	Mammography, annually Occult blood, annually Tonometry, annually	Influenza, annually

*Includes health risk and hearing assessment with education about exercise, nutrition, stress management, smoking, alcohol and drug abuse, seat belt use, repeated excessive exposure to the sun, and osteoporosis.

†After two consecutive negative results.

Source: Reprinted with permission from *Female Patient* (1986;11[2]:89), Copyright © 1986, PW Communications Inc.

routine mammography is still in a period of indecision on the part of both physicians and patients for a variety of reasons.

One of the reasons for the failure of mammographic screening to become the "Pap smear" of the breast is the inability to incorporate the study into the annual office examination. Expense and moderate breast discomfort dissuade many women from obtaining mammography on a routine basis.[8]

Of more importance than these reasons in discouraging routine mammographic screening for early breast cancer is the untoward fear that radiation from the procedure itself might contribute to the development of breast carcinoma. Such a phenomenon has never been shown to occur.[9] The radiation controversy regarding mammography that has appeared in the medical literature involves the age at which to start routine screening (under 50 versus over 50 years of age) and radiation risk calculations based on extrapolation of data from Hiroshima exposure, tuberculosis fluoroscopic exposure, and postpartum mastitis radiotherapy.[8]

Two major screening programs have been carried out in the United States to evaluate the usefulness of screening mammography in the detection of breast carcinoma. The first of these was initiated in 1963 by the Health Insurance Plan of Greater New York (HIP).[10] Thirty-one thousand women were screened by history, clinical examination, and mammography, with 31,000 women receiving no extra attention during the same period (1963-1968). The latter group served as controls. The major conclusion of this randomized trial was that breast cancer mortality could be reduced by 33% through the use of routine mammography screening. The increase in survival, however, was limited to women over 50 years of age, since no benefit over physical examination could be demonstrated between 40 and 49 years of age in the relatively small group of women (9,100) in that age group.[11]

The project concluded that any risk that resulted from radiation exposure during mammography was offset by the benefits of screening women older than 50 years of age. Below that age, although the risk increment was small, the risk-benefit balance was negative because of the absence of a demonstrated benefit (Table 3-2).[10]

Mammography in the HIP study was limited by the state-of-the-art equipment, which used a 3.2 rad mean breast dose compared with the 0.08 to 0.74 rad required today.[5,12] Examination was definitive in older women with fattier breasts but significantly limited in younger women with dense breasts.[8] Few invasive lesions under 1 cm or in situ carcinomas were identified.[11] Logically, mammography in the 1960s was less accurate than physical examination in women under age 50.

The second major screening program in the United States was the previously mentioned Breast Cancer Detection Demonstration Projects (BCDDP), which began in 1973. The program consisted of 27 projects, each of which voluntarily enrolled 10,000 asymptomatic women aged 35 to 74. The screening consisted of

Table 3-2 Breast Cancers Detected on Screening by Age Group and Modality

		Age at diagnosis		
Modality*	Total	40–49	50–59	60 or older
		Number		
Mammography only	44	6	27	11
Clinical only	59	19	26	14
Clinical and mammography	29	6	12	11
Total	132	31	65	36
		Percent†		
Mammography only	33.3	19.4	41.5	30.6
Clinical only	44.7	61.3	40.0	38.9
Clinical and mammography	22.0	19.4	18.5	30.6
Total	100.0	100.0	100.0	100.0

*Initial evidence for biopsy recommendation made independently by the two modalities.
†Percentages in this table may not add to 100.0 due to rounding.

Source: Reprinted with permission from *Cancer* (1977;39:2776), Copyright © 1977, JB Lippincott Company.

---

physical examination, mammography, and thermography on an annual basis for 5 consecutive years.[11] According to Beahrs and colleagues,[6] the Working Group to Review the Breast Cancer Detection Demonstration Projects, the BCDDP were primarily intended to answer operational questions related to the introduction of screening for breast cancer in a wide diversity of communities. The projects were not designed to answer scientific questions about the efficacy of screening. However, the results from the rounds of screening generated intense interest in the determination of whether the experiences could be used to measure the value of screening women under 50 years of age, and the contribution of mammography toward the reduction in breast cancer mortality among women at any age under screening conditions.

The BCDDP found nearly 50% of cancers in women under 50 years of age, as compared with the HIP study, in which only 20% were found in this age group (Figure 3-5).[13] Cancer detection rates for women of all ages in the BCDDP centers were nearly twice as high as those from the HIP program. Minimal cancers were found in 36% of cases as opposed to 12% in the HIP study.

An unfortunate difference between the BCDDP and the HIP study is that there was no control group in the former project. The researchers had no suitable comparison group and were therefore unable to determine when the cancers detected through screening would have been detected without screening and at which stage (Table 3-3).[6] The BCDDP data, therefore, do not include com-

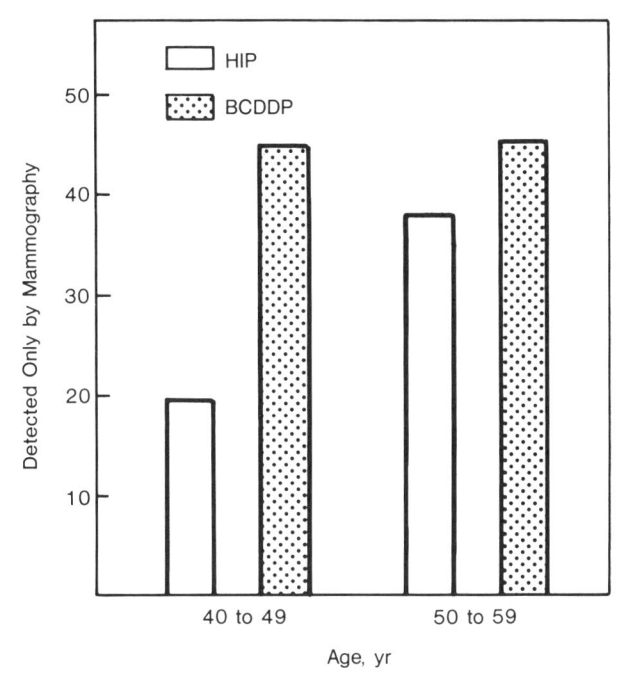

Figure 3-5 Detection of nonpalpable cancers according to patient age in HIP and BCDDP projects. *Source:* Reprinted with permission from *Journal of the American Medical Association* (1979;242[19]: 2108), Copyright © 1979, American Medical Association.

parative mortality rates in control and study populations. Although the BCDDP, unlike the HIP study, discovered minimal breast cancer with equal frequency in the 40- to-49-year age group as compared with the 50- to-59 age group, the lack of a control group led the Working Group to the conclusion that women in the program should undergo routine mammography screening between 40 and 49 years of age only when they have a personal history of breast cancer or a history of breast cancer in first-degree relatives (mothers or sisters).

Despite these drawbacks, the 280,000 women screened in the BCDDP clearly demonstrated that the combination of clinical examination and mammography can discover 20% to 30% of all cancers while they are non-infiltrating lesions, and 40% to 50% while still under 1 cm in size.[14]

The most recent major investigation into the efficacy of mass screening mammography took place in Sweden in 1977. It consisted of a randomized controlled trial that enrolled 163,000 women age 40 or older. The results to the end of 1984 showed a 31% reduction in mortality from breast cancer, and a 25% reduction in the rate of stage II or more advanced lesions among the invited group. It also

Table 3-3 Breast Cancers by Modality Findings and Histologic Evidence of Axillary Node Involvement among the Selected Age Groups of Screenees in the BCDDP (First Two Screenings)[a] and in the HIP Study (All Screenings)

	Percentages of breast cancers in			
	BCDDP screenees		HIP study screenees	
Parameters	40–49 yr. of age	50–59 yr. of age	40–49 yr. of age	50–59 yr. of age
Total	100.0	100.0	100.0	100.0
Modality with positive findings				
Mammography only	45.3	46.7	19.4	41.5
Mammography and physical examination	45.7	45.3	19.4	18.5
Physical examination only	8.0	6.6	61.3	40.0
Unknown	1.1	1.4	—	—
Axillary node status	100.0	100.0	100.0	100.0
Negative	58.7 [a]	61.5 [b]	67.7	69.7
Positive	18.5	19.0	22.6	25.8
Unknown	22.8	19.5	9.7	4.5

[a]Cancers detected (biopsy or aspiration recommended by the BCDDP) among women with the first screening by April 30, 1975, and cancers detected among these women with second screening by June 30, 1976.

[b]These percentages are heavily affected by the relatively large numbers of cases with unknown axillary node status, a significant proportion of which are noninfiltrating cancers. Adjustments to take this into account raise the figures by 8–10 percentage points. This factor has very little effect in the HIP study situation.

Source: Reprinted from *Journal of the National Cancer Institute* (1979;62[3]:641–709), National Institutes of Health, US Department of Health and Human Services.

---

demonstrated far more stage I cancers in the study group than advanced cancers (Table 3-4).[15]

The group found a 30% excess of invasive cancers in the study group compared with the control group (13.7 per 1,000 and 10.5 per 1,000, respectively), whereas the number of cancers in these groups on the HIP study had equalized 5 years after entry to the study. The researchers concluded that breast cancers are detected at a considerably earlier stage with modern mammography than they were with detection methods used 15 to 20 years ago, and this may be of considerable importance in mortality reduction. It reconfirms many of the benefits suggested by the BCDDP, which could not be proved because of the absence of a control group.

Because of the inability of the HIP study to effectively detect breast cancer in women younger than 50 years of age, and the National Cancer Institute's prohibition of mammography in the BCDDP for women under 50 unless there was a

Table 3-4 Breast Cancer Cases Diagnosed between the Date of Randomization and Dec. 31, 1984, in the Study and Control Groups by Age and Stage of Disease*

	Invasive cancer					Ductal in situ
	Total Invasive	Stage I	Stage II	Invasive ≤20 mm pNX§	Axillary Nodes Positive and/or Disseminated Disease	
Study group:						
Ever screened†	951	589	324	38	223	93
Never screened‡	117	27	85	5	61	5
Total study group	1068 (13.7)¶	616 (7.9)	409 (5.2)	43 (0.6)	284 (3.6)	98 (1.3)
Control group	595 (10.5)	209 (3.7)	376 (6.6)	10 (0.3)	253 (4.5)	15 (0.4)

*Women aged 40 to 70 at entry.
†Includes screen-detected and interval cancers.
‡Includes cancers among nonresponders and cancers diagnosed between randomization and invitation to screening.
§pNX: invasive tumor, size ≤20 mm, axillary nodes not examined histologically.
¶Figures within brackets denote no. per 1,000 women.

Source: Reprinted with permission from *Lancet* (1985:830), Copyright © 1985, The Lancet.

strong family history of breast cancer or a personal history of breast cancer, the media erroneously concluded that "mammography causes breast cancer."[8]

The issue of x-ray carcinogesis at mammographic doses is complex, and therefore not amenable to a three-page article in *The Ladies' Home Journal* or a two-minute spot at the end of the six o'clock news. Bailar, in his 1976 analysis, considered doses used in the 1960s, which were more than ten times higher than those used in modern mammographic equipment.[12,16] Even at the higher dose there are no data in human beings to establish a direct carcinogenic effect on the breast. Analysis of the possible risks were made by extrapolation from populations exposed to much higher doses, such as survivors of Hiroshima and Nagasaki, patients treated with radiation for postpartum mastitis, and women undergoing multiple fluoroscopic examination during therapeutic pneumothorax treatment of tuberculosis. Using a linear hypothesis to extrapolate data in these studies, as well as from animal models, which say that the risk per rad remains constant regardless of dose and can be extrapolated to zero from high dose, The National Research Council's committee estimated that six breast cancers per year per rad per 1 million women might be induced 10 years or more after exposure. In contrast, the annual incidence of naturally occurring breast cancer is almost 1,000 per million women (Figures 3-6 and 3-7).[9,17] It has been demonstrated, moreover, that the effect of radiation on breast tissue decreases significantly after 30 years of age.[8]

Risks based on extrapolation are hypothetical and subject to error. The radiation doses currently used are so small that their effect on human populations is probably immeasurable. The possible risk of radiation carcinogenesis should not be ignored, but it should be considered simultaneously with the potential benefits derived from the study in question. The National Research Council committee has

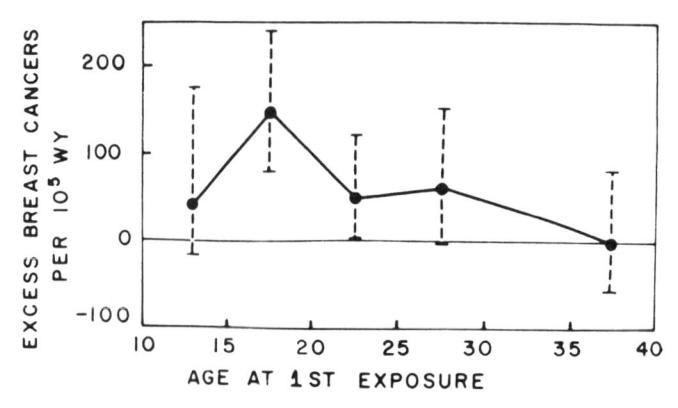

Figure 3-6 Excess breast cancer risk versus age at first exposure. *Source:* Reprinted from *Journal of the National Cancer Institute* (1977;59:823–832), National Institutes of Health, US Department of Health and Human Services.

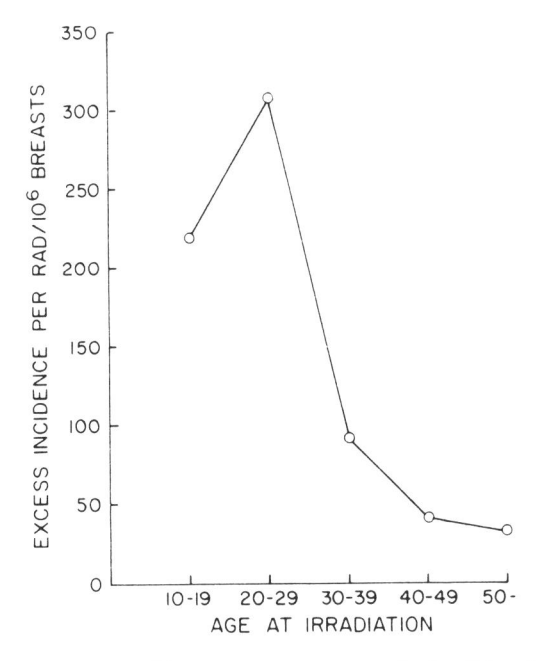

Figure 3-7 Excess breast cancer risk versus age at exposure for Swedish radiotherapy patients. *Source:* Reprinted from *Breast Carcinoma: Current Diagnosis and Treatment* (p 73) by SA Feig and R McLelland with permission of American College of Radiology, © 1983.

estimated that a 0.17-rad mean breast tissue dose, which is typical of today's equipment, might theoretically result in one excess cancer per year per million women.[9] Other activities that increase the chance of dying by one death per million persons per year are 400 miles travel by air, 60 miles travel by car, smoking three quarters of one cigarette, 1½ minutes of mountain climbing, and 20 minutes of being a man aged 60.[12]

Because of the media's negative interpretation of the medical data regarding mammography risk and benefits, women became aware of the procedure as one fraught with danger, rather than as one that could save their lives. The tragic consequences of these misconceptions and the numbers of advanced breast tumors that could have been detected much earlier through the use of mammography are immeasurable. In the field of medicine there is nothing blissful about ignorance. Despite the tremendous improvement in mammographic technique and the tenfold reduction in dose over the years, public paranoia regarding mammography will probably never be completely reversed. Clinical experience has shown that once patients have read frightening literature in the lay press, there is little that the medical sector can do to erase their fears and reverse their preformed opinions.

Breast self-examination and screening mammography are not competitive modalities in the detection of early breast carcinoma. Self-examination will always remain the first line of defense, as most breast cancers are detected by women in the privacy of their homes. Unfortunately many of these self-detected lesions are no longer localized. Mammography screening requires that a baseline examination be performed, with follow-up mammography at designated intervals in order to detect any changes suggestive of a growing cancer. In this way many breast cancers can be detected well before they become palpable lesions.[8]

The natural history of breast carcinoma involves the formation of an adenocarcinoma beginning in the ducts and invading the parenchyma (80%). The lesion begins in the upper outer quadrant (40% to 50%) and grows slowly, doubling its volume every 2 to 9 months in 70% of patients.[18] The doubling time of breast cancer is quite variable, according to Speroff, and an average doubling time is 100 days. At this rate it would take a single malignant cell 8 years to grow to a clinically detectable 1-cm mass. By the time the mass is clinically detectable, metastatic spread has already taken place in many women.[2] Rush[18] estimates that starting from a single cell, it takes 30 doubling times for a tumor to obtain a size of 1 cm—the smallest breast lesion then palpable on physical diagnosis. Therefore, even the fastest growing tumor may require 5 years before it becomes clinically detectable. It must be realized, however, that the growth rates of various histologic types are not always constant, varying with areas of necrosis within the tumor and hormonal changes in the patient. Growth rates are, however, quite consistent during the first 30 doublings.

The concept of the origin of the breast tumor in a single cell with increase in size by doubling suggests the long occult period that is probably present in many tumors before they are detected and treated. Cancer of the breast is often multicentric (15% to 40%), but each tumor probably starts from its own individual stem cell.[18]

A characteristic of malignant cells is marked lack of adhesiveness to adjacent tissue. Because of this as a small mass of tumor cells increases in size, increasing numbers of cells are shed into the intercellular spaces, where they are taken up by the lymphatics. At approximately the 20th doubling, the still-tiny tumor mass acquires its own blood supply by way of a network of new capillary formation. Tumor cells are then shed directly into the bloodstream and some cells entering the lymphatic network can cross over into the bloodstream by lymphaticovenous communication. Clinical data indicate that the implantation of metastatic cells from breast cancer seldom occurs until the primary lesion is larger than 0.5 cm in diameter, or about the 27th doubling.

The appearance of gross tumor in the axillary lymph nodes is an index of the failure of host resistance and indicates a greatly increased chance of dissemination of the malignant process. The chance of dissemination is roughly correlated with the number of nodes involved. As the size of the primary tumor increases and invades the surrounding glandular tissue, the accompanying fibrosis shortens Cooper's ligaments, producing the characteristic dimpling of the skin. Cords of tumor cells grow along the lymphatics, invading the skin itself. Before this invasion, localized edema of the skin develops, as many lymphatic avenues are blocked and drainage of fluid from the skin is impeded by tumor cells. Eventually the tumor cells replace the skin, which breaks down to form an ulcer. Blood vessels are invaded and tumor cells enter the circulation, passing into axillary or intercostal veins. They then scatter through the pulmonary vasculature into the lung parenchyma or up and down the vertebral column by way of the vertebral veins.

While the primary breast tumor extends toward the skin, tumor cells also pass by way of the lymphatic vessels from the upper outer quadrant to the axillary nodes, where they implant and continue to grow. As the axillary nodes enlarge, they are first shotty and fairly soft and then become firm and hard, since they are increasingly replaced by neoplasia. Eventually the nodes adhere to one another, thereby forming a large conglomerate mass. The tumor then breaks out of the lymphatic capsule, and the mass of nodes becomes fixed to the medial wall of the axilla. As the axillary nodes become obstructed with tumor, cells pass along the chain to the supraclavicular nodes, which then also enlarge. Malignant cells also travel by way of the right lymphatic trunk or the thoracic duct into the bloodstream, heart, and lungs. Systemic spread is the rule in breast carcinoma, and 95% of patients who die of uncontrolled breast cancer have distant metastases. Lung (65%), liver (56%), and bones (56%) are the most common metastatic sites.[18]

This review of the natural history of breast carcinoma leads one to the conclusion that the disease is a gradual process and that early detection is usually feasible. By means of monthly breast self-examination, annual physician breast palpation, and routine mammography of asymptomatic high- and low-risk women, carcinoma of the breast should never be allowed to run its natural course.

The National Cancer Institute Surveillance, Epidemiology, and End Results Program (SEER), 1977 to 1981, estimated that there would be 123,000 new cases of invasive breast carcinoma in 1986.[3] The probability of a newborn girl in the United States developing invasive breast cancer is 9.1%. In other words, about 1 out of 11 girls will develop this disease during her lifetime (Figure 3-8).[1]

The epidemiology of breast cancer seems to involve a crucial role for estrogen and prolactin in its etiology. The risk of breast cancer is determined by the intensity and duration of exposure of the breast epithelium to estrogen and prolactin. Age at menarche, age at menopause, age at first delivery, and postmenopausal weight have been clearly established as breast cancer risk factors by epidemiologic case-control studies (Figure 3-9).[19]

In an attempt to predict which women are most likely to develop breast carcinomas, high- and low-risk categories have been defined. They are also used to help determine the frequency of mammographic screening for an individual patient, as determined by the risk group into which she falls. The high-risk category of women for development of breast carcinoma includes several distinct

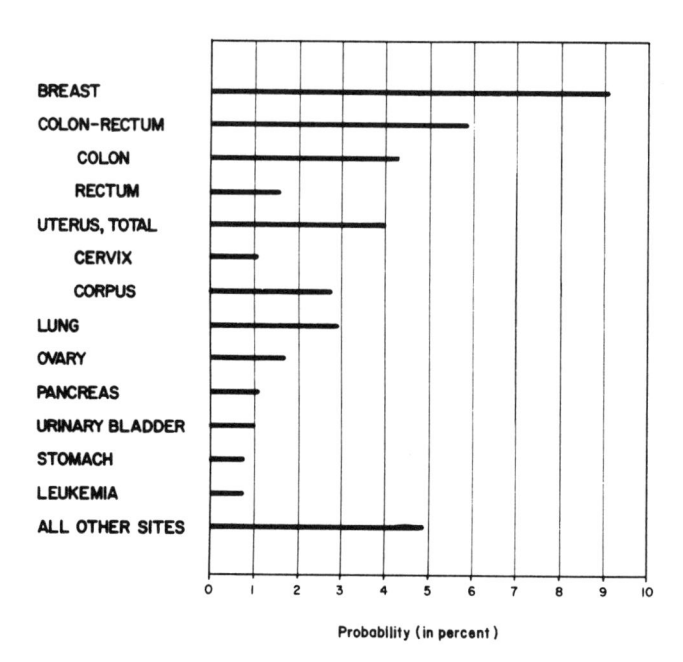

Figure 3-8 Probability at birth of eventually developing cancer by site in females: United States, 1978. Excludes carcinoma in situ and nonmelanoma skin cancer. *Source:* Reprinted from *Breast Carcinoma: Current Diagnosis and Treatment* (p 12) by SA Feig and R McLelland with permission of American College of Radiology, © 1983.

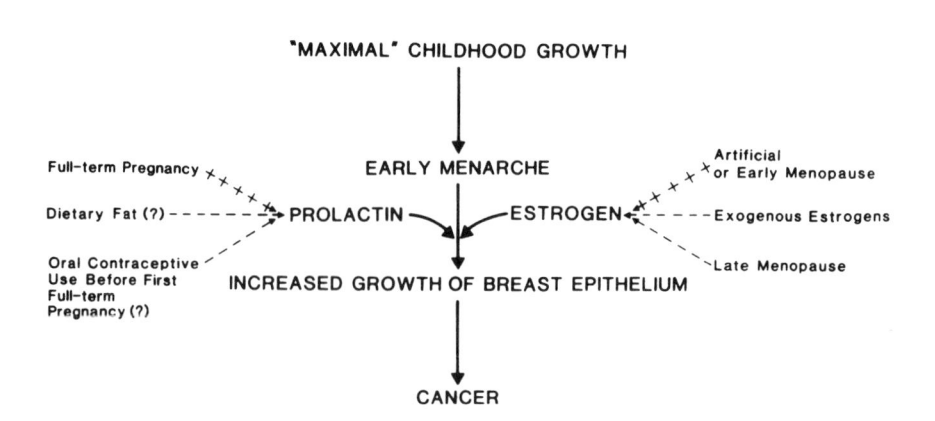

Figure 3-9 A model of the pathogenesis of breast cancer. *Source:* Reprinted from *Breast Carcinoma: Current Diagnosis and Treatment* (p 52) by SA Feig and R McLelland with permission of American College of Radiology, © 1983.

groups. Patients who have had a previous mastectomy for breast carcinoma have at least a 15% chance of developing cancer in the opposite breast, or as much as a fivefold increase.[8,20] Patients with a family history of breast cancer are also considered high-risk patients. Family members with a history of breast cancer and/ or ovarian cancer that occurred in the premenopausal or perimenopausal age group, relatives who have had breast cancer or malignant melanoma, and those with Peutz-Jeghers syndrome increase the breast carcinoma risk in the particular patient.[8]

These groups of patients share some genetic material, and the familial relationship most commonly thought of is that of first-degree relatives—mother, daughter, and sister. The risk in first-degree relatives is highest with premenopausal or bilateral breast disease, and even higher when both factors are present. Relatives of patients with postmenopausal cancer and unilateral cancer have only a 1.2-fold higher risk than the controls.

It has been estimated that if a mother has breast cancer, her daughter has a 25 times greater chance of developing cancer than does a woman without this family history. If both the mother and a sister have breast cancer, the chance is 40 to 50 times greater than would otherwise be expected. When a mother has breast cancer at an early age, especially under the age of 45, cancer in the daughter also tends to develop at an early age, sometimes in the 20s or 30s. There is a lesser but still increased risk for women whose more distant relatives, such as aunts, cousins, and grandmothers, have a history of breast cancer.[8]

Another risk group includes all women between the ages of 40 and 65. Many occult cancers are found among women in this particular age range. Breast cancer is almost unknown in the prepubertal woman and is very rare under the age of 20. From the age of 20 upward there is a gradually increasing incidence that plateaus between the ages of 45 and 55 at approximately 125 cases each year for every 100,000 females of the age range. After 55 the incidence begins to rise again sharply so that the annual risk of developing breast cancer for women 80 to 85 is twice as high as it is for women 60 to 65 (312 versus 153 cases per 100,000 women per year). It has been suggested that the plateau of incidence during the menopausal age period reflects the effect of a changing hormonal milieu in women at that time. Premenopausal breast cancer (age group 40 to 44) appears to be genetically influenced, whereas late breast cancer (age 60 to 69) is more closely associated with environmental factors, such as the amount of fat in the diet as well as obesity itself (Figure 3-10).[18]

In postmenopausal women the major source of estrogen is from the extraglandular conversion of androstenedione to estrone. This fact may also be the basis for the well-known association between obesity and the development of cancer of the endometrium. The actual site for the conversion in fat is not within the fat cell itself, but in the surrounding stromal tissue. Body weight, therefore, has a direct correlation with the circulating levels of estrone and estradiol. Also, obesity by an

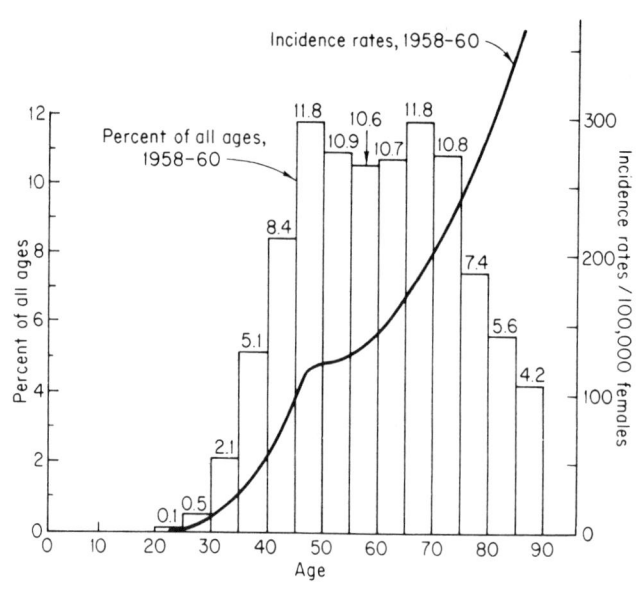

Figure 3-10 Newly diagnosed breast cancer among women, 1958-1960, percentage distribution and incidence rates by age. Note plateau in incidence between ages 45 and 55. *Source:* Reprinted from *Principles of Surgery,* ed 4 (p 531) by SI Schwartz et al with permission of McGraw-Hill Book Company, © 1984.

---

unknown mechanism suppresses sex hormone–binding globulin levels, thus increasing free and physiologically active forms of estrogen.[21] In addition, many obese women have large pendulous breasts that are extremely difficult to examine both by the physician and by self-examination at home. As a result, tumors in such breasts are usually larger before they are found.[8]

Another group of women who may be put into a high-risk category are those with a prominent duct pattern and excessive stromal connective tissue on their baseline mammogram, especially if the findings are inconsistent with the patient's age.[8] Wolfe formulated a classification of mammographic findings in order to predict the likelihood of development of breast carcinoma in the future.[20,22] It consisted of the following categories of mammographic findings:

Parenchymal Pattern	*Risk Level*
N1—A breast composed nearly completely of fat, with no ductal tissue or dysplastic elements present	Lowest
P1—Involvement with a prominent duct pattern of less than one fourth of the estimated breast volume, located in the retroareolar aspect	Low

P2—Prominent ducts involving one fourth or more of the estimated breast volume — High

DY—Sheetline areas of increased density (dysplasia) — Highest

This scheme, however, is somewhat controversial and should not be the sole determinant of the screening program for a particular patient.

Infertility and/or remaining unmarried constitutes yet another risk factor for the development of breast carcinoma. Single and nulliparous women have a 1.4 to 2.3 times greater risk of developing breast cancer than do parous women.[8] The protective effect of parity is also associated with age: those women with the first full-term pregnancy before age 20 have one half the risk of nulliparous women. Incomplete pregnancy before the first full-term pregnancy has no protective effect. It has been found that the first-trimester abortion, spontaneous or voluntary, before the first full-term pregnancy is actually associated with an increase in the risk of breast cancer.[19]

It appears that the first pregnancy has two effects on the risk of breast cancer. Hormonal changes of the first trimester of pregnancy cause an increase in the risk that is more than compensated for in the long term by carrying the pregnancy to term. This dual effect of the first pregnancy offers an explanation for the observation that if the first delivery is delayed to the mid or late 30s, the woman will experience an increase in risk beyond that of a woman who has never borne a child. An important clinical implication of the above discussion is that the increasing incidence of elective abortion as a form of post-facto contraception, especially among teenagers and young adults who have not experienced a complete pregnancy, may augment their risk for future development of breast cancer (Tables 3-5, 3-6, and 3-7).[19]

Regarding the use of oral contraceptives and the risk of breast carcinoma, most studies have yielded no indication of an association of breast cancer with pill usage. It is interesting to note that a protective effect toward benign breast disease

Table 3-5 Relative Risk of Breast Cancer by Age at First Full-Term Pregnancy (FFTP)

Age at FFTP	Relative Risk
Never	2.0
≤ 19	1.0
20–24	1.2
25–29	1.6
30–34	1.9
≥ 35	2.4

Source: Reprinted with permission from *World Health Organization Bulletin* (1970;43:209–221), Copyright © 1970, World Health Organization.

Table 3-6 Relative Risk of Breast Cancer in Relation to First-Trimester Abortion before the First Full-Term Pregnancy (FFTP)

Abortion Before FFTP	Cases	Controls	Relative Risk
Yes	24	17	2.4
No	139	253	1.0

Source: Reprinted with permission from British Journal of Cancer (1981;43:72–76), Copyright © 1981, Macmillan Press Ltd.

(fibroadenoma and chronic cystic disease) is associated with the progestin component of the pill.[23] There is concern, however, regarding the risk among young women who have postponed their first pregnancy through the use of oral contraceptives. In the Henderson, Pike and Ross study, women using oral contraceptives for at least 48 months before their first full-term pregnancy are at 2.3 times the risk for breast cancer than women with early full-term pregnancy.[19]

With regard to the use of postmenopausal estrogen replacement therapy, several studies have reported an elevated risk of 1.5- to 2-fold for long-term users, while other studies have shown no significant association between estrogen and the risk of breast cancer.[19,21] In a long-term prospective study by Gambrell, there has been no evidence that estrogen therapy increases the risk of breast cancer.[24] At the 15-year follow-up mark, there was a lower incidence of breast cancer in women using an estrogen-progestin combination than in women using estrogen alone. Progesterone is known to exert a protective effect on the development of endometrial carcinoma in menopausal women. For these reasons progesterone should be given intermittently to women on estrogen replacement therapy, even if the uterus has been removed.[21]

Table 3-7 Relative Risk of Breast Cancer in Relation to Use of Oral Contraceptives before First Full-Term Pregnancy

Duration of Oral Contraceptive Use (months)	Cases	Controls	Relative Risk
0	79	141	1.0
1–48	53	103	1.0
49–96	24	22	2.3
≥ 97	7	4	3.5

Source: Reprinted with permission from British Journal of Cancer (1981;43:72–76), Copyright © 1981, Macmillan Press Ltd.

One must consider, when evaluating the risk of development of breast carcinoma from oral contraceptives and/or postmenopausal estrogens, the benefits derived from these hormones. Protection from unwanted pregnancy and prevention of debilitating osteoporosis in the rapidly increasing numbers of postmenopausal women in this country today are goals that must be achieved despite the potential risks discussed earlier.

With regard to age at menarche and menopause, menarche before age 12 increases the risk as compared with menarche at age 15 years or older. Menstrual activity for 30 or more years also increases the risk.[8] Women whose natural menopause occurs before the age of 45 have one half the risk of breast cancer as compared with those whose menopause occurs after age 55. In addition, women with 40 or more years of active menstruation have twice the breast cancer risk of those with less than 30 years of menstrual activity. The risk of breast cancer development is markedly reduced by bilateral oophorectomy or pelvic irradiation. The effect is greater than that of natural menopause. Women with surgically induced menopause by hysterectomy and bilateral oophorectomy before age 35 have only 25% of the expected breast cancer rate.[19] Diabetes and endometrial carcinoma are also associated with an increased risk of breast cancer. Finally, for reasons that are not yet clear, the incidence of breast cancer throughout the world is greater among affluent women.[8]

The worldwide distribution of breast cancer incidence shows considerable variety. The incidence rates tend to be low in Asia and underdeveloped countries, intermediate in southern European countries, and high in North America, Scandinavian countries, and other Westernized locations (Figure 3-11).[1] The breast cancer incidence rates have increased from 1970 into the 1980s among both white and black women, although the increase is more pronounced among blacks. Being Jewish also increases the risk of breast cancer in the United States, as opposed to being gentile. Comparison of the incidence of breast cancer in the metropolitan areas of the United States indicates that the highest rates are found in the Northeast while the lowest incidence tends to be in the South. Since 1950 no country has shown a decreased incidence of breast cancer. The United States has also experienced an increase in rate, but it is not as rapid as that in many other countries.

Success in treating a human cancer is often measured in terms of the percentage of patients surviving 5 years after treatment was rendered. With regard to breast cancer, however, it is often difficult to establish whether or not a patient is free of the disease 5 years after treatment (Figure 3-12).[1] The risk of death from cancer of the breast continues to be higher than for the general population for at least 25 years after its removal, although the risk gradually diminishes with time. On the brighter side, there has been a startling increase in the 5-year survival in patients with operable breast cancer in the past century, regardless of the mode of therapy (Figures 3-13 and 3-14).[18] Breast cancer 5-year survival is naturally

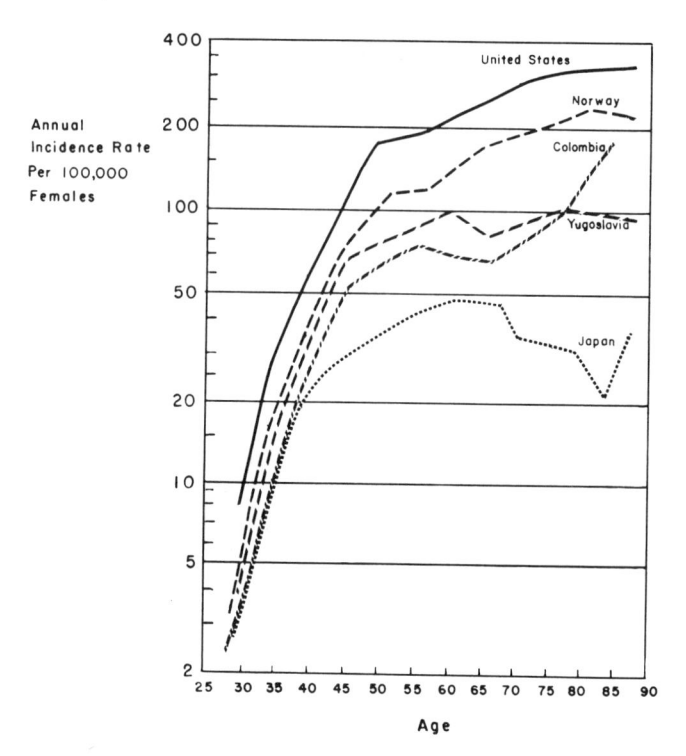

Figure 3-11 Female breast cancer incidence rates by age; selected areas, periods around 1970. Colombia (Cali), 1967-1971; Japan (averages of Miyagi; Prefecture, 1968-1971; Osaka Prefecture, 1970-1971; Okayama Prefecture, 1969); Norway, 1968-1972; United States, 1973-1976 (SEER); Yugoslavia (Slovenia), 1968-1972. *Source:* Reprinted from *Breast Carcinoma: Current Diagnosis and Treatment* (p 14) by SA Feig and R McLelland with permission of American College of Radiology, © 1983.

---

highest for stage I breast disease and decreases as the stage increases at the time of initial treatment.

The treatment of breast carcinoma has changed dramatically since the beginning of the century. The first historical reference to cancer of the breast appears in the Edwin Smith Surgical Papyrus (3000 to 2500 B.C.). After summarizing the clinical features of the disease, the author concludes that "there is no treatment." Breast cancer references are scattered and brief over the next 2,500 years. Celsus, a first-century Roman, spoke of the operation and recommended limiting it to early lesions: "None of these can be removed but the cacoethes (early lesion), the rest are irritated by every method of cure. The more violent the operations are the more angry they grow." Galen, in the second century, made the following clinical observation:

Mammography in the 1980s 61

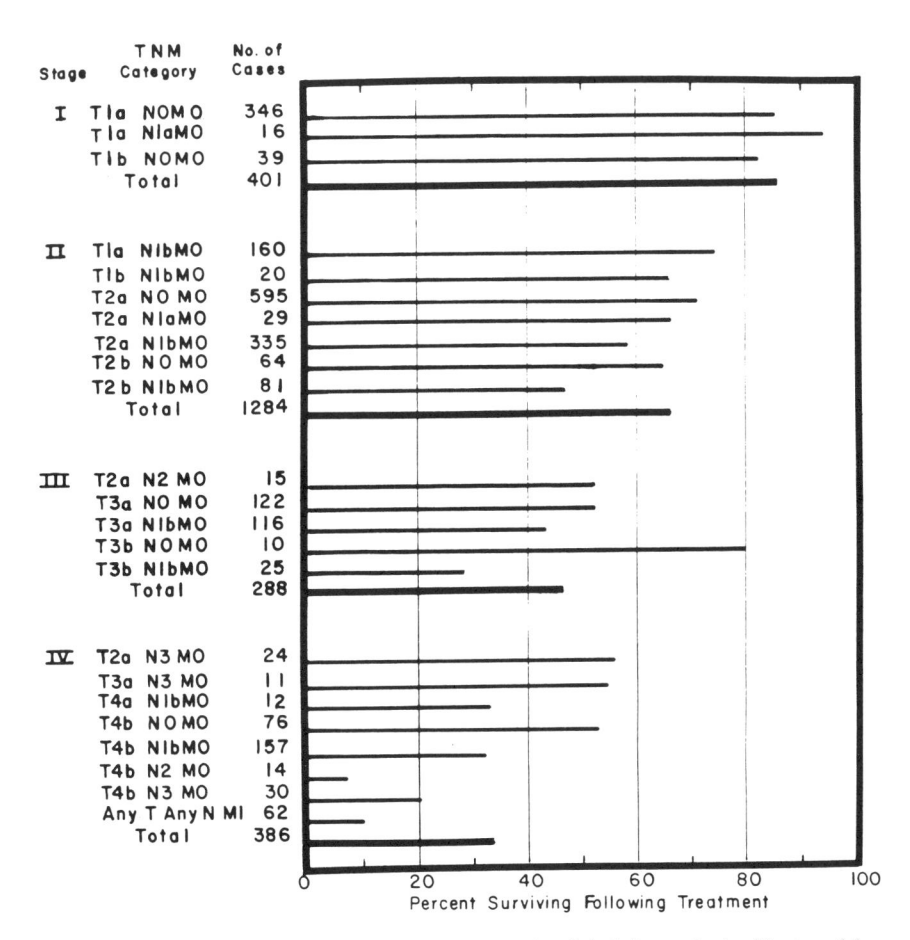

Stage	TNM Category	No. of Cases
I	T1a N0M0	346
	T1a N1aM0	16
	T1b N0M0	39
	Total	401
II	T1a N1bM0	160
	T1b N1bM0	20
	T2a N0 M0	595
	T2a N1aM0	29
	T2a N1bM0	335
	T2b N0 M0	64
	T2b N1bM0	81
	Total	1284
III	T2a N2 M0	15
	T3a N0 M0	122
	T3a N1bM0	116
	T3b N0M0	10
	T3b N1bM0	25
	Total	288
IV	T2a N3 M0	24
	T3a N3 M0	11
	T4a N1bM0	12
	T4b N0 M0	76
	T4b N1bM0	157
	T4b N2 M0	14
	T4b N3 M0	30
	Any T Any N M1	62
	Total	386

Percent Surviving Following Treatment

Figure 3-12 Breast cancer 5-year survival percentages under clinical-diagnostic classification of the Tumor, Node, Metastasis (TNM) system for staging, 1978 groupings. Based on white patients under age 65 at diagnosis surgically treated (by radical mastectomy if no evidence of distant metastasis) and initially treated 1940-1956. Cancers included are those defined histologically as infiltrating ductal carcinoma, scirrhous carcinoma, adenocarcinoma, and carcinoma not otherwise specified. Not included are unusual histologic types of breast carcinoma, papillary, lobular, colloid, or mucinous, or comedocarcinoma, for which there were too few cases to determine the applicability of the system. *Source:* Reprinted from *Breast Carcinoma: Current Diagnosis and Treatment* (p 31) by SA Feig and R McLelland with permission of American College of Radiology, © 1983.

We have often seen in the breast a tumor exactly resembling the animal the crab. Just as the crab has legs on both sides of his body, so in this disease the veins extending out from the unnatural growth take the shape of a crab's legs. We have often cured the disease in its early stages, but

62 THE GYNECOLOGIST AND THE OLDER PATIENT

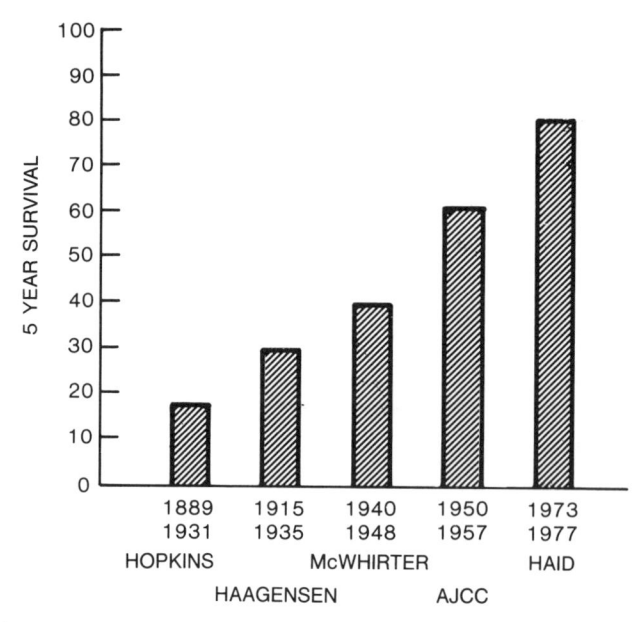

Figure 3-13 This graph illustrates the startling increase in 5-year survival in patients with "operable" (ie, stages I, II, and III) breast cancer in the past century regardless of the mode of therapy. The Hopkins series, the Haagensen series, and the American Joint Committee on Cancer series were treated by radical mastectomy; McWhirter's patients were treated with total mastectomy and radiation therapy; and those in the Haid series were treated with modified radical mastectomy, and in some patients adjuvant chemotherapy was used. *Source:* Reprinted from *Principles of Surgery,* ed 4 (p 545) by SI Schwartz et al with permission of McGraw-Hill Book Company, © 1984.

after it has reached a large size no one has cured it without operation. In all operations we attempt to excise a pathological tumor in a circle in a region where it borders on the healthy tissue.[18]

Despite Galen's discussion of operations for tumors, he attributed breast carcinoma to an excess of black bile, and logically an excision of a local outbreak could not cure the systemic imbalance. These Galenic theories dominated medicine until the Renaissance. Prominent physicians looked down on attempts at surgical removal as misdirected and futile. Surgical excision was recognized as rational therapy for breast cancer only when it was accepted that a cancer could arise in a part of the body as local disorder, as opposed to being part of a systemic imbalance. This new rationale was provided by Morgagni's study of gross pathology entitled "The Seats and Causes of Disease."[18]

Until recently radical mastectomy was the standard of treatment for operable breast cancer in the United States. The operation involves the removal of the entire breast with a generous portion of overlying skin, the underlying pectoralis major

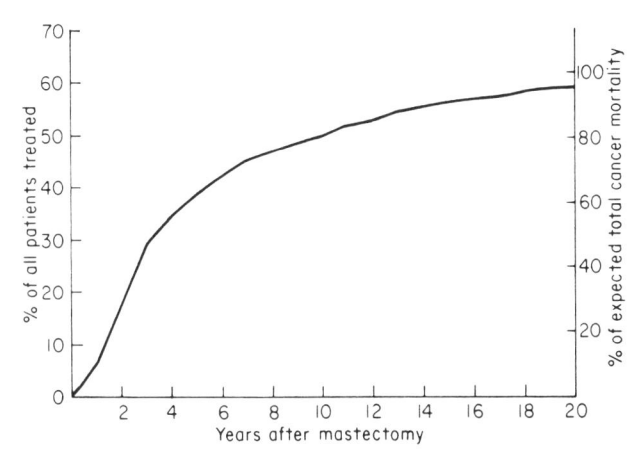

Figure 3-14 Mortality 20 years after treatment by radical mastectomy, 95% of expected mortality has been realized and over 40% of treated patients are still surviving. *Source:* Reprinted with permission from *Surgery, Gynecology & Obstetrics* (1966;122:1311), Copyright © 1966, Franklin H Martin Memorial Foundation.

and minor muscles, and the entire lymphatic fibrofatty contents of the axilla. This procedure evolved slowly from simple amputation of the breast as a treatment for breast carcinoma. LeDran, in the 18th century, repudiated Galen's humoral theory by stating that cancer of the breast was a local disease that was spread by lymphatics to regional nodes. In his operations enlarged axillary nodes were removed. In the 19th century Moore of Middlesex Hospital, England, emphasized wide removal of the breast, as well as the axillary contents in one block together with the breast, if he felt that there was neoplasm in the axilla. Banks, in 1877, supported Moore's concepts and advocated removal of axillary contents in one block with the breast whether there were palpable nodes present or not, since occult involvement of axillary nodes was so common.

Halsted, professor of surgery at Johns Hopkins Medical School, popularized what is now the radical mastectomy. His first operation was performed in 1882, and it was identical to that of today except that the pectoralis minor muscle was not removed. In 1894 Herbert Willy Meyer of New York duplicated Halsted's mastectomy and added the removal of the pectoralis minor muscle. Halsted later accepted this addition, and the modern radical mastectomy was soon widely adopted. For the next 50 years it was the only operation used by the well-trained surgeon for the treatment of breast cancer. Halsted considered a 6-cm mass to be "small." A tumor of this size is in marked contrast to the size of lesion capable of detection before surgery today.[18]

Since the late 1960s there has been controversy regarding the appropriate operation for patients with surgically resectable breast cancer. The debate was initially between the standard radical mastectomy and the simple mastectomy plus radiation therapy. It then involved radical mastectomy and total mastectomy alone, and finally radical mastectomy and partial mastectomy with or without radiation therapy. During the 1970s the modified radical mastectomy, which is essentially the same as the radical mastectomy except that the pectoralis major muscle is spared, increased greatly in popularity, which extended into the early 1980s. New Jersey surgeons in 1971 indicated that 75% would do radical mastectomy and 15% would do a modified radical operation for a 2-cm breast lesion. In 1977 surgeons in the same state indicated that 40% would do a radical mastectomy and 5% some other procedure. By 1982, however, 90% of these surgeons had opted for modified radical mastectomy for stage I breast cancers, but few were doing lesser procedures.[18]

In the second half of the 1980s there has been tremendous interest on the part of patients and physicians in conservative procedures designed to save the breast while not significantly compromising the ability to effect cure. An example is quadrantectomy, which involves removal of the quadrant of the breast containing the tumor, the overlying skin, and the fascia of the underlying pectoralis major muscle, as well as axillary dissection.[24] Other such procedures include local excision, or lumpectomy, with axillary dissection with or without radiation, and needle biopsy with external radiation as well as tumor implantation with radiation sources.[18]

When the standard Halsted radical mastectomy gave way to modified radical mastectomy in the 1970s, studies showed that there was no significant difference in survival. In addition, the modified radical mastectomy resulted in fewer complications and, cosmetically, less disfiguration. By the same token, the National Cancer Institute in Milan found that the treatment of "early breast cancer" (under 2 cm without palpable axillary nodes) with quadrantectomy, axillary dissection, and radiation therapy resulted in disease-free survival rates that were virtually identical to those of patients treated by radical mastectomy. Chemotherapy was used with either procedure if the axillary nodes were positive for tumor cells. Similar results are being reported in the United States with breast-conserving treatment plans. Radiotherapy lowers the local recurrence rates in patients who have undergone excisional biopsy or quadrantectomy, especially if the axillary nodes or surgical margins are positive (Figure 3-15).[25]

The discussion above brings us to the gist of why mammography should be an integral part of the health care of women today. With mammographic imaging, minimal breast cancer (tumors under 1 cm and in situ carcinoma) can be detected and promptly treated. Tumors of this size are too small to be detected by the hand of either the patient or the physician, as the smallest palpable lesion is 1 cm in size. The 5-year survival in patients with minimal breast cancer exceeds 90%.[18] With early detection of breast cancer by routine mammography both the patient's life and often her breast can be effectively spared. By the time a breast tumor is clinically palpable, a long occult period has passed during which many doublings

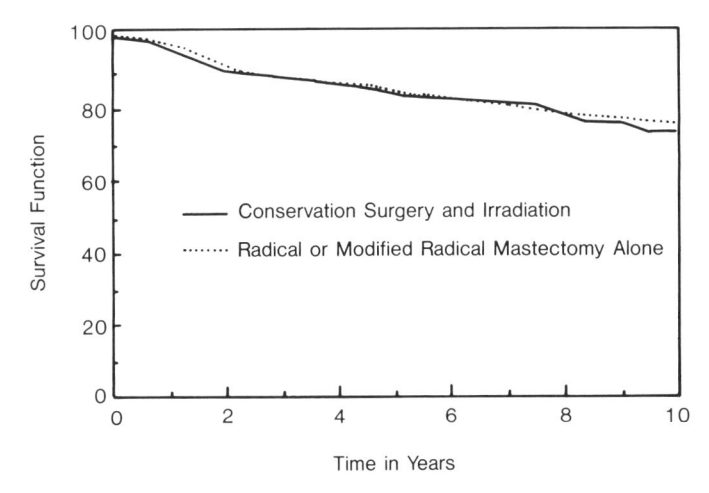

Figure 3-15 Disease-free survival rates of patients treated with conservation surgery and irradiation or with radical or modified radical mastectomy. *Source:* Reprinted with permission from *Cancer* (1984;53[3]:701), Copyright © 1984, JB Lippincott Company.

have taken place. Although clinical examination by the patient and her physician should never be replaced by any breast screening technique, mammography can significantly shorten this occult period and thereby detect the tumor at curable stage.

Some authors state that all breast cancers are a systemic disease in origin, although there are no data to support this thesis. Most information indicates that solid tumors begin as minute single or multiple-foci lesions in the anatomical site of origin. At some unpredictable time in its growth, distant spread occurs by way of lymphatic and blood vessels and by contiguous spread to nearby organs. It is obvious that if the cancer could be detected by some method of examination while still localized and adequately treated during this period, cure from breast cancer is possible (Figure 3-16).[26]

The evolution of mammography began in 1913 when Saloman, a surgeon, used x-rays to image gross mastectomy specimens. In 1930 a radiologist, Stafford Warren, reported the successful performance of mammography on patients. Unfortunately the exposure time of several seconds and the lack of breast compression, permitting motion, resulted in loss of detail, and his contemporaries were discouraged by the unpredictable quality of mammograms. The procedure was virtually abandoned in the United States until 1947, when Gershon-Cohen renewed mammographic investigation and, in association with Ingleby, correlated mammographic images with anatomy and pathology. The real clinical value of mammography became evident when Legorgne reported the typical mammographic appearance of carcinoma-associated calcifications and emphasized

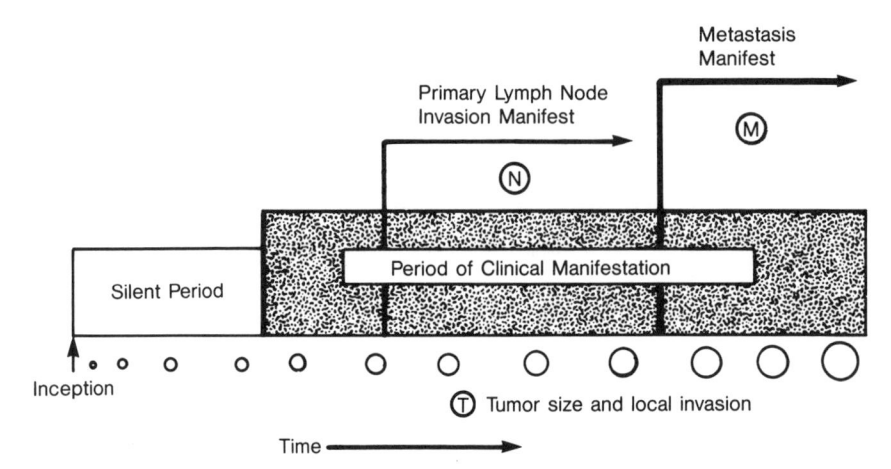

Figure 3-16 If a breast cancer can be detected during the silent period or when still localized through screening by use of physical examination and/or mammography and assuming adequate treatment, cure is likely, whereas later in the course of the disease the chance of cure is less. *Source:* Reprinted from *Breast Carcinoma: Current Diagnosis and Treatment* (p 304) by SA Feig and R McLelland with permission of American College of Radiology, © 1983.

their usefulness in diagnosing breast cancer. Nevertheless, except in a few centers, mammography continued to be impeded by lack of reproducible method for obtaining good images.[27]

In 1960 Egan reported the development of a high-milliamperage/low-kilovoltage method of producing dependable diagnostic quality in mammographic images on industrial x-ray film. The foundation was thereby laid to put mammography on trial as a screening tool for breast cancer detection. Also in the mid-1960s Gros, in France, substituted a molybdenum target for tungsten, thereby increasing the contrast between low-density breast structures—fat, parenchymal tissue, and calcifications. In addition, he initiated vigorous breast compression during exposures, resulting in elimination of motion artifacts, separation of mammary structures, and diminished scattered radiation. However, this improved image quality was associated with an increased surface exposure of 8 rads, compared with Egan's technique requiring 4 rads.

In 1969 the CGR Company introduced the Senograph, which was a mass-produced dedicated mammography unit. The mammograms from this unit provided another vast improvement in contrast, image sharpness, and reproduction of calcifications. The DuPont Company, in 1973, introduced the combined single-emulsion/high-definition intensifying screen for mammography, which they called the DuPont Lo-Dose I system. This screen permitted rapid automatic processing, shorter exposures, and reduced surface exposure from 8 rad to 1 rad.[6]

In 1975 the company introduced the Lo-Dose II unit, which required only 0.5 rad per film.

In 1972 xeromammography was introduced by Wolfe, representing another important advance. In this system a plate is charged with positive ions and, with the breast superimposed, is exposed to x-rays. Operating on the principle that x-rays dissipate a uniform electrical charge, the exposure results in a latent electrostatic image on the plate corresponding to the different densities within the interposed breast. The latent image within the processing equipment is transformed into a permanent blue and white image on paper, and the resulting images are of high quality, with skin exposures in the range of 1 to 2 rad. This superior image quality is due to an edge enhancement phenomenon that accentuates high-density structures, especially calcifications.[27] Less than 1 mm in diameter, clustered microcalcifications are strong indicators of malignant lesions and are often the only indication of early stage disease.[9]

Today's mammography units result in midline absorbed doses of 0.14 rad for film screen mammography and 0.6 to 0.9 rad for xeromammography, mere fractions of the doses required 20 years ago.[28] For comparison, a two-view standard chest x-ray uses 0.10 rad of radiation and an upper gastrointestinal series requires 10 rad.

At least three other methods of breast cancer detection have recently been popularized, partly in response to the fears people still retain toward mammography. These include thermography, ultrasonography, and transillumination, or diaphanoscopy. For purposes of completeness they are briefly reviewed here.

Thermography, according to the American College of Radiology, is a direct method of measuring temperature, either as discrete values or in the form of a visual image. Development of thermography has been encouraged because it is noninvasive and does not use ionizing radiation. There are many variations of thermographic technique, including telethermography, liquid crystal thermography, and computer-assisted thermography.[29] It has been in use clinically for more than 20 years, but its efficacy is still controversial. Theoretically thermography is an ideal screening test because it is simple, noninvasive, nonhazardous, and relatively inexpensive. The rationale behind thermography involves an increase in skin temperature in areas of inflammatory or neoplastic processes. If the temperature elevation reaches the skin surface by conduction or convection, emissions can be detected by infrared detectors (telethermography) or cholesteric crystals (contact or plate thermography).[9] Computer-assisted thermography uses discrete temperature measurements taken at standardized locations on each breast. These thermal measurements are entered into a computer program with one or more diagnostic pattern-recognition algorithms that are designed to calculate a "likelihood of malignancy" index. Thermographic detection of breast cancer, however, is not sensitive enough to be used as a reliable breast screening technique, since it has a high false-positive and false-negative rate. Its high false-negative rate, especially in women with occult early lesions, precludes its use as an independent screening technique. At this time thermography should be considered an experimental procedure with no established clinical indications.[29]

Breast ultrasonography has become a somewhat useful diagnostic method of imaging the breast. High-frequency sound waves produced by vibrations of an electronically stimulated crystal transducer pass into the breast and reflect off of tissue structures back to the transducer. There they can be reconverted to electrical signals, creating a cross-sectional image of the structures through which the sound has passed. No ionizing radiation is involved with ultrasound, and it has not proved to be hazardous to human health.[9] Breast ultrasound has been under investigation as a breast-imaging modality for more than 30 years, and a recent development of automated water-path scanning has resulted in a more reliable evaluation of the entire breast. The most important role of breast ultrasonography is to distinguish cystic from solid masses. Accuracy of 96th 100% has been reported, exceeding that of mammography and physical examination for this particular purpose. Its greatest clinical usefulness, therefore, involves cyst-solid differentiations for nonpalpable masses for which aspiration is impractical. This situation often occurs when noncalcified masses of indeterminate cause are detected by mammography.[30]

Breast ultrasound has also been used for breast cancer detection, but its sensitivity and specificity are not nearly as high as they are for cyst diagnosis. The sonographic differentiation of benign from malignant solid masses is not sufficiently reliable to help direct clinical decisions. Ultrasound is probably most helpful in the evaluation of uniformly dense breasts, as in young patients, in which noncalcified tumors may go undetected by mammography. Sonography, however, is relatively ineffective in detecting carcinoma of less than 1 cm in size, and a vast majority of cancers detected as only cluster microcalcifications by mammography are not visible on ultrasound. Malignancies are also difficult to detect sonographically in the fatty breast because the hypoecogenic pattern of most cancers is similar to that of normal fat. Because of these limitations, breast ultrasound is useful only when combined with x-ray mammography and physical examination. As previously mentioned, its primary usefulness is in making cyst-solid differentiations, especially in nonpalpable mammographically detected ambiguous masses for which aspiration is impractical, or in palpable breast masses that cannot be aspirated by clinical guidance or visualized radiographically. Ultrasound can demonstrate the true cystic nature of the latter lesion and guide successful aspiration and resolution of the mass, thereby avoiding surgery. Regarding nonpalpable masses detected by mammography, ultrasound or aspiration should be performed before biopsy to avert surgery on benign cysts.[9,30] Other uses for breast ultrasonography include evaluation of adolescent patients with symptomatic breast lesions, pregnant and breast-feeding patients with breast masses, inflammatory conditions of the breast such as mastitis and abscess, breast trauma, including hematoma and fat necrosis, recurrent masses in patients with fibrocystic disease, and in the augmented breast evaluation.[31]

The major limitation of ultrasound mammography is poor spatial resolution, which is at 2 mm with state-of-the-art equipment and which cannot reliably detect microcalcifications. Until technological improvements permit a substantial increase in the accuracy of diagnosing nonpalpable carcinomas, the role of ultrasonography will be limited to making cyst-solid differentiations.[31]

Breast transillumination, or diaphanoscopy, is a new adaptation of an old technique of shining light through the breasts. Cutler, in 1929, described the possibility of using visible light for the transillumination of breast lesions. He used high-intensity white light from a source that protected the patient from the associated heat, but the method was not efficacious because of lack of resolution and specificity. The concept has recently been resurrected with longer wavelengths of light in the far red and infrared part of the spectrum, using the breast as an optical filter, and thereby looking at tumor neovascularity. There is little scientifically documented information using this technique in the journals in this country. Transillumination techniques should be considered experimental as there is no well-documented evidence that they have any role in breast cancer screening at this time.[9]

Because of the significant improvement in technique, resolution, and diminished dosages of radiation, the American Cancer Society has revised its guidelines for mammography in younger asymptomatic women. In a statement entitled "Mammography Guidelines 1983," the following statement can be found:

> There has been remarkable improvement in the quality and diagnostic accuracy of mammography in recent years, concomitant with a marked reduction in the radiation dose—1 rad or lower at the mid-breast, using a two-view examination. Available information suggests that the risk of inducing breast cancer by the low doses now possible with modern mammography—if it exists at all—is minimal.
>
> Because of the detection of some palpable and small breast cancers and because of the reduced radiation exposures now possible with the optimum mammographic technique in carefully monitored equipment, a favorable benefit/risk ratio can now be expected in women beginning at age 40 and older.[32]

The most recent guidelines for detection of minimal breast cancer by the American Cancer Society appeared in *CA: A Cancer Journal for Clinicians* in the July/August 1985 issue. The guidelines recommend that a baseline mammography be obtained for all women between 35 and 40 years of age. Annual or biannual mammograms for all women between 40 and 49 are suggested, depending on the risk level of the individual patient. After age 50 annual mammography is recommended for all women (Table 3-8).[33]

In that same issue a survey of physicians was taken regarding the frequency with which they order mammography in a patient who has no personal history of cancer and who is asymptomatic. Although 94% of all physicians ordered Pap smears in

Table 3-8 Summary of American Cancer Society Recommendations for the Early Detection of Cancer in Asymptomatic People

Test or Procedure	Sex	Age	Frequency
Sigmoidoscopy	M & F	Over 50	After 2 negative exams 1 year apart, perform every 3-5 years.
Stool guaiac slide test	M & F	Over 50	Every year
Digital rectal examination	M & F	Over 40	Every year
Pap test	F	All women who are, or who have been, sexually active, or have reached age 18, should have an annual Pap test and pelvic examination. After a woman has had three or more consecutive satisfactory normal annual examinations, the Pap test may be performed less frequently at the discretion of her physician.	
Pelvic examination	F		
Endometrial tissue sample	F	At menopause, women at high risk*	At menopause
Breast self-examination	F	20 and over	Every month
Breast physical examination	F	20-40 Over 40	Every 3 years Every year
Mammography	F	35-39 40-49 50 and over	Baseline Every 1-2 years Every year
Chest x-ray			Not recommended
Sputum cytology			Not recommended
Health counseling and cancer checkup†	M & F M & F	Over 20 Over 40	Every 3 years Every year

*History of infertility, obesity, failure to ovulate, abnormal uterine bleeding, or estrogen therapy.
†To include examination for cancers of the thyroid, testicles, prostate, ovaries, lymph nodes, oral region, and skin.

Source: Reprinted from *Summary of Current Guidelines for the Cancer-Related Checkup: Recommendations* with permission of American Cancer Society, © 1988.

this type of patient, only 49% admitted to routinely ordering mammograms. Among the medical specialties, 68% of obstetricians-gynecologists ordered mammograms, whereas 45% of family practitioners and internists ordered them in women without symptoms of breast disease. Approximately 17% of obstetricians-gynecologists observed the American Cancer Society guidelines regarding mammography, whereas 9% of family practitioners and internists did so.[33]

The objections most frequently offered by physicians to routine mammography are that the study is too expensive to be ordered annually, or even at all, when there are no symptoms, and that it is undesirable to expose the patient to radiation from mammography if no specific symptoms exist. Some physicians felt that the yield was too low, that without a family history of breast cancer the test is unnecessary, and that it was necessary only if the patient has large breasts. Only 5% indicated that the asymptomatic patient would not cooperate in obtaining routine mammography if it were regularly ordered. Personal experience has found this rate to be much higher than 5%, as approximately one third to one half of women who are given an order for a mammogram will not have obtained it by the next annual office examination. The primary reason for this lack of cooperation in undergoing routine mammography is the aforementioned fear and paranoia that has persisted regarding the radiation involved.

With continuing physician reluctance to order routine mammography, it is little wonder that the American public retains its concerns regarding the test. A study entitled "Awareness, Opinion and Behavior Intention of Urban Women Regarding Mammography," by Berkanovic and Reeder, asked a representative sample of women living in Los Angeles what they had heard and what they believed about mammography and whether they would obtain a mammogram if their doctors advised it.[34] A striking 40% of these women said that they had never heard of mammography even after the procedure was described. Few of those who had heard of mammography had negative feelings about it, and 93% of the overall sample said that they would obtain a mammogram if their physicians recommended it. Among those women who had heard of mammography, 67% reported positive feelings, 12% had negative feelings, and 21% were neutral. Women with family members or friends who have had cancer were less positive about mammography. Again, personal experience has verified the last statement, as a tremendous anxiety builds up in family members of breast cancer patients, and the "what I don't know won't hurt me" attitude becomes a major blockade in convincing them to obtain annual mammography more regularly than the general population. The conclusion from this study was that the vast majority of women are likely to seek mammography if their physicians recommend it. Until the attitude of the physician toward mammography changes, most women will have to request the test during their annual examinations in order to detect a potential breast carcinoma at its earliest stage.

It is not the intent of this author to recommend mammography in lieu of self breast examination, physician examination, and other breast screening modalities. There are false-positive and false-negative rates for each of these techniques, and when used together, the individual patient stands the greatest chance of having an early breast cancer detected. The program outlined by the American Cancer Society for monthly breast self-examination over 20 years of age, breast examination by physician every 3 years between 20 and 40 years of age, and annually over age 40, with mammography as previously described will result in a significant improvement in the detection of early breast carcinoma, thereby diminishing the magnitude of surgery required to treat it. In addition, increased long-term survival will be an inevitable result of such a cancer detection program.

It is hoped that this chapter will dispel some of the unwarranted fears and misconceptions that have evolved along with mammography since its introduction in 1930. Only then will American women be afforded protection from advanced breast cancer that they deserve and enjoy much earlier detection than they have in the past. Low-dose mammography will probably never become the "Pap smear of the breast," but it should be viewed as a basic component of the periodic health examination of women today. The goal of both tests is really identical: to find cancer while it is still asymptomatic and before it jeopardizes the patient's life.

REFERENCES

1. Seidman H, Mushinski MH: Breast cancer: Incidence, mortality, survival, and prognosis, in Feig SA, McLelland R (eds): *Breast Carcinoma: Current Diagnosis and Treatment.* New York, American College of Radiology—Masson Publishing, 1983, pp 9–46.

2. Speroff L: Predicts ACOG will soon fully support cancer society's breast screening guidelines. *Ob Gyn News* 1986;21:1,22.

3. Holleb A (ed): *CA: A Cancer Journal for Clinicians* 1986;36:9.

4. Haagensen C, Bodian C, Haagensen D: The frequency of breast carcinoma, in *Breast Carcinoma: Risk and Detection.* Philadelphia, WB Saunders Company, 1981, pp 1–5.

5. Feig S: Low-dose mammography: Application to medical practice. *JAMA* 1979;242:2107.

6. Beahrs OH, Shapiro S, Smart S: Report of the working group to review the NCI/ACS Breast Cancer Demonstration Projects. *J Nat Cancer Inst* 1978;62:641–709.

7. Sutherland P, Gebhart R: A protocol for periodic health examinations. *Female Patient* 1986;11:89.

8. Martin JE: *Atlas of Mammograph: Histologic and Mammographic Correlations.* Baltimore, Williams & Wilkins, 1982, pp 1–12.

9. Kopans DB, Meyer JE, Sadowsky N: Breast imaging. *N Engl J Med* 1984;310:960.

10. Shapiro S: Evidence on screening for breast cancer from a randomized trial. *Cancer Suppl* 1977;39:2772.

11. Beahrs OH, Smart CR: The Breast Cancer Detection Demonstration Projects as viewed by the clinician, in Feig SA, McLelland R (eds): *Breast Carcinoma: Current Diagnosis and Treatment.* New York, American College of Radiology—Masson Publishing, 1983, pp 307–312.

12. Kalisher L, Feig S, McLelland R: *Mammography in Clinical Practice*. (Slides) Audiovisual Subcommittee, American College of Radiology.

13. Feig S: Mammographic screening: Benefit and risk, in Feig SA, McLelland R (eds): *Breast Carcinoma: Current Diagnosis and Treatment*. New York, American College of Radiology—Masson Publishing, 1983, pp 351–363.

14. Moskowitz M: Screening for breast cancer: How effective are our tests? *Breast Update II*. Orlando, Florida, Mt Sinai Med Ctr, 1984, p 3.

15. Tabar L, Gad A, Holmberg LH, et al: Reduction of mortality from breast cancer after mass screening with mammography. *Lancet* 1985 (April 13):829–832.

16. Bailar JC: Mammography: A contrary view. *Ann Intern Med* 1976;84:77.

17. Feig S: Low-dose mammography: Assessment of theoretical risk, in Feig SA, McLelland R (eds): *Breast Carcinoma: Current Diagnosis and Treatment*. New York, American College of Radiology—Masson Publishing, 1983, pp 69–75.

18. Rush B: Breast, in Schwartz S (ed): *Principles of Surgery*. New York, McGraw-Hill, 1983, pp 523-555.

19. Henderson MD, Pike MC, Ross RK: Epidemiology of breast cancer, in Feig SA, McLelland R (eds): *Breast Carcinoma: Current Diagnosis and Treatment*. New York, American College of Radiology—Masson Publishing, 1983, pp 51–59.

20. Homer M: *Early Detection of Breast Cancer by Baseline Mammography*. (Slides) Wilton, Connecticut, Medical Education Programs Ltd, 1982, pp 1–33.

21. Speroff L, Glass R, Kase N: *Clinical Gynecologic Endocrinology and Infertility*. Baltimore, Williams & Wilkins, 1983, pp 101–140.

22. Wolfe JN: Breast patterns as an index of risk for developing breast cancer. *Am J Radiol* 1976;126:1130–1139.

23. Wolfe JN: Risk for breast cancer development determined by mammographic parenchymal pattern. *Cancer* 1976;37:2486–2492.

24 Kalisher L, McLelland R, Feig S: Mammographic patterns and breast cancer risk, in Feig SA, McLelland R (eds): *Breast Carcinoma: Current Diagnosis and Treatment*. New York, American College of Radiology—Masson Publishing, 1983, pp 77–80.

25. Speroff L, Glass R, Kase N: *Clinical Gynecologic Endocrinology and Infertility*. Baltimore, Williams & Wilkins, 1983, pp 409–449.

26. Gambrell RD Jr: The menopause: Benefits and risks of estrogen-progestogen replacement therapy. *Fertil Steril* 1982;34:457.

27. Rosenfeld S: Management of Early Breast Carcinoma. Livingston, NJ, Dept Ob-Gyn, St Barnabas Medical Center. Paper presented. 1985.

28. Beahrs O: Comparative merits of mammography and physical examination, in Feig SA, McLelland R (eds): *Breast Carcinoma: Current Diagnosis and Treatment*. New York, American College of Radiology—Masson Publishing, 1983, pp 303–306.

29. Gold RH, Bassett LW: Mammography: History and state of the art, in Feig SA, McLelland R (eds): *Breast Carcinoma: Current Diagnosis and Treatment*. New York, American College of Radiology—Masson Publishing, 1983, pp 95–98.

30. Sadowsky NL: Xerography and film mammography. *Breast Disease Update II*, Orlando, Florida, Mt Sinai Med Ctr, 1984, p 12.

31. Policy statement on thermography for the detection of breast disease. American College of Radiology, 1983.

32. Policy statement on sonography for the detection and diagnosis of breast disease. American College of Radiology, 1984.

33. Cole-Beuglet C: The use of ultrasound in breast evaluation, in Sanders RC, James AE (eds): *The Principles and Practice of Ultrasonography in Obstetrics and Gynecology.* E Norwalk, Conn, Appleton-Century-Crofts, 1985, pp 603–615.

34. Mammography guidelines 1983: Background statement and update of cancer-related checkup guidelines for breast cancer detection in asymptomatic women ages 40-49. *CA* 1983;33:255.

35. Holleb A (ed): Survey of physicians' attitudes and practices in early cancer detection. *CA* 1985;35:195–213.

36. Berkanovic E, Reeder S: Awareness, opinion and behavioral intention of urban women regarding mammography. *Am J Public Health* 1979;69:1172.

Chapter 4

Dermatologic Lesions in the Elderly Gynecologic Patient

Roger Harrison Brodkin and Cynthia E. Saporito

Dermatologic diseases in the elderly gynecologic patient differ in a number of ways from those in the child and the premenopausal woman. This is particularly true regarding tumors and the sexually transmitted diseases as well as dermatoses that are more common in elderly women (eg, lichen sclerosus et atrophicus). For practical purposes dermatologic diseases are presented from a patient perspective as a complaint or as a physical finding rather than in a more classic textbook organization.

Itching of the anogenital area or the pubic area, groins, intertriginous areas, and buttocks is a common gynecologic complaint and may be caused by a number of dermatologic problems. Pruritic dermatoses include dermatitis, papulosquamous dermatoses, infections and infestations, and lichen sclerosus et atrophicus. Although a number of the vasculitides and tumors may be pruritic, the severity of the pruritus is less intense and less consistent. The history in this latter group is often more chronic and insidious, resulting in a prolonged period of delay between the onset of the lesions and symptoms and the seeking of medical help.

DERMATITIS

Contact dermatitis or pruritus may be caused by either irritants or allergens. Irritants produce contact dermatitis simply by their intrinsic capacity to be irritating to the skin, whereas allergens produce contact dermatitis by engendering the production of specific antibodies, which will then react with an otherwise harmless material to cause a similar inflammatory reaction. The most common irritant contact dermatitis in the elderly is moisture caused by urinary incontinence and by poor local hygiene. The alert patient is aware of the problem, and the diagnosis is easily made. Although there are numerous topical applications and preventive devices to deal with the problem of urinary dribbling, correction of the incontinence, usually by surgery, is the preferred treatment. Where this is not possible, frequent changes of underclothing, powdering, and use of bland emollients (eg, canned solid vegetable shortening or commercial skin lotions and creams) are helpful. Meticulous personal hygiene should always be stressed.

Allergic contact dermatitis is quite common. The most frequent causes are proprietary medications used to treat minor irritations, and toiletries used to treat excessive sweating and unpleasant odors. Antioxidants and accelerators in stretch garments and underclothing (rubber, Spandex, Lycra), analin dyes, and phenolic resins used in wet-strength tissues and no-wrinkle clothing are also common sources. Determining the cause in allergic contact dermatitis may be difficult. A particular chemical (eg, parachlorometaxylanol) may be present in numerous proprietary medications and toiletries, and the patient's medicine shelf may be filled with products containing a particular offending chemical. If recurrences are frequent, patch testing may be necessary. The course of contact dermatitis is variable. Acute exacerbations and remissions are commonly seen. Pruritus is often severe and may interfere with daily activities such as dressing, work, sleep, and social functions. Most commonly one finds clinical signs of acute inflammation, including erythema, edema, vesiculation, oozing, and crusting. The most important aspect of treatment is removal of the causal agent. Depending on the severity and extent of the dermatitis, warm tap water compresses, bland emollients, topical steroids, or a brief course of systemic steroids may be indicated.

Atopic dermatitis is usually not confined to the genitocrural area, but in elderly women localized atopic dermatitis in this distribution is not infrequently seen. A past personal history of "eczema" or a personal or familial history of atopic allergies (eg, hay fever, asthma, penicillin allergy) helps to make this diagnosis. The course of this disease is often chronic, recurrent, and relatively treatment-resistant. Pruritus is severe, and scratching is often worse during sleep. Erythema, edema, lichenification, pigmentary changes, and excoriations are frequently observed. Treatment mostly consists of the application of mild topical steroids. The mucous membranes are best treated with an ointment, while the hairy and glabrous skin is best treated with creams. These are often used in conjunction with compresses applied before the ointment or cream.

Chronic nonspecific dermatitis (neurodermatitis) is a dermatitis of unknown cause but is often presumed to be due to emotional or psychological stress. Its course is chronic and persistent with severe, intractable pruritus, and it is often treatment-resistant. Clinical findings usually include erythema, edema, lichenification, pigmentary changes, and excoriations. Hair loss from chronic, severe scratching may also be observed. Thick scaling in the moist folds becomes macerated and appears white (benign leukoplakia). Because the patient often volunteers a history of exacerbation during times of psychological stress, sometimes tranquilizers and sedatives are used. Steroid ointments are the treatment of choice. Because this dermatitis is chronic and tends to be treatment-resistant,

KOH mounts and cultures for fungi and yeast, as well as biopsy, are sometimes indicated. Potent topical steroids for a 2-week period followed by the prolonged use of a mild topical steroid in conjunction with tranquilizers and reassurance (many patients are afraid they have cancer or an infectious disease) is a conventional therapeutic plan for the management of this problem.

PAPULOSQUAMOUS DERMATOSES

Of the papulosquamous dermatoses, psoriasis is the most commonly seen in the elderly gynecologic patient. Lichen planus is uncommon and usually widespread in distribution, seldom being confined to the area below the umbilicus and above the knees. Pityriasis rosea is mainly a disease of younger people and much less common in the elderly.

Psoriasis is a chronic dermatosis of unknown cause and is often seen in the anogenitocrural area in the older aged patient. Symptoms are variable, but itching is usually found and is often severe. The scalp, elbows, and knees are the sites of predilection and should be examined to observe more characteristic lesions. The lesions of psoriasis are discrete, bright red, clearly defined papules and plaques. They are often thickly scaling and fissured, but depending on the patient's hygiene and local moisture, the heavy scale may be missing in the intertriginous areas. Treatment usually consists of topical steroids. Potent topical steroids must be used only intermittently to avoid side effects of striae and atrophy. Less potent topical steroids may have their efficacy increased with the addition of small amounts of salicylic acid, precipitated sulfur, or tar, either mixed with the steroid or used alternately.

Lichen planus, an uncommon dermatosis, is seen more frequently in adults and in the older age group. The cause is not known, but psychological stress and certain drugs have been causally implicated. Its course is chronic, often lasting for many months, and recurrences are common. Pruritus is a consistent complaint; however, excoriations are seldom found. The sites of predilection are the flexural aspects of the wrists and forearms, the legs, and trunk, often including the buttocks, lower abdomen, and groin. The mucous membranes are often involved, particularly the buccal mucosa of the mouth and seldom the labia and perianal areas. The lesions vary in size from a millimeter to a centimeter or more. They are discrete, polygonal, and purplish and present a distinctly violacious coloration. They are surmounted by a thin striated scale. The macerated scale may appear white and "lacey." Because this disease is often considered to be a manifestation of psychological stress, pressure, and tension, sometimes tranquilizers and reassurance are needed in treatment along with antihistamines and topical steroids.

INFECTIONS AND INFESTATIONS

In the elderly gynecologic patient, certain bacterial, fungal, yeast, and viral infections are seen in the genitocrural area. Infestation with lice and mites is also occasionally encountered. The common bacterial infections of the skin are mildly pruritic and not too common in the elderly female patient.

Impetigo vulgaris is caused by staphylococci and streptococci. It is usually seen as scattered follicular pustules, purulent crusts, and erosive plaques. Folliculitis often presents as follicular pustules, inflammatory papules and nodules, and abscesses. These eruptions are uncommon because of the maintenance of good hygiene and the rarity of shaving and waxing in this area in elderly females. Treatment consists of frequent washing with an antibacterial cleanser, and topical and oral antibiotics.

Tinea cruris is more common in males but is seen with some frequency in older females. Several dermatophytic fungi may cause this eruption, but *Trichophyton rubrum* is the most common. The course is stable and chronic. Symptoms of pruritus are annoying or moderately severe and tend to worsen in the summer. Irritant and allergic contact dermatitis is often superimposed with complaints of sudden worsening of a chronic pruritic intertrigo. The clinical lesions are distinctive, presenting as discrete, annular plaques with an active festooned border, showing erythema, edema, vesiculation, and crusting and a central area presenting scaling, thickening, and hyperpigmentation. Skin scrapings from the active border show long filaments with branching and segmentation. Culture on Sabouraud's agar is usually positive, with cottony white colonies after 2 weeks of incubation at room temperature. A variety of topical and oral fungicides are effective. Orally, griseofulvin is very effective but usually not necessary. The topical imidazoles are also highly effective, and their broad spectrum makes them effective against *Candida albicans* as well if there is some question in clinical diagnosis.

Monilial intertrigo is more common in the elderly gynecologic patient. It is caused by *C albicans*, and obesity, diabetes, and sweating are predisposing causes. In addition, debility and the administration of broad-spectrum antibiotics are also contributing factors. The course is acute and labile, worsening rapidly and sometimes seeming to remit. The symptoms are severe, with the acute onset of intense pruritus and burning, which may disturb sleep and render walking and sitting uncomfortable. The clinical signs are characteristic. In the genitocrural and intergluteal folds is a discrete, beefy red, moist, erosive plaque. The border presents a white macerated overhanging scale, and there are surrounding satellite pustules and small erosions. Skin scrapings should demonstrate pseudohyphae and budding spores, while culture on Sabouraud's or Nickerson's agar displays pasty colonies when incubated for 1 week. Treatment of monilial intertrigo is with topical nystatin (Mycostatin) or one of the imidazoles. This may be augmented with the use of oral nystatin if colonization of the gastrointestinal tract is suspected, or with vaginal tablets if vaginitis with discharge accompanies the intertrigo. In addition, compresses, control of diabetes, and weight reduction are often indicated.

The most common viral infection of the aged gynecologic patient is herpes zoster. Herpes simplex is seen less commonly and molluscum contagiosum is seen rarely. Genital warts are very rare.

Herpes zoster is caused by the zoster-varicella virus, which usually produces varicella as a primary infection in childhood and then remains latent in the dorsal nerve root and may recur as herpes zoster in adulthood. It occasionally involves a low sacral nerve. It runs a course of 1 to 2 months' duration in most cases. Itching is common in certain stages in the involved neurocutaneous segment, but this is usually overshadowed by pain, which may be intense and severe. Occasionally motor control of the bladder is impaired, and urinary incontinence and retention are sometimes seen. The clinical picture is distinctive. The lesions are distributed in a particular neurocutaneous segment and are distinctly unilateral, although generalized lesions are seen in rare instances. Within the involved cutaneous sensory nerve distribution are seen grouped vesicles, which first become pustules and then crusts or small ulcerations on an erythematous, edematous base. These gradually heal, usually without permanent scarring. Pain, paresthesias, and formications may persist, even after healing of the cutaneous lesions. Treatment depends on the severity of the pain. Topical therapy is of little benefit, but compresses and drying lotions (calamine lotion) or topical antibiotics (neomycin) are used to treat blistering and secondary infection. Oral analgesics and steroids, sedatives, and ketoconazole may be indicated if the pain is severe. The dose of oral ketoconazole must be doubled in treating herpes zoster, since that virus is less susceptible to this drug than the herpes simplex virus.

Herpes simplex infections are uncommon in the elderly gynecologic patient and are not usually sexually transmitted. They are seen in a recurrent form, however, in patients who suffer from chronic debilitating diseases. The course is more chronic in older people. The symptoms include itching and pain. Sites of involvement are the buttocks and crural folds. The lesions are discrete and confluent grouped vesicles or ulcerations. The diagnosis is best confirmed by culture, but cytologic and histologic techniques are also useful at times. Treatment consists of compresses and careful hygiene locally. Oral and topical acyclovir may be indicated in persistent or particularly distressing cases.

Scabies is caused by the mite *Sarcoptes scabiei* and is not rare in aged female patients, especially if they have been living in an institutional facility. The course is chronic with persistent, severe pruritus that typically worsens at night in the warmth of the bed. There are often similar cases in the household or institution among the patient's contacts. The groins, pubic area, and gluteal areas are the sites of predilection, but the hands, breasts, and axillae are also involved as sites of predilection and should be examined. In the involved areas one observes numerous red papules. The surface is often crusted or excoriated. Skin scrapings and KOH mounts show adult *Sarcoptes scabiei* eggs and feces. Treatment is very effective. The patient applies a product containing lindane or gamma benzene hexachloride for 24 hours over the entire skin. This is then washed off. Clothing and bed linens are changed. It is important to treat the patient's contacts so that reinfection is avoided. The treatment is often repeated after two to three days. Itching may take several days or weeks to totally subside.

Pediculosis pubis is also seen in elderly female patients and may be acquired sexually or through contact with toilet seats, clothing, or bedsheets harboring lice. Persistent, localized pruritus in the pubic area with visible lice and nits make the diagnosis obvious. Lindane and gamma benzene hexachloride are very effective in one application.

NONSYMPTOMATIC CONDITIONS

Vitiligo is common on the skin of the genital area but is often seen on the upper torso and extremities at the same time. The cause is unknown, but an autoimmune basis is suspected, since associated pernicious anemia, autoimmune thyroiditis, and other diseases have been found more commonly in these patients. The course of vitiligo is variable; it may be fixed and stable or progressive and spreading, or it may regress and disappear. The lesions show only pigment loss without clinical signs of inflammation, such as erythema, edema, vesiculation, or crusting, scaling, and thickening. The pigment loss may produce well-defined pink macules of varying size and configuration, often with a slightly hyperpigmented border and usually leaving pigmented hairs within the involved skin. Irregularly spotted pigmentation may be seen within the depigmented area. Treatment is not consistently or totally effective. Potent topical steroids and ultraviolet light B or A with or without psoralens topically or systemically are sometimes tried in severe cases. Reassurance that it is not cancer or contagious and may not spread widely is probably the best treatment.

Another, much rarer nonsymptomatic dermatosis is morphea, or the localized type of scleroderma. The cause is unknown. It never involves internal organs. The course is generally chronic and stable or very slowly progressive. The lesions may be solitary or multiple, large or small, and consist of well-defined atrophic plaques that may feel indurated and appear slightly depressed. The plaques are ivory with pale, violacious borders. Potent topical steroids have been used in treatment, even with occlusion. Intralesional steroids are also used. Treatment produces minimal benefit to the patient.

CONDITIONS THAT AFFECT THE VULVA

Senile atrophy of the vulva appears to be a condition resulting from diminished stimulation by lowered levels of ovarian hormones during the menopausal years.

Another theory has suggested that it is the end result of lichen sclerosus et atrophicus. It should also be remembered that if a person lives a long life, aging or senile changes are inevitable and not necessarily pathologic. As in normal aging, the skin and mucosa become thin and may have an erythematous and telangiectatic appearance. Thickening and hyperpigmentation have also been described, but these may be the result of scratching or rubbing. The elasticity of the tissues is diminished, the mucosa is dry, and loss of subcutaneous fat shrinks the normal anatomical appearance of the labia and clitoris. The clinical picture may be obscured by superimposed chronic nonspecific dermatitis or contact dermatitis. Treatment should include routine diagnostic tests for fungi and yeast. The patient must be reassured that malignancy and infection are not present. Instruction should be provided in good local hygiene. Tranquilizers or sedatives may be indicated. Topical treatment has included estrogen creams and estrogen and mild steroid ointments as well as anesthetics and antipruritics (mild concentrations of menthol phenol or camphor in an ointment or cream vehicle).

A group of persistent plaquelike lesions of the vulva constitute two important general diagnostic categories: vulvar dystrophies and carcinoma in situ. Paget's disease of the vulva occupies a special place in the latter group.

Vulvar Dystrophies

The dystrophic disorders of the vulva include two major forms: hyperplastic dystrophy and lichen sclerosus et atrophicus. There is also a mixed type that includes elements of both of these types. Cellular atypia is observed in the epithelium of the hyperplastic type and in the hyperplastic areas of the mixed type. This epithelial atypia consists of the finding of cells that lack maturation, nuclear polarity, and normal nuclear cytoplasmic ratio as well as showing numerous and abnormal mitotic figures. In carcinoma in situ these atypical cells are observed throughout the entire thickness of the epithelium, rather than in a limited and random distribution.

The causes of these vulvar dystrophies are not known. Their course is chronic with a tendency to gradual slow extension. Symptoms are variable and inconsistent. There may be no symptoms, or itching and irritation of mild or severe degree may be experienced by the patient. Carcinoma in situ and Paget's disease are also of unknown cause and may present a roughly similar appearance, behavior, and symptomatology.

Hyperplastic dystrophy can be found at any age but is more common under 50 years of age. This entity formerly included the various forms of leukoplakia. Approximately 50% of vulvar dystrophies are of this type. Areas of predilection include the clitoral prepuce, labia, and fourchette. Typically the lesion is a thickened or slightly indurated white plaque with a slightly rugose, scaly surface.

Areas of erythema and hyperpigmentation may also be seen, as well as excoriations. Ten percent of cases show significant cellular atypia or intraepithelial neoplasia, especially in the areas of the fourchette and perineum. The incidence of developing carcinoma in severe atypia has been reported to be from 10% to 25%. Treatment consists of creams and ointments containing steroids, estrogens, or antipruritics (menthol 0.25%, phenol 0.5%, camphor 0.5%). Scrapings and cultures for *C albicans* should be done, and biopsy is frequently indicated to determine the presence of cellular atypia if there is no response or an inadequate response to treatment. Areas that present severe atypia should be excised or destroyed by electrosurgery, cryosurgery, CO_2 laser, or scalpel. Careful follow-up is important.

Lichen sclerosus et atrophicus may be seen at any age from childhood to old age but is most common in postmenopausal females. This entity includes about 30% to 40% of the vulvar dystrophies. The torso and extremities may be involved in small or extensive areas of this dermatosis. The anogenital area is the site of predilection, often in an hourglass configuration surrounding the vaginal entroitus and anus. The lesion consists of a well-defined, bilateral, symmetrical area composed of small, coalescent, bone-white atrophic macules. Telangiectasia, comedones, and purpura are frequently observed within the lesion. A cigarette paper or parchmentlike surface may be seen. The atrophy may progress to atrophy of the labia minora, clitoris, and prepuce, and the marked fragility of the skin may result in painful fissures. The potential for malignancy in this disease is controversial, but epithelial atypia is rare and most practicing physicians are not concerned about the malignant potential of uncomplicated lichen sclerosus et atrophicus. Treatment is mainly effective in relieving symptoms. Topical corticosteroids have been used with success, but the risk of additional atrophy requires careful monitoring. Symptoms may also be relieved with 2% testosterone proprionate, progesterone ointment, 5% lidocaine ointment, or simple antipruritic ointments containing menthol, phenol, and camphor. Tranquilizers or antihistamines are also used. Reassurance is important.

Mixed dystrophy constitutes about 15% of this group. It consists of both former types with areas of hyperplastic dystrophy seen along with areas of lichen sclerosus et atrophicus. The different areas tend to behave in course and treatment response as they would if they were the entire lesion, except that in mixed dystrophy, hyperplastic lesions seem particularly predisposed to cellular atypia.

Carcinoma In Situ

Carcinoma in situ also presents as one or more persistent vulvar plaques (see Figure 4-1). Atypical cells are present throughout the entire thickness of the epithelium; however, there is no invasion through the basement margin. Car-

Dermatologic Lesions 83

Differential Diagnosis of Persistent Vulvar Plaques

- **Benign Dermatosis**
  - Psoriasis
  - (Chronic nonspecific dermatitis)
  - Tinea Cruris, etc.

- **Vulvar Dystrophy**
  - Hyperplastic dystrophy
    - with cellular atypia { mild, moderate, severe }
    - without cellular atypia
  - Lichen sclerosus et atrophicus
  - Mixed dystrophy
    - with cellular atypia { mild, moderate, severe }
    - without cellular atypia

- **Carcinoma in situ and Paget's Disease**

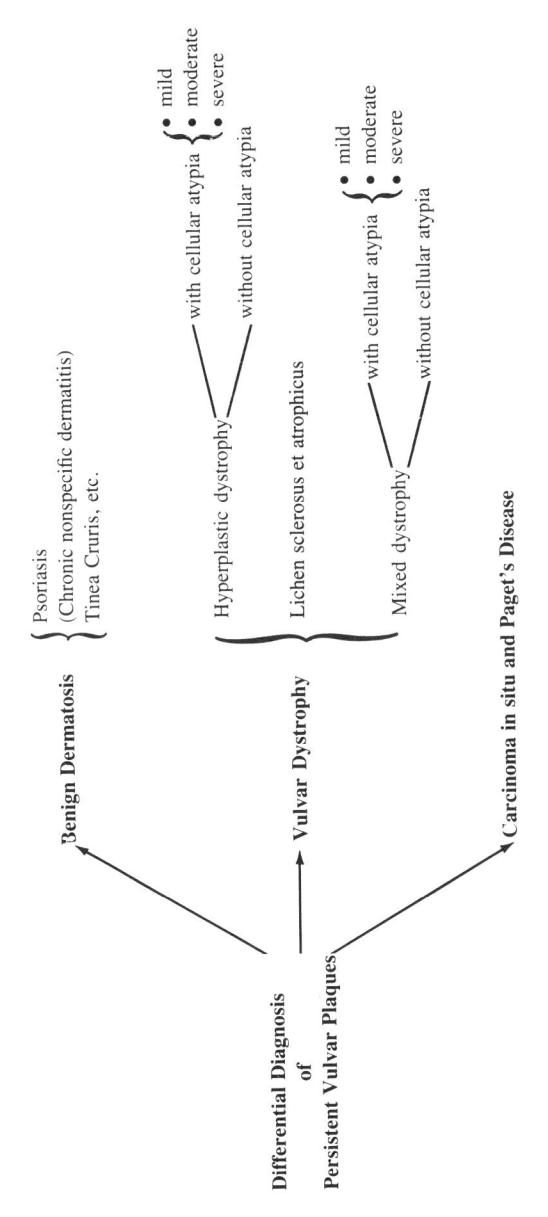

Figure 4-1 Differential diagnosis of persistent vulvar plaques.

cinoma in situ may be seen in dystrophic or normal epithelium. In nondystrophic epithelium it is becoming increasingly a disease of younger age groups and appears to be associated with human papillomavirus infection, especially types 11 and 16, and sexually transmitted diseases. This group formerly included entities bearing the name Bowen's disease, erythroplasia of Queyrat, and bowenoid papulosis, although controversy continues regarding the true malignant potential of this latter entity. It is not seen in elderly gynecologic patients. Carcinoma in situ may involve any area of the skin or mucosa of the external genitals or anus as well as the vagina and cervix. Examination of a patient with carcinoma in situ of the genital skin requires a meticulous search internally for associated similar lesions in the vagina and the anus. Here again, the lesions appear as solitary or multiple, discrete or coalescent, large or small papules and plaques. They may be white, pink, or red. The surface may be scaling, verrucous, erosive, or crusted and often presents combinations of these. Along with thorough clinical examination, colposcopy, toluidine blue staining, cytologic examination of scrapings, and biopsy are indicated, depending on the degree of suspicion clinically. Treatment consists of complete excision and careful, prolonged follow-up. Recurrence after treatment is quite common.

Paget's disease of the vulva also presents a persistent plaquelike lesion. It is rare but is seen in the elderly gynecologic patient. The cause is not known, but it is considered an apocrine gland carcinoma. Patients complain of persistent pruritus and irritation. The course is chronic and slowly progressive. The characteristic clinical appearance is of an asymmetric, well-defined, red or pink plaque. There may be areas of white macerated scale on the lesion, but a moist or crusted surface predominates. Commonly, however, it is insidious in its behavior and progresses unsuspected until treatment failure and frustration demand a biopsy.

Underlying adenocarcinoma is found in 20% of cases. Adenocarcinoma of the breast and gastrointestinal tract, as well as squamous cell carcinoma of the vulva and cervix, have been reported in association with Paget's disease of the vulva. Proper treatment includes appropriate evaluation of these possibilities as well as vulvectomy well beyond the visible borders of the lesion and deep into the subcutaneous fat. Prolonged follow-up is important.

TUMORS

Because of the great number of cell types and variety of structures that compose the skin, the large number and variety of tumors that may be found on the vulvae are difficult and complex in their classification. These tumors may traditionally be classified as benign or malignant, premalignant or pseudomalignant, nevoid, and so on. Further, they may be classified as solid or cystic and a number of other functional or morphologic categories.

Observation of the clinical signs, however, seems to be the most revealing means of classifying and diagnosing skin tumors in the elderly gynecologic patient. Most important is to determine the cell or structure of origin and the benignity or malignancy of the tumor from the clinical signs. Important benign tumors that arise from the cells of the surface epidermis are often warty, scaling, or pigmented. They include seborrheic keratosis, which is a common tumor in the elderly gynecologic patient, particularly in the intertriginous folds of the genitocrural region. Their cause is unknown, but a familial tendency is common. They are usually slow-growing or remain stable in size over a long period. If numerous, their presence may be annoying, but other than irritation and sometimes a complaint of an unpleasant odor when they are numerous, they are relatively nonsymptomatic. Lesions may be solitary or multiple and vary greatly in size and shape, measuring from 1 mm to several centimeters and being roughly oval in shape with a papillomatous, polypoid, digitate, or plaquelike configuration. Their color, too, is variable, ranging from light shades of yellow, gray, and tan to dark brown and coal black. Their surface is irregularly warty and covered with a thin scale, which presents a "waxen shine." Treatment consists most commonly of curettage and electrodessication or scissors excision for the smaller lesions. Larger lesions may be excised and sutured if a prolonged healing time is otherwise anticipated. The cure rate is high after treatment; however, individuals in whose family these tumors are common are disposed to develop new ones in the future.

Nevocytic nevi are occasionally seen in the genitocrural area of the elderly patient. Nevi present in the younger age group often involute in the later years of life. At times, however, they are seen as stable, nonsymptomatic, small papillomas. They are nonsymptomatic and generally not alarming to the patient, since they have been present for so many years. At times acute trauma may alarm the patient, or chronic irritation may call attention to their presence. The nevi are usually skin-colored or present areas of brownish hyperpigmentation. They are most often less than 1 cm in size and firm and discrete on palpation. Their shape is generally papillomatous and their surface is smooth. Treatment is most easily accomplished by scissors excision followed by electrodessication.

Benign tumors of the cells and structures of the dermis are often smooth-surfaced and skin-colored, and may be simple lumps or bumps. They are readily classified as solid or cystic. Solid tumors include lipoma, neurofibroma, hidradenoma papilliferum, clear cell hidradenoma, syringoma, leiomyoma, fibroma, and schwannoma or granular cell myoblastoma. Although there may indeed be differences in prevalence and incidence or growth rate or a variety of other subtleties of color and texture, physical signs are so few that clinical diagnosis is difficult and uncertain and often little more than a sophisticated guess or hunch. Biopsy and histopathologic study are much more important and necessary for accurate diagnosis. The treatment, therefore, is simple excision and biopsy.

Benign cystic tumors, too, present the same paucity of distinguishing physical signs that allow for accurate clinical diagnosis. Again, the smooth-surfaced lump or bump is all that the clinician may appreciate on examination. The cystic quality appreciated on palpation or transillumination, or the history of changing size to larger and smaller suggests nothing more than the existence of some type of cystic tumor. Other factors, such as location or age of the patient, may provide further clues in the specific diagnosis. In the elderly gynecologic patient one occasionally finds Bartholin's duct cysts, mesonephric or wolffian duct cysts, and canal of Nuck cysts presenting in this way.

The observation of a change in color in a dermal or subcutaneous tumor, either solid or cystic, may provide a further important clue to the specific diagnosis. In the solid tumors the red color of angioma simplex or cherry angioma, as well as in hemangiopericytoma, may reveal their vascular origin. Also, the distinctive buttery color of epidermoid cysts and sebaceous cysts is the clue to their specific nature. Cystic tumors, too, are usually treated by simple excision and biopsy.

There are also a number of mixed tumors of the skin in which both epidermal and dermal elements participate. This group, therefore, presents a lump or bump type of configuration with a distinctive surface change in color, roughness, and scaling. Fibroepithelial papillomas are common and often multiple and have a familial tendency. They are soft, papillomatous tumors with a surface that is often slightly warty or velvety and often hyperpigmented. They may be removed by scissors excision or electrosurgery under local anesthesia. Histiocytomas, too, present a scaling, rough, or verrucous and hyperpigmented surface. Palpation, however, reveals a discrete underlying, indurated, hard nodule in the dermis or subcutaneous tissue. These are treated by complete excision and suture, since removal only of the surface will be followed by prompt recurrence.

The pyogenic granuloma is a discrete, solitary, polypoid tumor that presents a surface that may be erosive and moist or crusted with a collar of scale or crust. Its bright red color reveals its highly vascular structure. This bright red or purplish color is also seen in the angiokeratoma, which is covered by a dull gray scaling and slightly verrucous surface epidermis. These lesions are best treated with curettage excision followed by electrosurgical destruction.

The premalignant tumors have already been discussed. Pseudomalignancies such as keratoacanthoma, pseudosarcomatous fasciitis, pseudolymphoma, and Spitz nevi are either rare in this age group or seldom found in this area of the skin.

Malignant tumors, too, may originate from the large number and great variety of cell types and structures. The physical signs that they present are equally numerous and varied. In general, they are nonsymptomatic and slow-growing. They may be smooth-surfaced, verrucous, scaling, superficially eroded, or deeply ulcerated. A variety of color changes may also be apparent, such as varying degrees of erythema or hyperpigmentation. The particular clinical feature, however, that suggests malignancy is determined from the disorganization of physical signs. This consists, for example, of a markedly irregular pattern of color, nodularity, vertical or lateral growth pattern, as well as the discreteness and smoothness of the borders. The same disorganized patterns that the histopathologist observes through the microscope are often reflected in the patterns of physical signs produced by these tumors.

Bowen's disease and Paget's tumor affecting the vulva have been previously covered.

Squamous cell carcinoma is seen in the genitocrural area of the elderly female, particularly on the vulva. The cause is not known, although human papillomavirus infection, chronic irritation, and poor hygiene have at times been suspected. These slow-growing tumors increase in size both laterally and vertically. They are nonsymptomatic, but drainage and bleeding are sometimes seen. The lesions are usually solitary and may present either as fungating, moist-surfaced papillomas or as ulcerations surrounded by an elevated, indurated edge. Squamous cell carcinoma is capable of metastasis to regional lymph nodes and to internal organs. For this reason the patient should be thoroughly evaluated generally for potential metastatic involvement. A complete physical examination as well as laboratory tests and x-ray studies may be indicated, depending on the patient's clinical complaints. Treatment consists of complete excision of the primary tumor, and if suspicious regional lymphadenopathy is found, a lymphadenectomy should be performed. The cure rate should be high if the tumor is treated early in its course when it is of a smaller size. Follow-up is important, to determine both the existence of metastatic lesions and the development of recurrent tumor.

Basal cell carcinoma is rare in the genitocrural area of older females. A number of causal factors have been cited in the general pathogenesis of the common type of basal cell carcinoma, including chronic, cumulative sun damage as well as the ingestion of inorganic arsenical agents, either from the environment or from material that was used medicinally many years ago. In the genitocrural area, however, the cause is not known. The lesions are very slow-growing, increasing their size by progressive centrifugal growth over a period of months or years. Eventually the surface becomes ulcerated, and bleeding, crusting, and nonhealing may occur. Pain and itching are not experienced. The lesions are generally solitary and consist of an ulceration of the skin with a serous or hemorrhagic crust on the surface. The margin is composed of closely set, translucent or pearly nodules traversed by visible telangiectasia. Superficial multicentric basal cell carcinoma presents a somewhat different clinical appearance, developing as a slowly enlarging, scaling, and erythematous plaque. The border appears discrete and thready, and small crusts may be seen along the border as well as on the surface of the tumor itself. Scaling and scar formation may also be visible on the surface of this type of basal cell carcinoma. Treatment consists of complete excision, which usually can be performed under local anesthesia with suturing to bring about rapid healing. The cure rate in this tumor should be 95% or better; however, patients should be followed for the development of new tumors as well as for possible recurrence of the old treated one.

Malignant melanoma is less common than the previous two tumors. The cause is not known; however, in general, malignant melanoma has been attributed to familial factors, particularly as part of the dysplastic nevus syndrome, and has been attributed to excessive cumulative sun damage. The course of malignant melanoma is variable, but generally it is a slowly and progressively growing tumor, in both its lateral and its vertical dimensions. It is nonsymptomatic, although early in its course it may present scaling and later there may be bleeding and ulceration. The tumor is generally solitary and discrete. The size is variable, depending on its duration and the rapidity of its growth. Its general appearance is most irregular and disorganized. The margins of the tumor show notching and variation from area to area. The color also varies from gray and tan to darker shades of brown, black, gray, and bluish black. The surface may show scaling, crusting, and ulceration. Treatment consists of thorough general physical examination, particularly with respect to regional lymphadenopathy, liver size, and so forth. Chest x-rays are routinely done, and other studies may be indicated, including electrocardiography, depending on the size, depth, and duration of the tumor, as well as other laboratory tests and x-ray studies when indicated by the patient's symptoms. Treatment consists of wide excision of the primary lesion, which may require a skin graft for coverage of the large and deep wound. Regional lymph nodes should be removed when involvement is suspected or when the tumor is at a deeper level or a greater thickness. The outlook for patients with malignant melanoma is always guarded, since metastases at times occur early in the course of this disease and may spread by the bloodstream as well as the lymphatic channels. Regular and prolonged follow-up is indicated in this tumor, since metastases and recurrences may appear many years after treatment of the primary tumor.

Bartholin's gland carcinoma is rare but is mainly found in the vulva of the older gynecologic patient. The cause is not known, and it appears as a slow-growing, nonsymptomatic nodule or mass. As growth continues it may produce ulceration of the overlying skin. The aggressiveness of the tumor depends on the cell type; however, many of these tumors eventually metastasize to inguinal lymph nodes and later to deep pelvic lymph nodes. Treatment consists of total wide excision, including contiguous lymph node areas in the cell types that metastasize to these lymph node areas.

Dermatofibrosarcoma protuberans is rarely found in the genitocrural area of the elderly female. Other soft tissue–site sarcomas, including neurofibrosarcoma, rhabdomyosarcoma, angiosarcoma, and epithelioid sarcoma, are also extremely rare and may generally be described in the same way. The cause is unknown, and the course is one of gradual, indolent, progressive growth. It is nonsymptomatic and usually presents as an irregularly bordered and nodular solitary plaque. The lesion is markedly indurated, and the borders are difficult to define clinically. The growth pattern, in both its nodularity and its irregular configuration, presents a distinctly disorganized appearance to the examiner. Treatment consists of wide excision of the primary tumor. General physical examination, laboratory tests, and x-ray studies are indicated for metastatic tumors, although metastases do not usually occur early in the course of this disease. Recurrences of the primary tumor are common, since it has the capacity to grow for a long distance into the surrounding, normal tissues without betraying its presence with clinically visible or palpable signs from the surface. Sometimes aggressive and mutilating surgery is required to control this rare tumor.

Metastatic carcinoma is seldom found in the genitocrural skin of the elderly female. A great variety of sites have been the source of metastatic tumors, and these have included the urethra, vagina, cervix, endometrium, and ovary. Breast, kidney, and lung tumors and melanoma have also been reported. These tumors seem to appear and grow rather suddenly and rapidly. They may be nonsymptomatic, or the patient may complain of pain. They may present as a solitary nodular tumor or a plaque studded with numerous small and irregular papillomatous lesions. They feel hard to palpation and are reddish or skin-colored. Ulceration is rare. Other than biopsy for diagnosis, treatment is generally not indicated, and because these lesions tend to occur late in the course of the primary tumor, treatment is often under way with chemotherapy.

Lymphomas and leukemias generally present as multiple, widespread nodular tumors, plaques, or erythroderma. Occasionally, however, a solitary nodular tumor will be seen as the first presenting sign of lymphoma or leukemia, and this is uncommon in the genital area of the elderly female. The tumors appear suddenly and grow rapidly. They may be skin-colored or varying shades of red. Their surface may be smooth or ulcerated, and they are hard on palpation. General physical examination, x-rays, and laboratory studies are indicated to determine the origin of this systemic malignant process, and treatment is generally with chemotherapy as well as local radiation therapy.

In the general care of the elderly gynecologic patient, the gynecologist in his or her role as a primary care physician, may be called on for advice on the management of dermatologic problems that do not necessarily involve the genitocrural areas. Melanotic freckle of Hutchinson is not a tumor of the female genitals, but is most common in the elderly female patient. It is most frequently located on the head and neck but may be seen on other sites. The cause is unknown. It is a slow-growing, nonsymptomatic lesion, spreading gradually centrifugally. The melanoma appears as a most irregular and disorganized lesion with a markedly notched and variable border and with a great variety in coloration, ranging from paler shades of yellow and tan to gray, brown, black, and bluish black. The surface may show subtle signs of scaling and crusting, particularly in larger lesions, and one or more black nodules may develop on this macule or plaque, but not until late in the course. Metastases occur after many years and generally appear in regional lymph nodes rather than develop by hematogenous spread. When regional lymph nodes are involved, the tumor again tends to remain stable for a relatively prolonged period in the regional lymph nodes before further spread to internal organs occurs. Treatment is a problem, since these tumors are often located on the face and are very large. Excision with primary closure or grafting is the treatment of choice when possible. Prolonged follow-up is required, since recurrences of the primary tumor after excision are common.

ALOPECIA

Another problem of great concern to the elderly gynecologic patient may be hair loss. It should be remembered that hair loss may be caused by a great variety of internal or local disorders. General internal conditions that are known to cause hair loss include the administration of certain drugs, particularly anticancer chemotherapeutic agents, as well as acute illnesses. Alopecia areata and a number of inflammatory scalp problems, such as psoriasis and atopic dermatitis, may also result in hair loss. Most commonly, however, female pattern alopecia, which

Table 4-1 Differential Diagnosis of Pruritus Vulvae

Pruritus—No inflammatory lesions	Contact pruritus—Indolent sensitizers Atopic pruritus Senile pruritus Psychogenic pruritus Systemic disease—Diabetes Drugs—Antibiotics
Dermatitis	Contact dermatitis—Allergic, Irritant Atopic dermatitis Chronic nonspecific dermatitis (Neurodermatitis)
Papulosquamous dermatoses	Psoriasis Lichen planus
Infections and Infestations	Bacterial—Impetigo, Folliculitis Fungal—Tinea cruris Yeast—*C albicans* Viral—Herpes simplex, herpes zoster Parasitic—Scabies, Pediculosis pubis, Tick
Tumors	Extramammary Paget's tumor Squamous cell carcinoma Basal cell carcinoma
Vulvar Dystrophies	Hyperplastic dystrophy Atrophic dystrophy Mixed dystrophy

Dermatologic Lesions 91

Table 4-2 Management of Pruritus Vulvae

I. History

    Personal and familial atopic allergies
    Psychic depression, sex life
    Drugs
    Mucosal dryness
    Systemic diseases
    Known topical allergies
    Previous dermatoses occurring on the skin

II. Physical Examination

    No signs of inflammation
    Inflammatory lesions
    Excoriations
    The search for more characteristic lesions in other areas of the skin on general dermatologic examination

III. Laboratory Tests

    Scraping (KOH mounts for fungi, yeasts and scabies; dry scraping for nits and lice; cytologic examination for herpes)
    Culture on Sabouraud's agar for fungi and *C albicans*; culture for bacteria; viral culture for herpes
    Biopsy (routine and special stains)

IV. General Laboratory Examinations

    CBC (complete blood cell count) and differential
    Blood chemistries
    Urinalysis

V. Treatment

    Specific trial of treatment
    Antibacterial antibiotics, antiviral antibiotics, antifungal antibiotics, antiyeast antibiotics
    Nonspecific treatment
    Topical and systemic steroids; topical menthol and phenol ointments
    Antihistamines
    Tranquilizers
    Topical scabicides

---

begins in middle age or earlier with diffuse thinning of the crown of the scalp without recession of the anterior hair line, is the most common cause. The management of these problems often requires careful diagnostic evaluation and testing beyond the training and interest of the gynecologist. However, the gynecologist, as any physician, should be sensitive to this problem and be sympathetic in assisting the patient to find help with what is often an exceedingly delicate and personally worrisome problem.

PRURITUS VULVAE

Pruritus vulvae is an utterly nonspecific complaint and may be caused by a large variety of specific dermatologic and gynecologic diseases (see Table 4-1). The specific diagnosis must be made by a careful history that includes evidence of personal or familial atopic allergies; past or concurrent dermatologic problems; contactants; current medications, etc., as well as clinical findings, such as type of skin lesions, discharge, etc., and laboratory studies that may include KOH wet mounts and culture for fungi and yeasts, blood glucose, biopsy, etc. (see Table 4-2). Attributing this complaint to senile changes in patients and utilizing empirical therapy with estrogens or antiyeast medication will lead inevitably to missing a specific diagnosis. This very common complaint must not be trivialized and sympathy must be properly mixed with methodical study to help the patient.

Chapter 5

Hypertension and Renal Diseases in Elderly Women

Michael Gutkin and Lawrence H. Byrd

INTRODUCTION

Hypertension is the leading cause of cardiovascular disease—stroke and heart disease—in older women. Hypertension is the brightest star in a constellation of risk factors for cardiovascular disease. All these risk factors should be reduced whenever possible. While moderate or severe hypertension should be treated with medication, in mild hypertension control of associated risk factors may be as important as control of blood pressure. In addition, the presence of pre-existing target organ damage is more important than the diastolic blood pressure in judging whether to prescribe medication. Antihypertensive therapy is more effective at reducing the incidence of stroke than that of myocardial infarction.

A brief outline is offered for the evaluation of blood pressure on physical examination, those circumstances that would benefit from consultation with an internist, an algorithm for treating the elderly hypertensive woman, and principles of therapy with commonly used agents.

High blood pressure can cause premature damage to the brain, heart, kidneys, and arteries—the "target organs."[1] Hypertensive postmenopausal women suffer from more strokes (cerebral thrombosis, hemorrhage, and embolism), transient cerebral ischemic attacks,[2] dementia,[3-6] angina pectoris,[7] myocardial infarction,[8] congestive heart failure,[9] renal insufficiency,[10] atherosclerosis of major arterial branches,[11] and thoracic and abdominal aortic aneurysm[12] than their normotensive counterparts. Lowering the blood pressure reduces the frequency of most of these complications.[13]

A blood pressure of 140/90 is used to divide patients into hypertensive and normotensive categories. This is an artificial distinction because even when blood pressure is below 140/90, higher pressures reduce life expectancy. Patients with 140 systolic have double the incidence of cardiovascular disease as in those with 100 systolic.[14]

The risk of premature vascular disease increases with the height of the blood pressure and the length of exposure to it. The life expectancy of a 45-year-old woman whose blood pressure is 150/100 is reduced by 8.5 years.[15] In patients over age 45, with systolic blood pressures of 110 to 129, the incidence of coronary heart disease is 2.8/1,000 patient years; with systolic blood pressures of over 150, the incidence is 11.1/1,000; and with systolic blood pressures of over 160, 13.8/1,000.[16]

Blood pressure, especially systolic blood pressure, rises with age in virtually all populations.[17] This is not desirable, and can be avoided. Those elderly patients who show little or no rise have a low rate of cardiovascular complications.[18] For purposes of this discussion, elderly is defined as age 60 and over, but the behavior of hypertension in the entire postmenopausal era is considered.

DETERMINANTS OF HIGH BLOOD PRESSURE

Blood pressure is the product of cardiac output and total peripheral resistance. Resistance is due to the friction between blood and endothelial cells during steady flow. This friction is mainly generated in the smallest blood vessels (arterioles and precapillary sphincters), where the blood vessel surface is greatest for a unit volume of blood. It dissipates the energy imparted to the blood by cardiac contraction. A proportion of systolic energy is needed to stretch the walls of large elastic blood vessels, to achieve the periodic acceleration of blood, and to overcome the internal friction (viscosity) of blood during pulsatile flow. This requires additional energy in healthy adults, about 15% of the total,[14] most of it spent in stretching the vessels. The sum of resistance to steady and pulsatile flow is characterized as impedance.

The increasing blood pressure seen with aging is due to rising impedance.[15,19] Impedance increases the most in the renal circuit.[20] Cardiac output remains normal in those elderly who are healthy,[21] have no evidence of ischemic heart disease, and are not institutionalized.[22,23]

CHANGES IN CIRCULATION WITH AGING

The aging circulation cannot regulate itself efficiently to prevent fluctuations in blood pressure. Both short-term and long-term buffering mechanisms are inefficient.

Short-term buffering is carried out by barostats (pressure regulators), which are located in the aortic arch and the bifurcation of the common carotid artery. It is their function to raise or lower a momentarily changed blood pressure by changing heart rate, myocardial contractility, and impedance. The aging process diminishes the function of these barostats by destroying their stretch receptors.[24] In addition, the heart does not accelerate well in aging patients, and often cannot raise its output properly in response to the demand of the barostats during hypotension.

Long-term buffering depends on renal and hormonal adjustments that vary the level of total exchangeable body sodium. Increasing total exchangeable sodium helps to promote long-term rises in blood pressure. Renal function declines faster with aging in patients with higher blood pressure.[25] The declining renal mass of the aged promotes sodium retention when there is abundant sodium in the diet. However, the ability to retain sodium is reduced in the elderly kidney when dietary intake is curtailed or when there are gastrointestinal losses.[26]

CHANGES IN RENAL FUNCTION WITH AGING

Deterioration in renal structure and function with aging affects the ability of elderly patients to maintain homeostasis and respond flexibly to medications, stress, illness, or alterations in diet, mobility, and environment.[27] Drug-induced illness and drug interactions are thus major problems in the aged. Adjustment of dosage of drugs like digoxin and aminoglycosides, which are excreted by the kidneys, must be based on creatinine clearance and not simply serum creatinine. Nomograms have been used to correct the serum creatinine for age, but even these approximations may be inaccurate.

There is an age-related decrease in the capacity to concentrate urine that is both central (impairment in vasopressin secretion) and renal (decreased capacity to elaborate maximally concentrated urine).[27] Consequently older patients require a large urine volume to excrete the obligatory daily solute load of approximately 600 mosm. But this necessary compensation is tenuous because the elderly may have impaired thirst perception and often cannot react to salt and water deprivation with effective conservation.

DEFINITIONS OF HYPERTENSION

Occasional rises in blood pressure may be viewed as a warning of more frequent rises in the future. Cardiovascular disease is more likely to occur when the elevated readings are present on a third consecutive weekly determination, and classification of the hypertension should rest on the most recent of the three.[28,29] The term labile hypertension is archaic. All hypertension is labile, and the higher the set point of the blood pressure, the greater the fluctuations around it.[30]

Borderline hypertension is defined as a blood pressure that is sometimes greater than 90 diastolic in the outpatient setting. A blood pressure of 154/92 on the first visit and 136/84 on the third would fall into this category. *Diastolic hypertension* is generally used to determine the scale of severity of fixed hypertension. *Mild hypertension* refers to a diastolic blood pressure of 90 to 104, *moderate hypertension* to a diastolic range of 104 to 114, and *severe hypertension* to a diastolic of 115 or greater. Seventy percent of hypertensives fall in the borderline or mild category.[31] *Systolic hypertension* may be *isolated* (no companion elevation of diastolic) or *disproportionate* (systolic greater than (2 × diastolic) − 15).

RISE OF SYSTOLIC BLOOD PRESSURE WITH AGE

One reason for the increasing systolic and decreasing diastolic pressure observed in the older members of civilized societies is the rigidity of their arteries.[32] The aorta and other arteries normally store some of the energy of left ventricular ejection by stretching, thereby reducing systolic blood pressure, and by returning energy to the circulation by rebounding during diastole. Another reason is increased stroke volume,[33] owing to bradycardia or to volume expansion from increased total exchangeable sodium.

WASTED CARDIAC WORK

High systolic pressure widens the vessels and causes more high-tensile strength elements to be recruited (Figure 5-1).[34–37] This makes the vessels even stiffer. At the peak of left ventricular ejection there is a large force applied to the vessel wall, which cannot stretch further. In these circumstances some of the systolic force is dissipated as heat and not returned during diastole.[38] This may double the 15% of cardiac energy that is normally wasted with each stroke.[39]

Wasted cardiac work contributes to the development of left ventricular hypertrophy,[40] which is a gateway for the development of hypertensive complications.[41] In its early stages it is reversible by antihypertensive therapy.[42] However, when the enlarging heart muscle outgrows its blood supply because of coronary atherosclerosis and arteriolosclerosis, hypertrophy becomes irreversible and marked by disorganization and fibrosis of muscle tissue.[43]

CARDIOVASCULAR DISEASE IN HYPERTENSIVE WOMEN

The Framingham (Mass) Study examined the incidence of cardiovascular disease in that community since 1949.[44] Systolic and diastolic hypertension had a

Hypertension and Renal Diseases 97

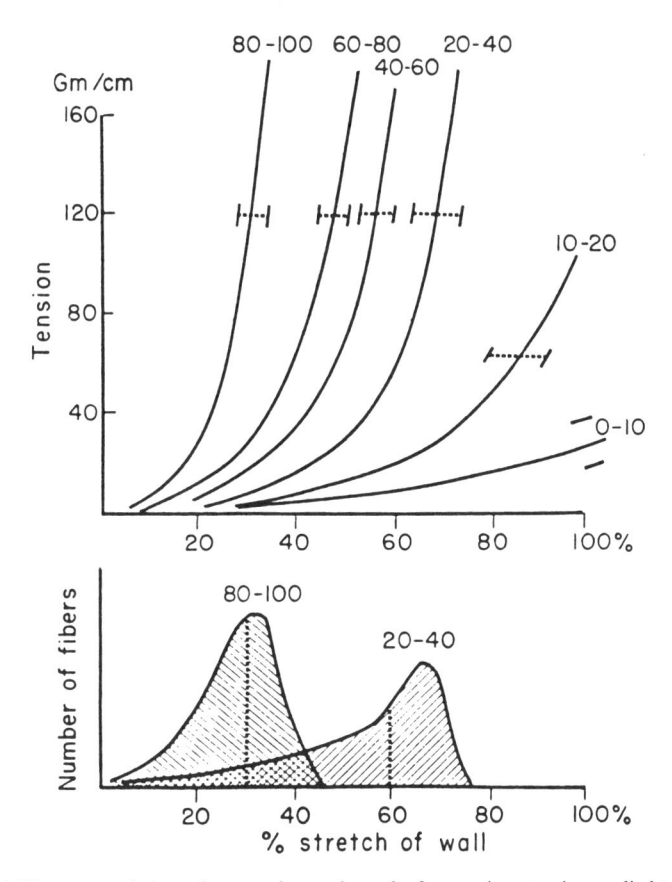

Figure 5-1 The top panel shows how much stretch results from a given tension applied to the large arteries of humans aged 0 to 100 years. Older blood vessels stretch (and therefore rebound) less in response to a given blood pressure than do younger ones. The bottom panel shows that in arteries from patients 80 to 100 years old, more collagen fibers are recruited at 30% stretch than in arteries from 20- to 40-year-old patients at 60% stretch. The areas under the curves represent the total amount of collagen in the arterial wall. *Source:* Reprinted with permission from *Canadian Journal of Biochemistry and Cell Biology* (1959;37:557–569), copyright © 1959, National Research Council of Canada.

---

formidable impact on the population's welfare. Seventy-five percent of all strokes and 75% of all myocardial infarctions occurred in subjects with high blood pressure. In a group of 30- to 62-year-old subjects followed for 18 years, about one third of the hypertensive subjects suffered an adverse cardiovascular event.[45] Even slightly abnormal blood pressures increased risk.[46] But certain attributes, other than diastolic hypertension per se, were also found to predispose the women in the study to heart disease and stroke. These "risk factors," compiled from the Framingham and other population surveys, are listed below.

RISK FACTORS FOR HEART DISEASE IN ELDERLY WOMEN

Age. The death rate increased by 7% per birthday anniversary in treated female patients with moderate hypertension.[47] The incidence of nonfatal cardiovascular complications was four times as high in a group over age 60 as in a matched group under age 50.[48,49]

Cigarette Smoking. The smoking habit raised mortality rates twofold (at any age) in treated hypertensive women.[50] In untreated hypertensive women smoking increased coronary events threefold to fourfold, effectively adding 5 years to their age.[51] Smoking even one to four cigarettes per day doubles the risk of coronary disease in women.[52]

Clinically Apparent Target Organ Damage. While other risk factors merely predict what might happen, established events point to the past as prologue. A history of myocardial infarction, angina pectoris, any electrocardiographic abnormality,[47–51,53,54] intermittent claudication,[11] elevated blood urea nitrogen,[47] proteinuria,[50] or grade II retinopathy[50] raises the death rate from cardiovascular disease by 100% in women. A previous myocardial infarction in a woman confers a 45% chance of death within 5 years and a 40% chance of another infarct within that time.[55] Echocardiographic evidence of left ventricular hypertrophy appears to be an independent risk factor for premature vascular events in women.[56]

Estrogens. Premenopausal women have relative immunity from coronary heart disease death.[56] After age 55 the incidence of coronary disease begins to rise, so that by ages 65 to 74 the female-male incidence ratio is 1:0. Women who have undergone surgical menopause, and who have not taken replacement estrogens, appear particularly vulnerable.[57] The coronary disease is likely to be relatively stable angina pectoris.[55] Replacement estrogen therapy in the postmenopausal woman does not increase,[58] or may even reduce, cardiovascular mortality rates.[59,60] After menopause, levels of atherogenic low-density lipoproteins rise; these are associated with coronary artery disease.[55,61]

Diabetes Mellitus. After adjusting for all other risk factors, diabetic elderly women have a 200% excess risk for coronary heart disease, equal in importance to that of hypertension, and their heart attacks tend to be severer.[62] The presence of diabetes removes the sex advantage of women in the incidence of myocardial infarction,[55,62,63] even when favorable levels of high-density lipoproteins are present.

Systolic Blood Pressure. The frequency of cardiac complications at any diastolic blood pressure is higher when systolic blood pressure is elevated.[31,33,47] When isolated systolic hypertension of 180 or greater is present in people aged 65 to 74, the risk of death from coronary disease is increased by two and one half times compared with those with lower systolic values,[45] and the fatality rate after myocardial infarction[64] rises dramatically. In a study of 191 females with a mean age of 80, the incidence of myocardial infarction was three times as high when isolated systolic hypertension (mean systolic blood pressure 181 mm Hg) was present compared with normotensive controls (mean systolic blood pressure 129 mm Hg).[64,65]

Antihypertensive Therapy as a Risk Factor. In several randomized prospective trials of antihypertensive therapy, mainly involving men, treatment could not be shown to reduce the incidence of fatal myocardial infarction,[13,49,53,64–67] or increase it, if ECG abnormalities were present at the start of treatment. Thiazide diuretics were implicated in this phenomenon, since these agents prevented the fall in cholesterol that was expected from dietary counseling[67] and caused hypokalemia and hypomagnesemia, which are risk factors for dysrhythmia.[53]

These findings have been widely publicized. But thiazide diuretics remain useful and should not be discarded thoughtlessly. The incidence of myocardial infarction in women is low, and this tends to moot the issue except in diabetics and smokers. Furthermore, in a very large and unselected population, the 8-year risk of coronary heart disease was lowered with thiazide treatment by an amount that would have been expected if thiazides had no adverse effect.[12] A large-scale European trial showed no apparent adverse effect of thiazide diuretics; there was no reduction in the overall incidence of myocardial infarction with antihypertensive therapy, but fatal infarction *was* markedly reduced.[51]

When clinical or electrocardiographic signs of myocardial ischemia are present, lowering the diastolic blood pressure below 85 mm Hg can produce a paradoxical increase in the risk of myocardial infarction in men or women.[68] The risk of this occurring is greatest when then untreated hypertension was severe.[69] Since thiazides are potent and are instrumental in lowering the blood pressure in patients with ischemic heart disease, they may have been innocent bystanders in a process of vigorous blood pressure reduction that led to myocardial infarction.

Family History. In women over age 60 family history of coronary artery disease is an unimportant contributor to the risk of myocardial infarction.[60,61,70]

Serum Cholesterol. The conveniently measured forms of cholesterol include the total cholesterol, the high-density lipoprotein–cholesterol fraction (thought to confer protection from coronary artery disease), and the low-density lipoprotein–cholesterol fraction (thought to confer susceptibility to coronary artery disease). The very low density lipoprotein fraction, which predominantly contains triglyceride, is not conveniently measured in clinical practice, but can be estimated by subtracting from the total cholesterol the sum of the high- and low-density lipoprotein fractions. Elevated serum triglycerides[71] and total cholesterol[72] are associated with coronary disease in older women. High-density lipoprotein–cholesterol appears to be protective; the proportion of total cholesterol that is high-density lipoprotein may be more important than the total[72,73] and should be more than 22%, with a low-density lipoprotein–cholesterol of less than 150 mg/dL.

Obesity. Obesity is an independent risk factor when it is present for 14 or more years in otherwise risk-free women of all ages.[74] Obesity is especially risky in women when the ratio of waist to hip circumference is greater than 0.8.[75] Being thin is not intrinsically risky. The diminished survival observed in thin people is probably the expression of preexisting disease or of cigarette smoking.[74–76]

Race. Data on whether black women over age 60 have greater risk for myocardial infarction than do white women are conflicting and inconclusive.[77,78]

RISK FACTORS FOR STROKE IN ELDERLY WOMEN

Age. Cerebral atherosclerosis is ubiquitous in the elderly. Fifty percent of all major cerebrovascular occlusions are not accompanied by infarcts, and 5% of all autopsies show recent encephalomalacia or recent intracranial occlusion.[79] Unlike myocardial infarction, stroke is as common in elderly women as in men.[80,81] The stroke rate rises as a logarithmic function of age,[82–84] and age is a more significant risk factor than systolic blood pressure in female patients of all ages.[50,51,83] There has been a gradual reduction in the incidence of stroke in the elderly women throughout the Western world, beginning before and accelerating since the advent of antihypertensive therapy and not entirely attributable to such therapy.[83–85]

Cigarette Smoking. Cigarettes have been noted as a risk factor for stroke mortality in elderly women.[86,87] Smoking is a more potent risk factor for stroke than is systolic blood pressure.[58]

Clinically Apparent Target Organ Damage. About one fourth of stroke victims will die of another stroke.[79] Forty percent of patients with transient cerebral ischemia develop stroke, half of them within 3 months of onset.[88] However, asymptomatic cervical bruits are not indicative of a higher rate of stroke in women.[89]

Heart Disease. Heart disease prevention is stroke prevention. One third of strokes occur in the 10% of the population having multiple coronary risk factors.[79,83] The rate of stroke in mild hypertensives of the Hypertension Detection and Followup Program who had evidence of heart damage was about three times as great as in those who did not have heart damage.[90] Electrocardiographic left ventricular hypertrophy (LVH) increases the risk of stroke sevenfold in women,[80,83] and stroke is more common when hypertrophy is discovered even earlier by echocardiography.[81] Atrial fibrillation increases the risk of stroke fivefold,[91] and increases stroke mortality[92,93] owing to embolism[94] or thrombosis.[92] Embolic strokes are more common in elderly women than in men.[93]

Estrogens. Estrogen use after the menopause does not predispose women to stroke,[95] and may protect them from it.[93]

Diabetes Mellitus. Diabetes mellitus is not as important a risk factor for stroke in the elderly woman as it is for myocardial infarction.[81,90]

Systolic Blood Pressure. Systolic hypertension is a principal risk factor for stroke[44,79,80,96] and lacunar infarcts[97,98] whether it accompanies diastolic hypertension[44,45,83] or is isolated (Figure 5-2). But increased systolic blood pressure may be a risk factor for stroke only in those patients with heart disease.[95]

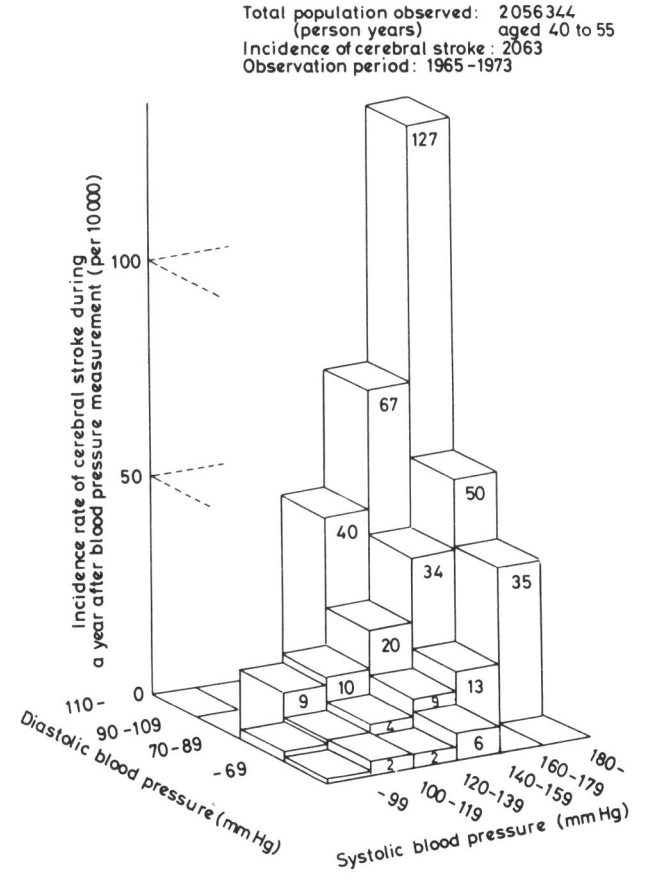

Figure 5-2 The rate of stroke in 230,000 Japanese railway workers, representing more than 2 million patient years. Rising systolic blood pressure has a profound influence on the risk of stroke at a given diastolic blood pressure. *Source:* Reprinted from *Mild Hypertension: Natural History and Management* (p 58) by F Gross and T Strasser (eds) with permission of Churchill Livingstone, © 1979.

Serum Cholesterol. Serum cholesterol and triglycerides show no association with stroke or with stroke mortality[83,86] in women.[51,85]

Race. Stroke rates in black hypertensive women and white hypertensive women appear to be equal.[90,99]

Diet. A high potassium intake (over 75 mmol/day) may protect against stroke in normotensive and hypertensive elderly women.[100]

HIGH-RISK PATIENTS

The authors arbitrarily define a high-risk patient as a woman who has clinically apparent target organ damage, diabetes mellitus, a low-density lipoprotein-cholesterol level of over 200 mg/dL, longstanding obesity with a waist-hip ratio of over 0.8, a systolic blood pressure of over 180 mm Hg, or a cigarette smoking habit.

THE PRINCIPLE OF MULTIPLE RISK FACTORS

Vascular disease develops in a multifactorial setting (Figure 5-3).[101] In order to prevent cardiovascular disease in hypertensives it is important to lower serum

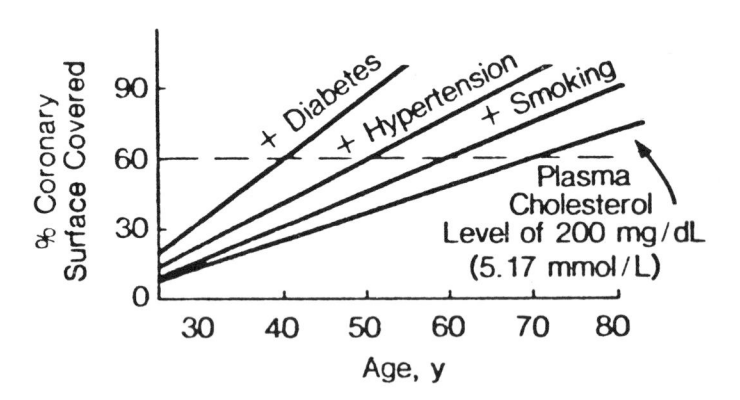

Figure 5-3 Age, smoking, hypertension, and diabetes conspire in an additive fashion to cover the surface of the coronary arteries with atheromata. At any given plasma total cholesterol level and age, eliminating the three other risk factors can lessen the risk of coronary disease. In some patients with mild blood pressure elevations, correcting diabetes and smoking habits, and lowering cholesterol levels could have an impact equal to that of lowering the blood pressure with drugs. At 60% of the coronary surface covered, the risk of clinical coronary artery disease is markedly enhanced (dashed line). *Source:* Reprinted with permission from *Journal of the American Medical Association* (1986;256:2856), Copyright © 1986, American Medical Association.

cholesterol, eliminate cigarette smoking, and improve abnormal glucose tolerance by maintaining ideal body weight. In patients with mild or borderline hypertension the control of associated risk factors is sometimes the primary goal, whose importance outweighs the benefit of reducing blood pressure with drugs.

Multiple risk factors for cardiovascular disease tend to coexist in hypertensives more often than predicted by chance alone,[70] and each risk factor amplifies the importance of the other (Figure 5-4). For example, diabetes, smoking, and age

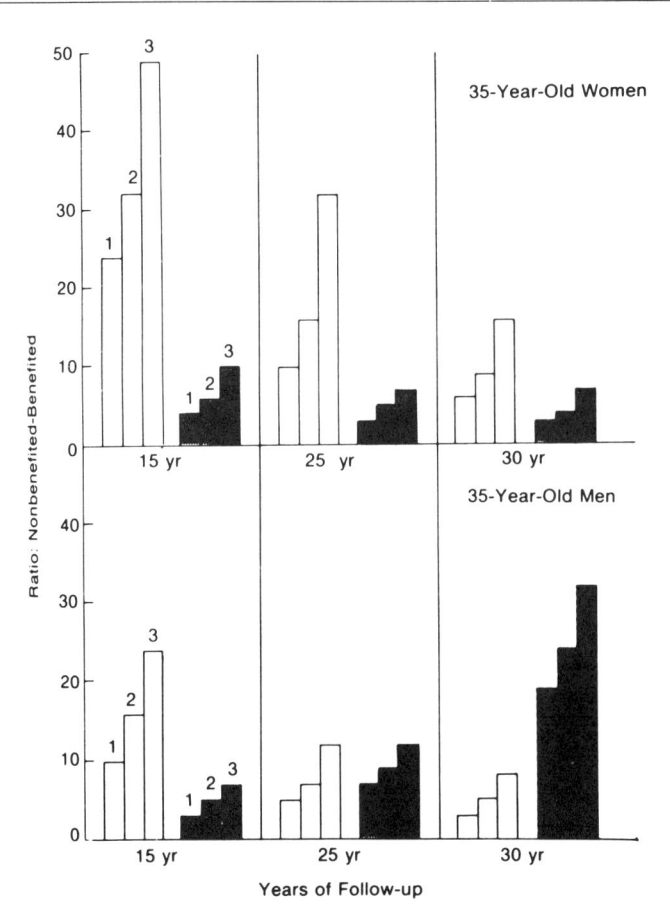

Figure 5-4 Risk of cardiovascular disease developing in 15, 25, and 30 years in high-risk (shaded bar) and low-risk (open bar) 35-year-old women. Column 3 represents the benefits of lowering systolic blood pressure from 165 to 135 mm Hg for the period of observation. Sixteen low risk patients would have to be treated with no benefit for 30 years in order to benefit 1. For high risk the ratio is 7 to 1. *Source:* Reprinted with permission from *Archives of Internal Medicine* (1985;141:1585), Copyright © 1985, American Medical Association.

significantly increase coronary and stroke risk in women with a positive family history of heart disease,[70,102] but family history is unimportant in the absence of these other risk factors.

Hypertension is the strongest single risk factor for coronary artery disease[103] and stroke[80] in women. When there are multiple other risks, can we compensate for them by lowering the blood pressure more aggressively? The answer is a tentative yes. The risk of stroke, for example, falls progressively in high-risk patients as diastolic blood pressure is lowered into the 80s and 70s.[46,51,104]

Lowering diastolic pressure into the 80s and 70s also has the potential to compensate for coronary risk factors.[105] When the diastolic blood pressure of the 40- to 60-year-old male is less than 80 mm Hg, he is only 80% as likely to have a myocardial infarction or suffer sudden death as his companion with a diastolic pressure of 80 to 88. The benefit of a diastolic blood pressure of less than 80 versus 80 to 88 is comparable to the benefit of having an average serum cholesterol of 206 mg/dL compared with one of 229 mg/dL and about 40% as beneficial as being a nonsmoker versus being a smoker. The benefit of treating 60-year-old women who are thin and who smoke is far greater than the benefit of treating nonsmokers. Their additional risk from smoking can be completely eliminated by more vigorous antihypertensive therapy.[106]

When the total number of risk factors is small, the benefit of antihypertensive therapy is also small. Let's look at 35-year-old women in a Framingham low-risk category (no ECG LVH, nonsmoker, normal glucose tolerance, normal cholesterol) who have a systolic blood pressure of 165 (Figure 5-4). If all were given a hypothetical blood pressure medication that had no adverse effects, worked perfectly, and permanently lowered their systolic blood pressure to 135, and this cohort was followed for 30 years, 15 such patients would have to be treated in order to prevent a premature end point in 1.[107] The benefits of treating high-risk female patients are more apparent (right panel).

THE BENEFIT OF ANTIHYPERTENSIVE THERAPY: RANDOMIZED PROSPECTIVE TRIALS

The higher the blood pressure, the worse the prognosis. Can antihypertensive drug therapy improve the outlook?

Several randomized prospective trials of antihypertensive therapy were designed to answer this question. They were conducted in populations with varying characteristics—some older, sicker, and with severer hypertension than others. These studies generated a scale of population attributes to which an individual patient can be compared.

The Veterans Administration (VA) Cooperative trial examined the result of antihypertensive therapy in men with mild, moderate, or severe hypertension.[13]

The trial served as a paradigm for later studies involving women. The important features were as follows:

- Patients were entered into the trial after their elevated blood pressures persisted for 2 to 4 months on no medication.
- Patients were randomly assigned to drug or placebo treatment.
- Drug treatment was most effective at preventing further rises in blood pressure.[104]
- There was a high morbidity and mortality rate of the drug-treated group compared with that of the community at large; that is, successful treatment did not completely eliminate excess morbidity.
- The benefit of treating diastolic blood pressure of 105 or over with drugs was so obvious that drug therapy is now standard therapy for moderate and severe hypertension.
- The benefits of treating mild hypertension were uncertain.

This study showed that antihypertensive therapy could reduce cardiovascular disease in a population of hypertensives, but that the chance of preventing a complication in a single individual could be small. To deal with this problem, the authors introduce the term "treatment efficiency." This term helps the physician judge whether the discomfort and expense of drug therapy is worthwhile in an individual patient.

$$\text{Efficiency of "x" treatment (\%)} = (\text{event rate* expected} - \text{event rate* observed})$$

or

$$\frac{\text{Reduction in adverse events by "x" treatment}}{\text{Patient years of treatment}}[106]$$

Sample Calculation: In the European Working Party on High Blood Pressure in the Elderly (EWPHBPE) Trial,[108] 424 men and women were randomized to placebo treatment and 416 to drug therapy. In the placebo group there were 19 instances of severe rise in blood pressure over an average of 3 years, representing 15 events/1,000 patient years of treatment. In the drug-treated group there were only two episodes of severe rise in blood pressure over an average of 3.4 years, representing one event/1,000 patient years of treatment. For preventing severe rise in blood pressure, then, treatment efficiency was $\frac{(15 - 1)}{1,000} \times 100 = 1.4\%$ per

---

*Event rate = number of observed adverse events/per patient years of observation.

year. In other words, about 71 patients would be treated per year with drugs to prevent 1 patient from having a severe rise in blood pressure (1/71 = 1.4%).

The VA Cooperative Study showed high treatment efficiency. Trials of mild hypertension showed less dramatic results. When their populations were comparable in age, entry blood pressure, risk factors for cardiovascular disease, and blood pressure control, differences in treatment efficiency depended on whether patients with established cardiovascular complications were included or excluded from the trial.

Table 5-1 describes the entry characteristics of patients in the various trials. Note that their risk factors (smoking, serum cholesterol, age, womanness) were similar except in two crucial regards: age (the EWPHBPE entered no one under age 60) and the presence of preexisting disease. The High Blood Pressure Detection and Follow-up Program (HBPDFP) and EWPHBPE trials were the only ones that admitted a substantial number of patients with mild hypertension who had preexisting disease (13% and 35% respectively).

TRIALS THAT COMPARED DRUG WITH PLACEBO TREATMENT

In all drug versus placebo trials there was significant reduction in the incidence of the collective complications of hypertension (stroke or transient ischemic attack, angina, myocardial infarction or worsening ischemia on ECG, congestive heart failure, or worsening hypertension) with treatment. The single complication that was most frequently reduced was worsening hypertension, with a treatment efficiency ranging from 1.4%[108] to about 4%.[49]

The Australian National Blood Pressure (ANBP) trial and the Medical Research Council (MRC) trial examined low-risk populations with relatively low blood pressure (Table 5-1). In the men and women of those trials the treatment efficiency for avoiding events other than rising blood pressure was only between 0.15%[109] and 0.73%.[49] In other words, the number of low-risk patients—male or female—who would have to receive drug therapy in order to avoid an adverse event in one patient per year (other than rising blood pressure) was between 805 and 150. Between 1,000[109] and 2,000[49] *women* had to be treated with drugs to avoid one stroke per year (treatment efficiency of 0.1% and 0.5% respectively). The most obvious benefit of drug treatment in the women of these trials was the prevention of higher blood pressure (treatment efficiency 2.1%).[109] In the elderly women of the ANBP, treatment efficiency was up to 7.5% in smokers.[106] Otherwise, there was no benefit of treatment to elderly women.

In the older and higher-risk EWPHBPE group, treatment efficiency for all end points other than rising blood pressure was 3.3%, so that about 30 patients were

Table 5-1 Antihypertensive Therapy Trials

Name of Trial	Average Age on Entry	Percentage of Females	Number Entered Mean Length of Observation	Inclusion of Patients with Prior Coronary Disease	Stroke	Medication	Diabetes	Final Diastolic BP (DBP) Drug/Placebo	Percentage Removed for Rise in DBP Placebo/Active
Trials with Placebo Controls									
Australian National Blood Pressure Trial[49,106,110]	50	50	3,427 / 4 years	Excluded	Excluded	Excluded	Excluded	88/93	12/0 (>110 DBP)
Medical Research Council Trial[109]	52	43	17,279 / 5.5 years	Excluded (recent)	Excluded (recent)	Excluded	Excluded	85/92	12.5/3 (>109 DBP)
European Working Party on High Blood Pressure in the Elderly Trial[108]	72	70	840 / 4.5 years	Excluded (congestive heart failure)	Excluded (cerebral hemorrhage)	Included	Excluded	85/90	1.5/0.1 (>119 DBP)
Trials That Compared One Kind of Treatment with Another									
High Blood Pressure Detection and Follow-up Program[80,111,112]	50	54	10,940 / 5 years	Included	Included	Included	Included	83†/88*†	N/A
International Prospective Primary Prevention Study of Hypertension[51]	52	50	6,357 / 4 years	Excluded	Excluded	Included	Excluded (insulin-dependent)	89/90‡	N/A

*Control group was treated less intensively by practitioners in the community.
†For participants with entry diastolic BP not over 104.
‡Control group was treated without using beta blockers.

committed to drug therapy per year to prevent one adverse effect. Treatment efficiency for stroke was greater than that for myocardial infarction.

The placebo groups in these trials did surprisingly well. Those placebo-treated patients whose blood pressure exceeded a certain threshold, or who suffered complications, were started on treatment. This winnowing out process left a healthier remnant, whose blood pressure fell with time. Almost half became normotensive, usually within 4 months.[49] In the MRC trial 68% of the placebo group had diastolic blood pressures of less than 90 at one time or another, and thus would be considered to have borderline hypertension.[109] In the EWPHBPE the fall in blood pressure of the placebo group—from 182/101 at entry to 167/90 at 7 years—probably reflected survival of those with lower blood pressure and lower likelihood of cardiovascular complications.

TRIALS THAT COMPARED ONE TYPE OF TREATMENT WITH ANOTHER

In the International Prospective Primary Prevention Study of Hypertension (IPPPSH) study, which examined the special benefits of beta blockers in antihypertensive therapy, patients who had mean blood pressures of 171/108 were entered if they were free of preexisting target organ damage. Treatment, which included thiazide diuretics, lowered the incidence of myocardial infarction and stroke in men and women. There was no special advantage to using beta blockers in women.

The HBPDFP trial examined a more challenging question: Will cardiovascular events be more noticeably diminished in a group that receives more frequent, methodical, and effective antihypertensive therapy?[90,111] The group that received more effective therapy in special centers was known as the "stepped care" (SC) group. The group that received less effective therapy, from community practitioners, was known as the "referred care" (RC) group. The diastolic blood pressures of the RC group were about 5 mm Hg higher during treatment.

The SC group enjoyed a lower rate of stroke (treatment efficiency 0.7% for the group with entry diastolic blood pressure of 90 to 94, 1.3% for the diastolic group 95 to 99, 2.9% for the diastolic group 100 to 104) and myocardial infarction (treatment efficiency of more vigorous therapy 0.1%).[112] But for women aged 55 to 74 with mild hypertension, treatment efficiency for prevention of stroke by more versus less vigorous therapy was only 0.16%.[90] For white women more vigorous therapy appeared to have no effect on the rate of cardiovascular events.

The HBPDFP study included mild hypertensives with established target organ damage. Two percent of the entrants had a history of stroke, 5% of myocardial infarction, and 7% of diabetes mellitus. Thirty-three percent of the deaths were noted in the 13% of patients who already had established target organ damage on entry. By contrast, the mortality rate of the *placebo-treated* group of the ANBP was lower than that of the *more intensively drug-treated group* of the HBPDFP because the ANBP entrants had a low incidence of established target organ damage on entry. Had patients with target organ damage also been excluded from the HBPDFP, the mortality rates for the treated groups in both studies would have been about the same.[112]

The *placebo* group of the MRC trial, with an average diastolic blood pressure of 92, had a lower rate of stroke than the *more intensively drug-treated* group of the HBPDFP, with an average diastolic blood pressure of 88. This is because the MRC study excluded those with established target organ damage from the start.[109] The Glasgow study reached similar conclusions.[47]

High-risk patients have the largest reduction of stroke morbidity rates from drug therapy. It has been shown that patients who have already suffered one stroke can avoid a second by means of antihypertensive therapy, if their blood pressure is well controlled[113] or if they have no ECG LVH.[84] In those trials that included patients who were stroke-prone because of target organ damage at entry, the stroke rate was reduced to that in the community at large by antihypertensive therapy, in men and women of all ages[90] or women aged 60 to 69.[50] Reduction in stroke mortality was greater than the reduction in myocardial infarction[50,108,111]

IMPLICATIONS OF FINDINGS FOR MILD HYPERTENSIVES

The presence of preexisting target organ damage or associated cardiovascular risk factors is more important than the diastolic blood pressure in judging whether to give drugs to mild hypertensives. This is especially true when the diastolic blood pressure is under 95 mm Hg.[64,92] Therefore, the most vigorous treatment should generally be offered to those who have had a recognizable end point. Drug treatment should also be directed to those high-risk patients having any one of the associated risk factors of smoking, longstanding obesity, diabetes mellitus, or systolic blood pressures over 180 mm Hg. But drug treatment offers vanishingly small advantage to a low-risk elderly female whose diastolic blood pressure remains below 95 mm Hg on repeated and prolonged observation.

When we decide to use drugs, how low must we bring the blood pressure of patients with mild hypertension to achieve morbidity and mortality rates similar to those of the community at large? For myocardial infarction, the issue is uncertain. As regards stroke, the diastolic blood pressure should be less than 90 mm Hg and probably about 80 mm Hg. In the high-risk groups of the HBPDFP the stroke rate of the SC group (more intensively treated) approached that in the community. The diastolic blood pressure of this group was in the 80s over the course of treatment. In the IPPPSH population there was a logarithmic fall in cerebrovascular disease with fall in blood pressure, so that when diastolic blood pressure was maintained at

83 mm Hg, the stroke rate was 0.8/1,000 years, a rate about one tenth that of patients maintained at 93 mm Hg. In the Glasgow study failure to reduce the diastolic blood pressure to less than 90 mm Hg over a 5- to 6-year interval was associated with accelerated mortality, the increase rising sharply as diastolic blood pressure escalated to a higher range.[47]

Antihypertensive therapy does not eliminate the risk of stroke.[114,115] In 12 hypertensives cerebral blood flow was measured before and after their blood pressures were lowered to about 150/90 with drugs. Cerebral blood flow was depressed before treatment. After an initial rise in cerebral blood flow with drug therapy, there was a secondary fall in four patients by 3 years' treatment. All four then proceeded to develop transient cerebral ischemia, multiinfarct dementia, or atherothrombotic brain infarction while under treatment.[114]

Similar examples of the "failure" of antihypertensive therapy to prevent target organ damage are available as regards the failure to prevent declining renal blood flow during treatment,[116] the worsening of arteriolonephrosclerosis during treatment,[117] and the weak effect of antihypertensive therapy in diminishing the rate of myocardial infarction. This has led to the discussion of "irreducible risk"[47,118] during antihypertensive therapy. But the prevention of myocardial infarction may be difficult when serum cholesterol is above a certain threshold, and should not rest on antihypertensive therapy without attention to other risk factors (antihypertensive therapy may be especially effective in reducing infarct rates when the systolic blood pressure is over 180 mm Hg).[118]

Furthermore, the fact that some patients escape the benefit of antihypertensive therapy may simply mean that their blood pressures were not brought low enough[115]; that there were peculiarities of certain agents that limit their effectiveness (examples: the failure of propranolol to lower myocardial infarction rates in smokers in the MRC trial,[109] the failure of hydralazine to prevent left ventricular hypertrophy[119]; or that by the time their mildly elevated blood pressures were regarded as worthy of treatment, they had already suffered cardiovascular complications that could have been avoided by early detection.[81]

The chance that blood pressure will worsen to levels of 110 diastolic with no drug treatment rises to 12.5% in low-risk groups with the mildest blood pressures.[64,109] This has the most profound implications for those low-risk hypertensives who are not receiving drugs because treatment efficiency is expected to be low. Such patients must be offered close follow-up, and treatment should begin if they have developed moderate or severe hypertension.

To date, the benefits of drug treatment for isolated systolic hypertension remain unproved,[32] but there is suggestive evidence that an isolated systolic blood pressure of over 180 mm Hg justifies treatment.[12,45,120]

BLOOD PRESSURE TREATMENT IN THE VERY OLD

There is uncertain benefit to antihypertensive therapy in patients aged 80 years or older. This population has been observed to show a declining incidence of hypertension with advancing age.[112,121-123] It is not clear whether a falling blood pressure with advancing age is a physiologic or a pathologic phenomenon. Part of the reason for this decline may be the advent of heart disease, such as myocardial infarction, congestive heart failure, and atrial fibrillation, which may cause a falling blood pressure.[124-128]

Although acceleration of atherosclerosis was prominent in hypertensives who were in the seventh or eighth decade of life, little difference was seen in the severity of atherosclerosis between hypertensives and normotensive subjects in their ninth decade.[129,130] With increasing duration of follow-up there was a declining advantage of more intensive versus less intensive therapy in patients aged 68 to 77,[131] and no beneficial effect of drug therapy on worsening hypertension in patients 85 or older.[130] In another[132] study no reduction in mortality or other adverse cardiovascular events could be proved. Treatment of high blood pressure is of definite benefit to populations 60 to 69 years old, less benefit to populations in their 70s, and of uncertain benefit to populations in their 80s.

MEASUREMENT OF BLOOD PRESSURE

Blood pressure is the most easily obtained index of severity, and it should be determined with care. The mercury manometer is the standard. If the column of mercury is lowered by 2 mm per heartbeat, readings to the nearest 1 mm Hg can be obtained. Such accuracy is important in mild hypertensives, in whom small blood pressure changes as the result of treatment are expected. Unfortunately, in a patient with a wide pulse pressure, this can mean two or more minutes spent on each blood pressure determination! Considering the number of determinations necessary on the first visit, it would be advisable to enlist the assistance of a well-trained, patient nurse. The brachial artery should be palpated while the manometer is inflated, to the point where it collapses. The earliest Korotkoff sound before an auscultatory gap will not be missed if the manometer is inflated to 30 mm Hg above the disappearance of the pulse.[133]

In large prospective surveys of antihypertensive therapy, patients' blood pressures were determined after a 10- to 15-minute interval in a comfortable ambiance, not smoking, with an empty bladder, and with no interaction between examiner and patient, such as talking or pantomime. The blood pressure was taken with a cuff appropriate in size to the patient's arm, using mercury sphygmomanometers in a way that allowed determination of blood pressure to the nearest 1 mm Hg. In order to extrapolate the results of these surveys to the individual, similar conditions should be extended to the patient in the office.

The blood pressure should be determined sitting, in both arms, in duplicate, and the mean of two determinations recorded. A large adult cuff should be used for arms over 31 cm in diameter and a 10-cm "pediatric" cuff should be available for the woman with arm circumference under 25 cm.[133] Differences in blood pressure of more than 10 mm Hg systolic or diastolic between the two arms may signify either subclavian stenosis, in which case a bruit may be heard in the supraclavicular fossa, or axillary stenosis, in which a bruit, if present, is more likely heard in the infraclavicular region.[134] Subclavian steal is more common as a result of left subclavian stenosis than of right, and can be detected by simultaneous palpation of right and left radial arteries, whereupon a perceptible delay in pulse on the side of the steal is often evident.[135] There is no such delay in the presence of simple subclavian stenosis.

Blood pressure should then be determined supine and erect. There is a high incidence of orthostatic hypotension in the elderly, signifying volume depletion or autonomic insufficiency. Rises in diastolic blood pressure of more than 10 mm Hg on assuming the standing-from-lying posture suggest a high incidence of future cardiovascular events and help to define the urgency of treatment.[136] A total of three sitting determinations on different days are desirable, as it is the blood pressure that is found after the patient has become acclimatized to the procedure and surroundings that most accurately predicts adverse events.

The remainder of the physical examination should then proceed, with special emphasis on the peripheral pulses, including auscultation for bruits, the retinal vasculature, the heart and lungs, abnormal abdominal pulsations or masses, and femoral bruits.

Symptoms of headache, visual disturbance, chest pain, palpitation, shortness of breath, or back pain in a patient with an abnormally pulsatile aorta should be evaluated by internal medicine consultation. Certain findings on history or physical examination call for immediate or prompt treatment (Table 5-2). Their treatment may consist of bed rest in the hospital (in these circumstances rest at home is not adequate) or the acute administration of rapidly acting drugs that lower blood pressure acutely and reliably in the outpatient setting, or both. When these historical or physical features are directly attributable to the blood pressure, treatment is urgent. When they are primarily referable to a specific organ (example: angina pectoris), therapy of such complications should be started. In either instance, consultation with an internist is advised.

Table 5-2 Complications of Hypertension That Require Immediate Treatment

- Fresh retinal exudates (cotton wool spots) with or without papilledema
- Transient neurologic or visual disturbance
- Severe headache without obvious cause
- Dyspnea or proteinuria without past history of cardiac or renal disease
- Angina pectoris
- Congestive heart failure
- Intermittent claudication
- Abdominal aortic aneurysm over 5 cm

Table 5-3 Signs of Secondary Hypertension

- Onset of diastolic hypertension after age 55, especially when severe
- Hypokalemia (less than 3.7 mEq/L) not provoked by drugs, or hyperkalemia
- Any two of the triad of headache, palpitation, and sweating
- Proteinuria or abnormal urinary sediment
- Retinal hemorrhages or exudates
- Smoking history
- Blood urea nitrogen over 25 mg/dL, serum creatinine over 1.8 mg/dL (60–69 years) or over 1.2 mg/dL (70 or older)
- Signs of sleep apnea; polycythemia (hematocrit over 52%)
- Diastolic abdominal bruit, or systolic bruit radiating to the flanks

---

At least 80% of elderly women with hypertension display no apparent underlying cause for their elevated blood pressures. Findings that should alert the gynecologist to the presence of secondary hypertension (primary chronic renal disease accounting for 5%, and renal artery stenosis, pheochromocytoma, aldosterone-producing adrenal adenoma, and Cushing's syndrome accounting for the remainder) are listed in Table 5-3. Most of these may be suspected on the basis of history and physical and sequential multiple analysis, including blood urea nitrogen, glucose, creatinine, uric acid, electrolytes, a complete blood count, a urinalysis, and electrocardiography.

Sleep apnea is being recognized with increasing frequency in hypertensive patients. This abnormally frequent interruption of regular breathing can be present even if the hypertensive subject is not obese. It may be due to anatomical factors occluding the airway in supine posture (obstructive sleep apnea) or to an abnormal central nervous system response to the apneic episodes commonly present in normals (central sleep apnea). Such patients complain of feeling poorly rested on awakening, are heard to snore loudly at night, have a dry mouth on awakening, and have daytime somnolence, often falling asleep at the job or at the wheel. Daytime arterial oxygen desaturation and high hematocrits may be present. The hypertension is related to high blood viscosity and arterial desaturation as well as other unknown factors, perhaps related to persistent autonomic responses to nighttime desaturation and obesity. The syndrome may respond dramatically even to small degrees of weight loss or to positive nasal airway pressure.[137,138]

AMBULATORY BLOOD PRESSURE MONITORING

Hypertensives show both a higher blood pressure set point and larger fluctuations around the set point. These fluctuations may be provoked by the process of blood pressure determination.[139] The practice of ambulatory blood pressure

Table 5-4 Nonmedicinal or Behavioral Therapy

Advantage	Disadvantage
Low cost	Discouraged patient doesn't return
Low morbidity	Difficult to judge compliance
Corrects other risk factors simultaneously	Duration of beneficial effects unknown

monitoring has identified differences between office and usual daily blood pressure, and several studies provide strong evidence that ambulatory blood pressure better defines cardiovascular risk.[140] This is especially relevant to hypertension in the elderly female. In women over age 60 the average disparity between office and ambulatory blood pressure is 30 mm Hg (higher in the office).[141,142]

What is not known is whether infrequent severe rises in pressure can cause premature vascular damage. If this pattern persists on the ambulatory monitor, it may be justified to search for target organ damage, using such sophisticated techniques as echocardiography for left ventricular wall thickening, submaximal exercise testing for silent coronary disease, and para-aminohippuric acid clearance for reductions in renal blood flow.

All hypertension should be treated in some fashion, but drugs are not the only available measure. Aerobic exercise may induce substantial falls in blood pressure.[143] Normalizing body weight can have potent effects to lower blood pressure and may eliminate the need for drugs.[144] Sodium restriction[145] should be advised if the patient eats salty food or adds salt to her food. In some patients calcium supplementation is effective.[146]

A danger of such behavioral therapy is that it places a large burden of the responsibility for treatment on the patient's shoulders. The patient may not return for follow-up because of her actual or perceived failure to comply with recommended measures (Table 5-4).

The first consideration in drug therapy is to remove drugs that cause hypertension. Alcohol in equivalent quantities of greater than 30 g of absolute ethanol/day, cold remedies containing sympathomimetic amines, nonsteroidal anti-inflammatory agents, corticosteroids, and abuse of nonprescription drugs (cocaine, over-the-counter anorectics) or foods (licorice) can substantially elevate blood pressure.[147] Preliminary evidence suggests that replacement estrogens can do the same, and that naturally occurring compounds may be preferable to the conjugated equine variety.[148]

RECOMMENDATIONS FOR TREATING THE ELDERLY HYPERTENSIVE WOMAN

1. Rule out secondary hypertension.
2. Address any associated risk factors for cardiovascular disease that can be reduced, and any behavioral causes of hypertension. Try to get the patient to

stop smoking, stop drinking, use less salt, and lose weight. Lower her cholesterol, if the low-density lipoprotein–cholesterol exceeds 150 mg/dL or the ratio of high-density lipoprotein to total cholesterol is less than 22% in a patient with a low-density lipoprotein level over 150 mg/dL. Prescribe a moderately low sodium, low saturated and total fat diet.[149]
3. Treat all patients with a diastolic blood pressure of 105 and above with drugs, and with health advice concerning associated risk factors.
4. For patients with diastolic blood pressures of 90 to 104 mm Hg, observe blood pressure monthly for 4 months, or classify the blood pressure using an ambulatory blood pressure monitor. If the diastolic blood pressure remains over 90 mm Hg, use drugs when:
   a. the systolic blood pressure is over 180 mm Hg.
   b. there is established evidence of cardiovascular disease, cerebrovascular disease, diabetes mellitus, hypercholesterolemia, obesity (body weight over 130% of ideal for 14 or more years[86]), cigarette smoking (especially in a thin patient),[106] or left ventricular hypertrophy. In these patients, lower diastolic blood pressure to 80 mm Hg, if possible, and systolic to less than 180 mm Hg.
   c. the patient will not return for follow-up because she has mistaken the absence of drug treatment for the absence of a problem.
   d. there are symptoms of hypertension.
   e. there is an upward trend in diastolic blood pressure on three successive vists at 2-month intervals.
   f. the patient prefers drug therapy to observation (but understands that the benefit to be gained by drug therapy is small).
5. Patients with diastolic blood pressures of 90 to 104 mm Hg who are not committed to drug therapy should be followed with an internist. They should be monitored for incipient target organ damage by:
   a. obtaining a baseline echocardiogram and ambulatory blood pressure reading, and repeating them periodically. If there is increased left ventricular mass or high blood pressure on the monitor during the working day, begin drug treatment.
   b. in smokers, obtaining a submaximal treadmill exercise test. If it shows evidence of myocardial ischemia, start treatment.
   c. offering a program of regular aerobic exercise and dietary control of body weight, serum cholesterol, and sodium intake (Table 5-5).
   d. determining blood pressure quarterly. If diastolic blood pressure is over 104 mm Hg on each of 2 successive weeks, start drug therapy. If patients are reluctant to return for monitoring of their blood pressure, teach them to determine their own with a reliable instrument at home, or repeat ambulatory blood pressure monitoring.

Table 5-5 Means of Judging Compliance with Behavioral Therapy

Treatment	Response
Low fat hypocaloric diet	Weight—total body fat*
Sodium restriction	24-hour urinary sodium
Exercise	Resting bradycardia, anaerobic threshold, maximum oxygen consumption, total body fat

*Measured by skinfold thickness or electrical impedance.

DRUG THERAPY

Drug therapy in the elderly hypertensive is complicated by several factors.

1. A tendency toward orthostatic hypotension because of reduced plasma volume and defective baroreceptor reflex sensitivity,[150] particularly amplified in the postprandial state.[151]
2. Reduced drug excretion because of diminished kidney and liver function, placing older patients at greater risk for developing adverse drug reactions.
3. Frequency of concomitant, associated illnesses, such as diabetes mellitus, heart disease, and pulmonary disease. This creates a larger potential for antihypertensive agents worsening a concomitant illness, or interacting unfavorably with another required medication.
4. A higher incidence of cerebral arterial disease and cerebral atrophy make central side effects such as confusion or sedation more common.

In general, the smallest effective dose of a single drug is the ideal therapy, but this is not always possible. It is especially important to check blood pressure in lying and standing positions, in order to detect undesirable orthostatic falls.

Factors That Affect Compliance

Drug therapy of hypertension is complicated by a variety of factors in the elderly, but compliance certainly looms as one of the most important. In addition to the usual problems of treating an often asymptomatic process and the relative likelihood of some adverse drug effects, the physician is also faced with memory lapses, inadequate supervision and support, and already complex drug regimens required for other common ailments of the aged. It is thus desirable to simplify the antihypertensive regimen as much as possible. However, despite all these potential handicaps, compliance is not a "lost cause" in attempting to treat older hypertensives. Several studies suggest that the elderly patient is indeed a suitable candidate for antihypertensive therapy.

Orthostatic Hypotension

Because of baroreceptor dysfunction, rapid adjustment to changes in posture may be impaired, and orthostatic hypotension occurs in the elderly. In fact, a morbid decrease in blood pressure on standing is common. Caird and coworkers[152] studied nearly 500 ambulatory, community-dwelling people over age 65 and found systolic pressure drops of 20 mm Hg or more in 24%. This tendency becomes more marked after age 75 and especially in the postprandial state.[151] Because such orthostatic blood pressure falls can predispose to dangerous syncope or near syncope (especially hazardous in older women with osteoporosis and a tendency toward hip fracture), and because the older hypertensive frequently has defective baroreflexes, a reduced cardiac output, and a reduced plasma volume, the ideal antihypertensive agent for her would not aggravate any of these.

Thiazide Diuretics

The thiazide diuretics are generally effective and well tolerated in an elderly population. Their favorable hemodynamic effect depends on reduction of total body sodium by about 250 mEq, a deficit that will be maintained as long as the patient adheres to a no-salt-added diet (2 g sodium). The thiazides act to reduce blood pressure by diminishing peripheral resistance (in 80% of cases) or a mixed effect on peripheral resistance and cardiac output.[153] Some of their unfavorable effects—glucose intolerance, hypercholesterolemia, hypokalemia, hyperuricemia—could theoretically diminish the patient's prognosis to such a degree that lowering the blood pressure results in no net gain to the patient.[154] These adverse effects, and lack of drug potency observed during treatment, can be averted by maintenance of ideal body weight, reduced total and saturated fat intake, and reduced sodium intake.

As long as the sodium deficit induced by thiazides persists, their action persists, and renal compensatory mechanisms come into play to prevent progressive sodium loss. Consequently neither should a long-acting thiazide have any special advantage, nor should the patient expect a large urinary volume as reassurance that the drug is working. Generic hydrochlorothiazide, in its proper dose range of 25 to 100 mg/day, costs less than $50 per year and there is no advantage to more expensive preparations. The related compound chlorthalidone may be more appropriate in high-risk patients with resting ECG abnormalities. Loop diuretics (furosemide, bumetanide), which work by reducing cardiac output, are not substitutes for the thiazides.

The smallest effective dose of thiazide should be used, and the biochemical effects of the drug monitored by repeating a CBC, electrolytes, blood urea nitrogen, glucose, cholesterol, and uric acid twice yearly, and a serum magnesium and urinalysis yearly. Hypokalemia (to less than 3.1 mEq/L) can cause malignant ventricular dysrhythmia.[155] When the patient undergoes psychological or physical trauma (eg, hospitalization), the associated epinephrine release can drive an already depressed potassium down to dangerously low levels.[156] Drug-induced hypokalemia may be a hint that the patient suffers from primary aldosteronism. Combining the thiazide with triamterene or amiloride can improve this problem. Oral potassium supplements are expensive, can cause gastrointestinal symptoms, and may even result in hyperkalemia if the patient is taking nonsteroidal anti-inflammatory agents. Hypokalemia can be avoided by making sure the patient's sodium intake is restricted. Hyponatremia is an indication to reduce the dose, as it can cause severe neurologic derangement.[157]

Thiazides appear to promote a larger loss of extracellular fluid volume in older than in younger patients, a factor that predisposes to hyponatremia. Diuretic-induced volume depletion can lead to azotemia. If the patient is otherwise asymptomatic, a rise in the blood urea nitrogen to 25 mg/dL is acceptable.

Hypomagnesemia should be corrected, as it might be responsible for sudden death in patients with ischemic heart disease, and because magnesium deficiency opposes the reduction in peripheral resistance afforded by thiazides.[158] Oral magnesium oxide, 200 to 400 mg/day, usually suffices.

After a 1-year period on treatment, the dose of medication should be reduced to determine the minimum amount that is effective. This "step-down" approach enables the physician to see whether behavioral measures have assumed an increasing role in antihypertensive therapy.

Calcium Antagonists

A class of drugs called calcium antagonists (calcium entry blockers) was discovered and shown to lower blood pressure in hypertensive patients more than 20 years ago. There has been a recent surge of enthusiasm for these agents, which include nifedipine, verapamil, and diltiazem. They are available worldwide and have been proved safe and efficacious in long-term therapy.

These drugs are the closest thing to an "ideal antihypertensive agent" to treat hypertension in older individuals. Their desirable features include favorable hemodynamic effects (lowering of peripheral resistance, preservation or elevation of cardiac output, relaxation of stiff great vessels, and improvement in coronary and peripheral blood flow), and absence of salt and water retention, orthostatic hypotension, undesirable metabolic effects, and central side effects.[159] One of their most beneficial effects for an older hypertensive patient is their ability to allow an increase in arterial compliance.[160] The only other oral agents that have been shown to share that property of dilating large arteries are angiotensin-converting inhibitors and nitrates.

Older age is associated with up to a 90% response rate to calcium antagonists.[161] Race is also a powerful predictor of response: blacks, for example, tend to respond very well to calcium antagonists probably because of their low plasma renin profile.[162] Hence, on the basis of available information, calcium antagonists are proposed as first-line therapy for older hypertensives as an alternative to diuretics as the traditional cornerstone of therapy. This is particularly true for women with concomitant conditions that are benefited by calcium antagonists, such as coronary artery disease, peripheral vascular disease, chronic lung disease, and vertebrobasilar insufficiency. Whereas diuretic-induced plasma volume contraction potentially compromises blood flow to vital organs, calcium antagonists tend to preserve and even improve cardiac, cerebral, and renal blood flow despite the fall in blood pressure.[163,164] Calcium antagonists tend to lower systolic blood pressure in proportion to pretreatment pressure. Accordingly, they usually do not lower blood pressure excessively and are unlikely to induce hypotensive episodes that could adversely effect cerebral and coronary perfusion in older patients. Diuretic-induced metabolic side effects (hypokalemia, hyperglycemia, hyperuricemia, hyperlipidemia, and stimulation of the sympathetic nervous system and renin-angiotensin system) have not been encountered with calcium antagonists. These agents can be used alone or readily combined with other drugs, including diuretics, methyldopa, clonidine, or beta blockers, when deemed necessary.

In general, the limiting side effects of these drugs in an older population are constipation, headache, palpitations, atrioventricular block, and ankle edema.

Angiotensin Blockers

Captopril and enalapril are newer agents that block the enzyme responsible for conversion of inactive angiotensin I to the powerful pressor peptide angiotensin II (angiotensin-converting enzyme [ACE]). These ACE inhibitors, so-called, have several advantages: they do not cause orthostatic hypotension, central nervous system side effects, or metabolic disturbances that would tend to negate the cardiovascular benefit conferred by their antihypertensive effect.[165] They are well tolerated, even by older patients, and can be effective even in low doses. They can specifically relax large arteries, which is a distinct advantage in older patients with predominant systolic hypertension. They have three potential adverse effects of note: proteinuria, neutropenia, and a hemodynamically induced form of declining renal function. The first two are exceedingly uncommon, but the latter occurs in about 25% of patients with bilateral renal artery stenosis.[166]

Beta Blockers

Beta blockers have traditionally been used commonly in older patients with hypertension, frequently in combination with a diuretic. The authors contend that they should be prescribed less frequently. Beta blockers have been found to be relatively ineffective in patients with low renin typing, commonly found in older patients.[167] In fact, Drayer and colleagues[158] demonstrated a paradoxical rise in blood pressure in many such patients treated with propranolol. In addition, the lowering of cardiac output in older patients may be particularly undesirable and can lead to congestive heart failure.

Older patients are also those prone to develop bradycardia because of underlying sinus node dysfunction. Beta blockers can lead to worsening claudication, Raynaud's phenomenon, and even impending gangrene in patients with peripheral vascular disease. This is probably due to the reduction in cardiac output and blockade of β_2-mediated skeletal muscle vasodilation, resulting in unopposed alpha-mediated vasoconstriction. In the authors' experience, beta blockers with β_1-selectivity or intrinsic sympathomimetic effect do not truly protect against this adverse effect.

When these drugs are used, dosages should be minimized because of reduced excretion by the liver and kidneys in older patients. In addition, insulin-requiring diabetics should receive only β_1-selective agents, in order to avoid blocking the physiologic sympathetic response to hypoglycemia mediated by β_2-receptors that acts as a warning to the patient that he or she is having an insulin reaction.[168]

Centrally Active Agents

These agents include methyldopa, clonidine, and guanabenz. Such agents have been commonly used in older patients, but their use tends to be limited by central nervous system side effects, such as lethargy, depression, and sleep disturbances. They should be used at low doses in aged patients, especially at initiation of therapy (ie, methyldopa 250 mg twice a day, clonidine 0.1 mg twice a day).

Other Agents

Direct vasodilators (eg, hydralazine and minoxidil) are generally less desirable in an older population, in whom the risk of coronary artery disease is higher.

Minoxidil is especially difficult to use in female patients because it causes hirsutism. These agents generally cannot be used alone, and usually are given in conjunction with an anti-adrenergic agent and a diuretic. A new agent called labetalol, a combined alpha and beta blocker, can be used in selected patients, but its tendency to cause orthostatic hypotension limits its appeal in an older population. Certain agents should be avoided altogether or used with the utmost caution: guanethidine (severe orthostatic hypotension, diarrhea), reserpine (depression, peptic ulcer), and prazosin (first-dose syncope, orthostatic hypotension).

PSEUDOHYPERTENSION

There are at least three types of pseudohypertension in older people. One is based on the fact that indirect cuff blood pressure measurement may significantly overestimate true direct intra-arterial readings. This phenomenon is explained by the inability of the air-filled bladder of the sphygmomanometer to compress a stiff, calcified brachial artery.[169,170]

A second type of pseudohypertension has become apparent from ambulatory blood pressure monitoring. In this procedure, readings are taken in the "real world," at home and work, rather than in the artificial and anxiety-provoking setting of a doctor's office or clinic. The authors' experience in nearly 600 patients monitored by this method demonstrates a remarkable degree of "white coat" hypertension in older women.[142] A third type occurs when a blood pressure cuff that is too small for the size of the patient's arm is used.

RENAL DISEASE IN THE AGED

The biological price of aging includes progressive deterioration of renal structure and function. Numerous anatomical and physiologic alterations occur. After the age of 30, glomerular filtrate and renal blood flow rates decline in a linear fashion, so that values in octogenarians are only half to two thirds those measured in young adults. Renal mass similarly declines, and the incidence of sclerotic glomeruli increases with advancing age.[27] Accordingly, the aging kidney is at high risk of eventual failure when the functioning nephron number is further reduced by acquired renal disease. No specific kidney disease has been identified that is totally confined to the geriatric population. The types of kidney disease that tend to predominate in the aged include vascular and atheroembolic disease, obstructive uropathy, systemic disease with renal involvement, and intrinsic renal disease.[171] The aged are particularly prone to nephrotoxic injury by radiocontrast administration or aminoglycosides.[172]

There is a high incidence of urinary tract infections in the aged, with an incidence reaching 50% in women aged 70 to 79.[173] Moreover, there is a lack of association between bacteriuria and symptoms in the elderly, requiring the physician to have a high index of suspicion.[173] There is also a tendency to hyperkalemia in the aged, often related to reduced activity of the renin-aldosterone axis.

Acute renal failure in the aged female is most often related to hypotension, dehydration, surgery, infection, radiocontrast, and drugs. Although obstructive uropathy is less common in aged females than in males, it is not uncommon with carcinoma of the cervix, and may also be seen with ovarian and breast carcinomas, uterine prolapse, and fibromyoma. Renal atheroembolism is not uncommon, and may present a clinical picture difficult to differentiate from vasculitis: fever, hematuria, high erythrocyte sedimentation rate, eosinophilia, hypocomplementemia.[174] Primary renal disease in the elderly may present as the nephritic or the nephrotic syndrome. There appears to be a relatively higher incidence of idiopathic crescentic glomerulonephritis and of membranous nephropathy in patients over age 60. It should also be noted that diabetic nephropathy has become the second leading cause of end-stage renal disease, affecting a large number of aged patients as well as younger ones. Improvements in hemodialysis and peritoneal dialysis have occurred and offer broader options for aged patients with chronic renal failure, but renal transplant is generally avoided in the elderly.

Because the kidney is one of the endocrine glands that regulates calcium metabolism (producing 1,25-dihydroxycholecalciferol), age-related deterioration in renal function may lead to metabolic bone disease and fractures. The elderly female is especially noted to be in negative calcium balance, constantly losing bone mass. Controversy exists as to the relative importance of calcium and estrogen supplementation in an aging female population at risk for osteoporosis.[175,176]

REFERENCES

1. Gordon T, Kannel WB: Multiple contributions to coronary risk: Implications for screening and prevention. *J Chronic Dis* 1972;25:561–569.

2. Doyle AE: Vascular complications of hypertension, in Robertson JIS (ed): *Handbook of Hypertension.* New York, Elsevier, 1983, vol. 1, pp 365–377.

3. Wilkie F, Eisdorfer C: Intelligence and blood pressure in the aged. *Science* 1972; 172:959–962.

4. Wilkie F, Eisdorfer C, Nowlin JB: Memory and blood pressure in the aged. *Exp Aging Res* 1976;2:3–16.

5. Organic mental impairment in old people: editorial. *Lancet* 1981;2:561–562.

6. Babikian V, Ropper AH: Binswanger's disease: A review. *Stroke* 1987;18:1–12.

7. Levy RI, Feinbeib M: Risk factors for coronary artery disease and their management, in Braunwald E (ed): *Heart Disease.* Philadelphia, WB Saunders, 1980, p 1249.

8. Kirkendall WM, Hammond JJ: Hypertension in the elderly. *Arch Intern Med* 1980; 140:1155–1161.

9. The Framingham Study: An epidemiological investigation of cardiovascular disease. DHEW publication No (NIH) 74-599. Government Printing Office, 1974.

10. Wollam GL, Gifford RW Jr: The kidney as a target organ in hypertension. *Geriatrics* 1976;31:71–79.

11. Gordon T, Kannel WB: Predisposition to atherosclerosis in the head, heart and legs, the Framingham Study. *JAMA* 1972;221:661–666.

12. Shea S, Cook EF, Kannel WB, et al: Treatment of hypertension and its effect on cardiovascular risk factors: The Framingham Heart Study. *Circulation* 1985;71:22–30.

13. Veterans Administration cooperative study group on antihypertensive agents. Effects of treatment on morbidity in hypertension. *JAMA* 1970;213:1143–1152.

14. Kannel WB, McGhee D, Gordon T: A general cardiovascular risk profile: The Framingham Study. *Am J Cardiol* 1976;38:46–51.

15. Freis E: Age, race, sex and other indices of risk in hyperthyroidism, in Laragh JH (ed): *Hypertension Manual*. New York, Dun-Donnelley, 1973, p 33.

16. Lew EA: High blood pressure, other risk factors and longevity: The insurance viewpoint, in Laragh JH (ed): *Hypertension Manual*. New York, Dun-Donnelley, 1973, pp 61–63.

17. Winkelstein W Jr, Kantor S: Some observations on the relationship between age, sex and blood pressure, in Stamler J, Stamler R, Pullman TN (eds): *The Epidemiology of Hypertension*. New York, Grune & Stratton, 1967, pp 70–79.

18. Dyer AF, Stamler J, Shekelle R, et al: Hypertension in the elderly. *Med Clin North Am* 1977;61:513–529.

19. Brandfonbrener M, Landome M, Shock NW: Changes in cardiac output with age. *Circulation* 1955;12:557–566.

20. Wesson LG: *Physiology of the Human Kidney*. New York, Grune & Stratton, 1969, p 98.

21. Lakatta EG: Cardiovascular reserve and aging, in Horan MI, Steinberg GM, Dunbar JB, et al (eds): *Blood Pressure Regulation and Aging. An NIH Symposium*. New York, Biomedical Information Corp, 1986, pp 51–78.

22. Tzankoff SP, Norris HA: Effect of muscle mass decrease on age-related BMR changes. *J Appl Physiol Respir Environ Exerc Physiol* 1977;43:1001–1006.

23. Rodehoffer J, Gersetenbeith G, Becker LC: Exercise cardiac output is maintained with advancing age in healthy human subjects: Cardiac dilatation and increased stroke volume compensate for a diminished heart rate. *Circulation* 1984;69:203–213.

24. Wood AJJ: Hypertension in the elderly: Pharmacotherapy, in Horan MJ, Steinberg GM, Dunbar JB, et al (eds): *Blood Pressure Regulation and Aging. An NIH Symposium*. New York, Biomedical Information Corp, 1985, p 218.

25. Lindeman RD, Tobin JD, Shock NW: Association between blood pressure and the rate of decline in renal function with age. *Kidney Int* 1984;26:861–868.

26. Epstein M, Hollenberg NK: Age as a determinant of renal sodium conservation in normal man. *J Lab Clin Med* 1976;87:411–417.

27. Brown WW, Davis BB, Spry LA, et al: Aging and the kidney. *Arch Intern Med* 1986; 146:1790–1796.

28. Sowers JR, Zawada EF: Hypertension in the aged, in Zawada EJ, Sica DA (eds): *Geriatric Nephrology and Urology*. Littleton, Mass, PSG Publishing, 1985, pp 265–281.

29. Onyer J, Weber M, DeYoung J, et al: Circadian blood pressure patterns in ambulatory hypertensive patients. *Am J Med* 1982;73:493–499.

30. Mancia G: Blood pressure variability at normal and high blood pressure. *Chest* 1983;2(suppl 2):317–418.

31. Epstein FA: An epidemiological view of mild hypertension, in Gross F, Strasser T (eds): *Mild Hypertension: Natural History and Management*. Tunbridge Wells, Engl, Pitman Medical Publishers, 1979, pp 4–6.

32. Avolio AP, Chen SG, Wang RP, et al: Effects of aging on changing arterial compliance and left ventricular load in a Northern Chinese urban community. *Circulation* 1983;68:50–58.

33. Adamopoulos PN, Chrysant SG, Frohlich ED: Systolic hypertension: Nonhomogenous diseases, in Laragh JH (ed): *Topics in Hypertension*. New York, Yorke Medical Books, 1980, chap 17.

34. Roach MR, Burton AC: The reason for the shape of the distensibility curves of arteries. *Can J Biochem Physiol* 1957;35:681–690.

35. Simon AC, Safar ME, Levinson JA, et al: Action of vasodilating drugs on small and large arteries of hypertensive patients. *J Cardiovasc Pharmacol* 1983;5:626–631.

36. Simon AC, Levenson J, Bouthier JD, et al: Effects of chronic administration of enalapril and propranolol on the large arteries in essential hypertension. *J Cardiovasc Pharmacol* 1985;7:856–861.

37. Learoyd BM, Taylor MG: Alterations with age in the viscoelastic properties of human arterial walls. *Circ Res* 1966;18:278–292.

38. Bader H: Dependence on wall stress in the human thoracic aorta on age and pressure. *Circ Res* 1967;20:354–361.

39. Nichols WW, Conti CR, Walker WW, et al: *Circ Res* 1977:40;451–458.

40. Gerstenblith G, Fredericksen J, Yin FCP, et al: Echocardiographic assessment of a normal adult aging population. *Circulation* 1977;56:273–378.

41. Castelli WP: CHD risk factors in the elderly. *Hosp Pract* 1976;11:113–115.

42. Tarazi RC: Regression of left ventricular hypertrophy by medical treatment: Present status and possible implications. *Am J Med* 1983;75(suppl 3A):80–86.

43. Wikman–Coffelt J, Parmley WW, Mason DT: The cardiac hypertrophy process: Analysis of factors determining pathological vs physiological development. *Circ Res* 1979;45:697–707.

44. Kannel WB, Dawber TR, Sorlie P, et al: Components of blood pressure and risk of atherothrombotic brain infarction: The Framingham Study. *Stroke* 1976;2:327–331.

45. Kannel WB, Gordon T, Schwartz MJ: Systolic versus diastolic blood pressure and risk of coronary heart disease: The Framingham study. *Am J Cardiol* 1971;27:335–346.

46. Dyer AR, Stamler J, Shekelle RB, et al: Hypertension in the elderly. *Med Clin North Am* 1977;61:516–529.

47. Isles CG, Walker LM, Beevers GD, et al: Mortality in patients of the Glasgow blood pressure clinic. *J Hypertens* 1986;4:141–156.

48. Veterans Administration Cooperative Study Group on Antihypertensive Agents: Effects of treatment on morbidity in hypertension. *Circulation* 1972;45:991–1004.

49. Management Committee: The Australian therapeutic trial in mild hypertension. *Lancet* 1980;1:1261–1267.

50. Bulpitt CJ, Beevers DG, Butler A, et al: The survival of treated hypertension patients and their causes of death: A report from the DHSS Hypertensive Care Computing Project (DHCCP). *H Hypertens* 1986;4:93–99.

51. The IPPPSH Collaborative Group: Cardiovascular risk and risk factors in a randomized trial of treatment based on the beta blocker oxprenolol. The international prospective primary prevention study in hypertension. *J Hypertens* 1985;3:379–392.

52. Willett WC, Green A, Stampfer MJ, et al: Relative and absolute risks of coronary heart disease among women who smoke cigarettes. *N Engl J Med* 1987;317:1303–1319.

53. Kuller LH, Hulley SB, Cohen JD, et al: Unexpected effects of treating hypertension in men with electrocardiographic abnormalities: A critical analysis. *Circulation* 1983;73:114–123.

54. Schatzkin A, Cupples LA, Heuren T, et al: Sudden death in the Framingham Heart Study. *Am J Epidemiol* 1984;120:888–889.

55. Kannel WB, Hjortland MC, McNamara PM, et al: Menopause and risk of cardiovascular disease: The Framingham Study. *Ann Intern Med* 1976;85:447–452.

56. Kannel WB: Role of blood pressure in cardiovascular disease: The Framingham Study. *Angiology* 1975;26:1–14.

57. Colditz GA, Willett WC, Stampfer MJ, et al: Menopause and the risk of coronary heart disease in women. *N Engl J Med* 1987;316:1105–1110.

58. Pfeffer RI, Whipple GH, Dwosaki TT, et al: Coronary risk and estrogen use in postmenopausal women. *Am J Epidemiol* 1978;107:479–487.

59. Hillner BE, Hollenberg JP, Parker SG: Postmenopausal estrogens in prevention of osteoporosis. Benefit virtually without risk if cardiovascular effects are considered. *Am J Med* 1986;80:1115–1128.

60. Barrett–Connor E, Khaw K: Family history of heart attack as an independent predictor of death due to cardiovascular disease. *Circulation* 1984;69:1065–1069.

61. Knopp RH, Walden CE, Heiss G, et al: Prevalence and clinical correlates of beta-migrating very low density lipoprotein. *Am J Med* 1986;81:493–502.

62. Kannel WB: Lipids, diabetes and coronary heart disease: Insights from the Framingham Study. *Am Heart J* 1985;110:1100–1107.

63. Lerner DJ, Kannel WB: Patterns of coronary heart disease morbidity and mortality in the sexes: A 26-year followup of the Framingham population. *Am Heart J* 1986;111:383–390.

64. Helgeland A: Treatment of mild hypertension: A five-year controlled drug trial. *Am J Med* 1980;69:725–732.

65. Smith WM: Treatment of mild hypertension. Results of a ten-year intervention trial. US Public Health Service Hospitals Cooperative Study Group. *Circ Res* 1977;40(suppl 1):98–105.

66. Multiple Risk Factor Intervention Group: Coronary heart disease death, nonfatal acute myocardial infarction and other clinical outcomes in the multiple risk factor intervention trial. *Am J Cardiol* 1986;58:1–13.

67. Lasser N, Grandits G, Caggiula AW, et al: Effects of antihypertensive therapy on plasma lipids and lipoprotein in the multiple risk factor intervention trial. *Am J Med* 1984;76(suppl 2A):52–65.

68. Cruickshank JM, Thorp JM, Zachorios FJ: Benefits and potential harm of treating high blood pressure. *Lancet* 1987;1:581–584.

69. Stewart I McDG: Relation of reduction in pressure to first myocardial infarction in patients receiving treatment for severe hypertension. *Lancet* 1979;1:861–865.

70. Khaw K, Barrett-Connor E: Family history of heart disease is a modifiable risk factor. *Circulation* 1986;74:239–244.

71. Kannel WB, Castelli WP, Gordon T, et al: Serum cholesterol, lipoproteins and the risk of coronary heart disease. *Ann Intern Med* 1971;74:1–12.

72. Castelli WP, Garrison RJ, Wilson PWF, et al: Incidence of coronary heart disease and lipoprotein cholesterol levels. The Framingham Study. *JAMA* 1986;256:2834–2838.

73. Castelli WP: Epidemiology of coronary heart disease: The Framingham Study. *Am J Med* 1984;76(suppl 2A):4–12.

74. Hubert HB, Feinleib M, McNamara PM, et al: Obesity as an independent risk factor for cardiovascular disease: A 26-year followup of participants in the Framingham heart study. *Circulation* 1983;67:968–977.

75. Barrett–Connor E: Obesity, atherosclerosis and coronary artery disease. *Ann Intern Med* 1985;103(pt 2):1010–1019.

76. Bloom E, Reed D, Yano K, et al: Does obesity protect hypertensives against cardiovascular disease? *JAMA* 1986;256:2972–2975.

77. Gillium RF, Liu KC: Coronary disease mortality in United States blacks, 1940-1978: Trends and unanswered questions. *Am Heart J* 1984;108:728–732.

78. Tyroler HA, Heyden S, Bartel A, et al: Blood pressure and cholesterol as coronary heart disease risk factors. *Arch Intern Med* 1971;128:907–914.

79. Kannel WB: Current status of the epidemiology of brain infarction associated with occlusive arterial disease. *Stroke* 1971;2:295–318.

80. Kannel WB, Wolf PA, Verter J: Manifestations of coronary disease predisposing to stroke: The Framingham Study. *JAMA* 1983;250:2942–2946.

81. Casale PN, Devereux RB, Milner M, et al: Value of echocardiographic measurement of left ventricular mass in predicting cardiovascular morbid events in hypertensive men. *Ann Intern Med* 1986;104:173–178.

82. Kurtzke JF: Cerebrovascular Survey Report. National Institute of Neurologic and Communicative Disorder and Stroke, rev ed, 1985, pp 1–34.

83. Wolf PA, Kannel WB, Verter J: Current status of risk factors for stroke. *Neurol Clin* 1983;1:317–343.

84. Hypertension Stroke Cooperative Study Group: Effect of antihypertensive therapy on stroke recurrence. *JAMA* 1974;229:409–418.

85. Bonita R, Beaglehole R: editorial. Does treatment of hypertension explain the decline in mortality from stroke? *Br Med J* 1986;292:191–192.

86. Khaw K, Barrett–Connor E, Suarez L, et al: Predictors of stroke associated mortality in the elderly. *Stroke* 1984;15:244–248.

87. Nakayama Y: Epidemiological research in Japan on smoking and cardiovascular disease, in Schettler CA, Gotto Y, Hato G, et al (eds): *Atherosclerosis IV. Proceedings of the Fourth International Symposium*. New York, Springer-Verlag, 1977.

88. Wolf PA, Kannel WB, Verter J: Current status of risk factors for stroke. *Neurol Clin* 1983;1:317–343.

89. Heyman A, Wilkinson WE, Heyden S, et al: Risk of stroke in asymptomatic persons with cervical arterial bruit. *N Engl J Med* 1980;302:838–841.

90. Hypertension Detection and Followup Program Cooperative Group: Five-year findings of the hypertension detection and followup program: III. Reduction in stroke incidence among persons with high blood pressure. *JAMA* 1982;247:633–638.

91. Sage JI, van Vitent RL: Risk of recurrent stroke in patients with atrial fibrillation and non-valvular heart disease. *Stroke* 1983;14:537–540.

92. Britton M, Gustafsson C: Non-rheumatic atrial fibrillation as a risk factor for stroke. *Stroke* 1985;16:182–188.

93. Kane WC, Aronson SM: Cardiac disorders predisposing to embolic stroke. *Stroke* 1970;1:164–172.

94. Kannel WB, Abbott RD, Savage DD: Coronary heart disease and atrial fibrillation: The Framingham Study. *Am Heart J* 1983;106:389–396.

95. American Canadian cooperative study group: Persantine aspirin trial in cerebral ischemia: III. Risk factors for stroke. *Stroke* 1986;17:12–18.

96. Rosenberg SH, Fausone V, Clark R: The role of estrogens as a risk factor for stroke in postmenopausal women. *West J Med* 1980;133:292–296.

97. Shekelle RB, Ostfeld AM, Klawans HL: Hypertension and the risk of stroke in an elderly population. *Stroke* 1974;5:71–75.

98. Mohr JP: Lacunes. *Neurol Clin* 1983;1:201–221.

99. Solberg LA, McGarry PA: Cerebral atherosclerosis in Negroes and Caucasians. *Atherosclerosis* 1972;16:141–154.

100. Khaw KT, Barrett–Connor E: Dietary potassium and stroke-associated mortality. *N Engl J Med* 1987;316:235–240.

101. Colandrea M, Friedman GD, Nichaman MZ, et al: Systolic hypertension in the elderly. An epidemiologic assessment. *Circulation* 1970;41:239–245.

102. Kannel WB, Blaisdell FW, Gifford R, et al: Risk factors in stroke due to cerebral infarction. *Stroke* 1971;2:423–428.

103. Kannel WB, Castelli WP, Gordon T: Serum cholesterol, lipoproteins, and the risk of coronary heart disease. *Ann Intern Med* 1971;74:1–12.

104. Veterans Administration cooperative study group on antihypertensive agents: III. Influence of age, diastolic pressure, and prior cardiovascular disease; further analysis of side effects. *Circulation* 1972;45:991–1004.

105. Relationship of blood pressure, serum cholesterol, smoking habit, relative weight and ECG abnormalities to incidence of major coronary events: Final report of the pooling project. *J Chronic Dis* 1978;31:201–306.

106. The Management Committee of the Australian national blood pressure study: Prognostic factors in the treatment of mild hypertension. *Circulation* 1984;69:668–675.

107. Madhavan S, Alderman MH: The potential effect of blood pressure reduction on cardiovascular disease: A cautionary note. *Arch Intern Med* 1985;141:1583–1586.

108. European working party on high blood pressure in the elderly: Mortality and morbidity results from the European working party on high blood pressure in the elderly trial. *Lancet* 1985;1:1349–1354.

109. Medical research council working party: MRC trial of treatment of mild hypertension: Principal results. *Br Med J* 1985;291:97–104.

110. Management Committee: Treatment of mild hypertension in the elderly. *Med J Aust* 1981;2:398–402.

111. Hypertension detection and followup program cooperative group: Five-year findings of the hypertension detection and followup program. *JAMA* 1979;242:2562–2571.

112. Hypertension detection and followup program cooperative group: The effect of treatment on mortality in "mild" hypertension: Results of the hypertension detection and followup program. *N Engl J Med* 1982;367:976–980.

113. Carter A: Hypotensive therapy in stroke survivors. *Lancet* 1970;1:485–489.

114. Meyer JS, Rogers RL, Mortel KF: Prospective analysis of long term control of mild hypertension on cerebral blood flow. *Stroke* 1985;16:985–990.

115. Black DG, Heagerty AM, Bing RF, et al: Effects of treatment for hypertension on cerebral hemorrhage and infarction. *Br Med J* 1984;289:156–159.

116. Aukell M, Hartford M, Wikstrand J: Renal function before and after withdrawal of long term treatment in primary hypertension, in *Abstracts American Society of Hypertension*. Thorofare, NJ, Charles Slack, 1986, p 33.

117. Morduchowicz G, Boner G, Ben–Bassat M, et al: Proteinuria in benign nephrosclerosis. *Arch Intern Med* 1986;146:1513–1516.

118. Bulpitt C: Prognosis of treated hypertension, 1951-1981. *Br J Clin Pharmacol* 1982; 13:73–79.

119. Sen S: Regression of cardiac hypertrophy: Experimental animal model. *Am J Med* 1983;75(suppl 3A):87–93.

120. Samuelsson OG, Wilhelmsen LW, Svardsudd KF, et al: Mortality and morbidity in relation to systolic blood pressure in two populations with different management of hypertension: The study of men born in 1913 and the multifactorial primary prevention trial. *J Hypertens* 1987;5:57–66.

121. Holme I, Waaler HJ: Five-year mortality in the city of Bergen according to age, sex, and blood pressure. *Acta Med Scand* 1976;200:229–239.

122. Miall WE, Brennan DJ: Hypertension in the elderly: The South Wales study, in Onesti G, Kim K (eds): *Hypertension in the Young and Very Old*. New York, Grune & Stratton, 1981, pp 227–283.

123. Rose GA, Blackburn H: *Cardiovascular Survey Methods*. Geneva, World Health Organization, 1968.

124. Fuller JH, McCartney P, Jarret RJ, et al: Hyperglycemia and coronary heart disease. The Whitehall Study. *J Chronic Dis* 1979;32:721–729.

125. Agner E, Morck HI: Arterial hypertension in 70–80-year-old men and women. From the Glostrup population studies. *Acta Med Scand* 1980;suppl 646:19–24.

126. Aronow WS, Starling L, Etienner F, et al: Risk factors for coronary artery disease in persons older than 62 years in a long term health care facility. *Am J Cardiol* 1980;57:518–520.

127. Rajala P: Blood pressure and mortality in the very old. *Lancet* 1983;2:520.

128. Lindholm L, Schersten B, Thulin T: High blood pressure and mortality in the elderly. *Lancet* 1983;2:745–746.

129. Hammon EC, Garfinkel L: Coronary heart disease, stroke and aortic aneurysm: Factors in the etiology. *Arch Environ Health* 1969;19:167–182.

130. Kuramoto K, Matsushita S: The treatment of mild hypertension in the elderly, a prospective study using multiple regression analysis. *Jpn Circ J* 1985;49:1144–1149.

131. Borhani NO: Eight-year followup of participants in the hypertension detection and followup program: Persistence of reduction in blood pressure and mortality in a treated hypertensive population, in *Abstracts American Society of Hypertension*. Thorofare, NJ, Charles Slack, 1986.

132. Kuramoto K, Matsushita S, Juwajima I, et al: Prospective study on the treatment of mild hypertension in the aged. *Jpn Heart J* 1981:75–85.

133. Burch GE, DePasquale NP: *Primer of Clinical Measurement of Blood Pressure*. St Louis, CV Mosby, 1962, p 58.

134. Kurtz KJ: Dynamic vascular auscultation. *Am J Med* 1984;76:1066–1074.

135. Berguer R, Higgins R, Nelson R: Noninvasive diagnosis of reversal of vertebral artery blood flow. *N Engl J Med* 1980;24:1349–1351.

136. Sparrow D, Tifft CP, Rosner B, et al: Postural changes in diastolic blood pressure and the risk of myocardial infarction: The Normative Aging Study. *Circulation* 1984;70:533–537.

137. Kales A, Cadieux RJ, Shaw LC, et al: Sleep apnea in a hypertensive population. *Lancet* 1984;2:1005–1008.

138. Lombard RM, Zwillich CW: Medical therapy of obstructive sleep apnea. *Med Clin North Am* 1985;69:1317–1336.

139. Mancia G, Bertinieri G, Grass G, et al: Effects of blood pressure measurement by the doctor on patient's blood pressure and heart rate. *Lancet* 1983;2:695–697.

140. Sokolow M, Perloff D, Cowan R: Contribution of ambulatory blood pressure to the assessment of patients with mild to moderate elevation of office blood pressure. *Cardiovasc Rev Rep* 1980;1:295–303.

141. Fry J: The natural history of hypertension: A case for selective non-treatment. *Lancet* 1974;2:431–433.

142. Byrd L, Novembre C, Krieger J, et al: Ambulatory blood pressure monitoring: Role of sex and age (unpublished data).

143. Kiyonaga A, Arakawa K, Tanaka H: Blood pressure and hormonal responses to aerobic exercise. *Hypertension* 1985;7:125–131.

144. Stamler R, Stamler J, Grimm R, et al: Nutritional therapy for high blood pressure. *JAMA* 1987;257:1484–1491.

145. Morgan T, Adam W, Gillies A, et al: Hypertension treated by salt restriction. *Lancet* 1978;1:227–230.

146. Resnick LM, Muller FB, Laragh JH: Calcium regulating hormones in essential hypertension. Relationship to plasma renin activity and sodium metabolism. *Ann Intern Med* 1986;105:649–654.

147. Messerli FH, Frohlich ED: High blood pressure—a side effect of drugs, poisons and food. *Arch Intern Med* 1979;139:682–687.

148. Jespersen CM, Arnung K, Hagen C, et al: Effects of natural estrogen therapy on blood pressure and renin angiotensin system in normotensive and hypertens menopausal women. *J Hypertens* 1983;1:361–365.

149. Grundy SM, Bilheimer D, Blackburn H, et al: Rationale of the diet heart statement of the American Heart Association: Report of the nutrition committee. *Circulation* 1982;65:839A–854A.

150. Sowers JR, Zawada EJ: Hypertension in the aged, in Zawada EJ, Sica DA (eds): *Geriatric Nephrology and Urology*. Littleton, Mass, PSG Publishing, 1985, pp 265–281.

151. Lipsitz LA, Nyquist RP, Weil JY, et al: Postprandial reduction in blood pressure in the elderly. *N Engl J Med* 1983;309:81–83.

152. Caird FI, Andrews GR, Kennedy RD: Effect of posture on blood pressure in the elderly. *Br Heart J* 1973;35:527–530.

153. van Brummelen P, Man in't veld AJ, Schalekamp MA: Hemodynamic changes during long term thiazide treatment of essential hypertension in responders and nonresponders. *Clin Pharmacol Ther* 1980;27:328–336.

154. Grimm RH, Leon AS, Hunninghake DB, et al: Effects of thiazide diuretics on plasma lipids and lipoproteins in mildly hypertensive patients. A double blind controlled trial. *Ann Intern Med* 1981;94:4–11.

155. Hollifield JW: Thiazide treatment of hypertension: Effects of thiazide diuretics on serum potassium, magnesium and ventricular ectopy. *Am J Med* 1986;80(4A):8–12.

156. Brown MJ, Brown DC, Murphy MB: Hypokalemia from beta 2-receptor stimulation by circulating epinephrine. *N Engl J Med* 1983;309:1414–1419.

157. Arieff AI: Effects of water, acid-base and electrolyte disorders on the central nervous system, in Arieff AI, DeFronzo RA (eds): *Fluid, Electrolyte and Acid-Base Disorders*. New York, Churchill Livingstone, 1985, p 969.

158. Drayer JIM, Keim JH, Weber MA, et al: Unexpected pressor responses to propranolol in essential hypertension. *Am J Med* 1976;60:897–902.

159. Buhler FR, Bolli P, Erne P, et al: Position of calcium antagonists in antihypertensive therapy. *J Cardiovasc Pharmacol* 1985;7(suppl 4):521–527.

160. Levenson J, Simon A, Safar ME, et al: Large arteries in hypertension: Acute effects at a new calcium entry blocker, nitrendipine. *J Cardiovasc Pharmacol* 1984;6:S1006–S1010.

161. Ben-Ishay D, Leibel B, Stessman J: Calcium channel blockers in the management of hypertension in the elderly. *Am J Med* 1986;81(suppl 6A):30–34.

162. Hansson L, Aoki K, Buhler FR, et al: International views of the use of calcium antagonists in the treatment of hypertension. *J Cardiovasc Pharmacol* 1985;7(suppl 4):545–548.

163. Loutzenhiser RD, Epstein M: Renal hemodynamic effects of calcium antagonists. *Am J Med* 1987;82(suppl 3B):23–28.

164. Bertel O, Marx BE, Conen D: Effects of antihypertensive treatment on cerebral perfusion. *Am J Med* 1987;82(suppl 3B):29–36.

165. Veterans Administration cooperative study group on anti-hypertensive agents: Low dose captopril for the treatment of mild to moderate hypertension. *Arch Intern Med* 1984;144:1947–1952.

166. Hollenberg NK: Renal hemodynamics in essential and renovascular hypertension: Influence of captopril. *Am J Med* 1984;76(suppl 5B):22–28.

167. Gavras I, Gavras H, Chobanian AV, et al: Hypertension and age: Clinical and biochemical correlates. *Clin Exp Hypertens* 1982;7:1097–1106.

168. Lager I, Blohme G, Smith U: Effect of cardioselective and nonselective beta blockade on the hypoglycemic response in insulin dependent diabetics. *Lancet* 1979;1:458.

169. Masoro E: Other physiologic changes with age, in Masoro E (ed): *Epidemiology of Aging.* DHEW publication No. (NIH) 75-711. Government Printing Office, 1975, pp 137–155.

170. Spence JD, Sibbald WJ, Cape RD: Pseudohypertension in the elderly. *Clin Sci Mol Med* 1978;55:3995–4025.

171. Frocht A, Fillit H: Renal disease in the geriatric patient. *J Am Geriatr Soc* 1984;32:28–43.

172. Byrd LH, Sherman RL: Radiocontrast-induced acute renal failure a clinical and pathophysiologic review. *Medicine* 1979;58:270–278.

173. Boscia JA, Kobassa WD, Abrutyn E, et al: Lack of association between bacteriuria and symptoms in the elderly. *Am J Med* 1986;81:979–982.

174. Cosio FG, Zager RA, Sharma HM: Atheroembolic renal disease causes hypocomplementemia. *Lancet* 1985;2:118–121.

175. Walls of the blood vessels and their function, in Burton AC: *Physiology and Biophysics of the Circulation.* Chicago, Year Book Medical Publishers, 1965, chap 7.

176. Fukuda Y, Sakuma K, Hashimoto T: Long term observations of blood pressure in 32,000 workers of the Japanese National Railways, in Gross F, Strasser T (eds): *Mild Hypertension: Natural History and Management.* Tunbridge Wells, Engl, Pitman Medical Publishers, 1979, pp 57–66.

177. Grundy S: Cholesterol and coronary heart disease: A new era. *JAMA* 1986;256:2849–2858.

Chapter 6

Gastroenterology and the Aging Gastrointestinal Tract

William C. Sloan

INTRODUCTION

The increasing age of our population is readily visible. It is estimated that 23 million persons—11% of our population—are over 65 years of age. This figure may increase by 16% over the next 25 years.

Gastrointestinal complaints in an aging population are extremely common and account for much of what ails our aging gynecologic clientele. This chapter covers dysphagia, jaundice, the role of endoscopy, and ulcer disease as they relate to an elderly population.

DYSPHAGIA

Dysphagia is a significant symptom in any age group. The inability to swallow solids, liquids, or both must be thoroughly investigated to clarify the etiology of this symptom complex so that proper therapy may be promptly instituted. Because the elderly are particularly vulnerable to nutritional deficiencies, prompt investigation is indicated.

The esophagus is lined by striated muscle in the upper fourth and smooth muscle for the remainder of the organ. There is an upper sphincter and a lower one, and peristalsis propagates from the pharynx through the lower esophageal sphincter area. A swallowing center is located in the brain, which coordinates the motor activity of the esophagus, and the brain stem nuclei of the 5th, 7th, 10th, and 12th cranial nerves are involved in this control mechanism. With age, there are alterations of the esophageal smooth muscle, and nonpropulsive repetitive esophageal contractions can therefore occur. The vagus nerve (cranial nerve X) may be responsible also for age-related changes in the esophagus. These include weak, noncoordinated contractile waves with alterations in the lower esophageal sphincter relaxation mechanism. Such changes have been called presbyesophagus when seen in the elderly, but they are poorly understood and difficult to treat.

Neurologic causes of dysphagia are common in the elderly. They result in dysphagia for both solids and liquids rather than for solids alone. Both Parkinson's disease and cerebrovascular accidents may lead to global or total dysphagia to all nutrients. Myasthenia gravis with muscle weakness, ocular signs, and a positive response to the administration of Tensilon should also be considered. Rarely myopathy, myositis, and metabolic disease may also cause dysphagia of a similar type.

Many mechanical entities can lead to dysphagia, especially in the aged population. Zenker's diverticulum can cause halitosis and vomiting soon after eating. This entity may lead to aspiration pneumonia. It may require surgery consisting of ligation of the diverticulum and myotomy of the hypertrophic upper esophageal sphincter muscle, felt to be the most likely cause of this outpouching of the proximal esophagus.

Carcinoma of the esophagus is an all-too-common cause of dysphagia, mainly to solids, in the elderly. Progressive dysphagia with marked weight loss is seen. Smoking, alcoholism, and prior caustic ingestion seem to predispose to this tumor. Results of therapy are extremely poor, but recent studies have held some promise of survival with an aggressive approach to chemotherapy.

Reflux esophagitis may be subtle in the aging. A typical history of heartburn and reflux symptoms may not be easily elicited. Many elderly patients will present with vague symptoms of dyspepsia and with profound anemia and dysphagia resembling that seen in a carcinoma. After radiographic evaluation and endoscopic biopsy, a benign stricture may be found that can be treated with dilatation. Measures to treat reflux include elevation of the head of the bed, antacids, and histamine (H_2) blocking agents. Peristaltic stimulating agents, such as metoclopramide, can be used also. Abstinence from smoking, alcohol, and aspirin-containing agents is also mandatory. Periodic dilatations may be required to maintain lumen patency of the esophagus.

The elderly frequently take multiple medications. Such drugs can include potassium tablets, aspirin, tetracycline, quinidine, and iron. These agents can cause esophagitis and subsequent stricture formation if they are taken before bedtime in a semihorizontal position with an inadequate amount of fluid. A careful history will usually clarify this unusual but fairly difficult to treat cause of dysphagia.

Rarely cervical arthritis may be severe enough to produce large, protruding osteophytes that then impinge on the posterior esophageal lumen, leading to progressive dysphagia. This condition may require surgery if it significantly interferes with nutrition.

Enlarged vessels such as the aorta can press on the lower esophageal area and result in progressive dysphagia. Cardiac chamber enlargement may produce the same type of impairment.

Achalasia may also present in the elderly. This disorder is frequently longstanding and is associated with dysphagia to both solids and liquids. Marked esophageal dilatation may be seen. There is an absence of peristalsis in the body of the esophagus and failure of the lower esophageal sphincter relaxation mechanism with swallowing. Treatment is by pneumatic dilatation or surgery. There is an increased risk of esophageal carcinoma as well in these patients.

Rarely scleroderma may also present with esophageal dilatation and decreased peristalsis involving the smooth muscle portion of the esophagus. This entity may also periodically require esophageal dilatation to relieve the strictures that occur in the evolution of scleroderma of the esophagus.

Evaluation of any swallowing problems should first include a careful history and physical examination. Radiographic evaluations should then follow with barium studies and cine-esophagogram, if needed, to clarify any potential motility disorder. Endoscopic studies with biopsies should then follow, if indicated. On occasion motility studies will be needed to further clarify the nature of the disorder.

Dysphagia should never be regarded as a functional complaint in any age group unless a complete evaluation has been done to assess its cause and to plan a proper approach to therapy. Rewards will be most forthcoming in any age group but particularly in the elderly, in whom nutrition plays such a critical role in the maintenance of general health.

JAUNDICE

Jaundice presents a set of particular problems in the elderly. The differential diagnosis rests essentially between medical causes for icterus as distinguished from surgical causes. Failure to distinguish between these two categories can be catastrophic, as the therapeutic approach is quite different between the two.

The history remains a fundamental tool in evaluating the jaundiced patient. Many elderly patients are on multiple drugs that can cause icterus. Laxatives, sedatives, sulfa drugs, and any multiplicity of other agents must be considered in evaluating these individuals. Exposures to recent toxins and other jaundiced individuals must be clarified. Hepatitis in the elderly may be subtle in its presentation. It may present with signs and symptoms that suggest a malignancy—weight loss, fatigue, and right-sided abdominal pain may be present. Fever may be misleading, as well as joint pain, which may also accompany the jaundice. Other medical causes of this condition, such as congestive heart failure, alcoholism, cirrhosis, and lymphomas of the liver, must also be considered. A history of prior blood transfusions must be carefully sought, particularly with the frequency of open heart surgery in the elderly population and its attendant risks to the acquisition of hepatitis.

The physical examination of the jaundiced patient may also serve to significantly confuse. The presence of abdominal masses and nodularity of the liver may suggest tumor masses or advanced cirrhosis. Ascites is an important finding, and a diagnostic paracentesis should always be done to sample the abdominal fluid. Encephalopathy is common in the elderly patient with compromised liver function as well.

Liver function tests may help to clarify the clinical picture. High hepatic enzymes suggest primary hepatitis. Elevated alkaline phosphatase levels may indicate hepatic or bone involvement, and further testing must then be done to clarify this abnormality. An elevated gamma-glutamyl transpeptidase with an increased alkaline phosphatase as well points to a hepatic source. The level of the bilirubin is of little help in distinguishing the cause of the jaundice. Various serologic tests are now available to pinpoint the prior exposure that the patient may have had to both A and B hepatitis. Unfortunately such tests do not exist for non-A, non-B hepatitis.

Surgical causes for jaundice predominate in the elderly. Gallstones and their potentially associated common duct calculi are common causes for icterus in this age group. The classic triad of fever, chills, and right upper quadrant pain may be absent. Vague symptoms of fever, malaise, and confusion may exist in the biliary diseased patient. Carcinoma of the pancreas and the biliary tree must also be considered. Finally, metastasis of the liver is all too common in the geriatric population.

The 1980s have seen rather dramatic advances in the evaluation and care of the jaundiced patient. Grey scale and real-time ultrasonography has been perfected so that the liver, gallbladder, and pancreas may be rapidly and clearly imaged. Computed tomography has come of age to further delineate the liver and its surrounding organs. These techniques can identify a mechanical or surgical cause of the jaundice and can guide the surgeon appropriately to relieve this condition. Endoscopic techniques such as retrograde cholangiopancreatography can also be used. Therapeutic tools to extract stones from the common bile duct and to place stents for obstructed ducts are also rapidly becoming commonplace. Percutaneous transhepatic cholangiography can also be used to palliate an obstructed biliary duct.

Thus the elderly jaundiced patient represents a challenge to the gastroenterologist. With the careful evaluation of such an individual and with the proper application of both diagnostic and therapeutic measures, considerable improvement can be achieved.

GASTROINTESTINAL ENDOSCOPY

Gastrointestinal endoscopy has progressed dramatically since the early 1970s. Flexible endoscopes have markedly altered the approach to both the diagnosis and therapy of gastrointestinal complaints.

Elderly patients present a particular challenge to the endoscopist. Often they are frail and present with vague histories, with insufficient data as a result. The elderly may be taking multiple medications as well, which may significantly alter the clinical picture.

Upper intestinal endoscopy may be safely done in the elderly. Very thin lumen endoscopes now exist that are essentially pediatric in size. They can be passed under direct visualization into the cervical esophagus to visualize the entire organ and then passed down through the stomach and into the duodenum. Minimal doses of tranquilizers are necessary to sedate the patient, and on occasion no sedation should be used. The entire examination can be done in less than five minutes with good visualization of the upper digestive tract and with minimal patient discomfort. Esophagitis, varices, gastritis, ulcers, and neoplasms of the upper gastrointestinal tract may be readily visualized and, if necessary, biopsy specimens may be obtained.

Radiographic studies of the upper digestive tract may also be accomplished, but this may be difficult in the elderly. Poor patient cooperation may prevent adequate studies from being carried out. False-positive appearances may be present on barium meals that only can be clarified by direct visualization of the involved organ system. Strictures of the esophagus may also require endoscopic clarification and biopsy. Multiple pathologic lesions, such as ulcers, hernias, and varices, may be seen on x-ray, all in the same patient, and hence, endoscopic clarification may be required to determine which is the offending pathologic entity causing the patient's discomfort.

In patients with dysphagia, endoscopy is extremely important. Webs, rings, and early neoplasms may not be appreciated by both single and, on occasion, double contrast studies.

In the presence of upper intestinal bleeding, endoscopy is critical to clarify the problem and plan effective therapy. Endoscopy should be the study of first resort to avoid barium ingestion, which may subsequently interfere with the use of angiography. In addition, recent advances involving the use of heater probes and lasers will now allow direct application of therapeutic techniques through the endoscope to control bleeding sites.

Lower esophageal pathology also lends itself quite well to flexible endoscopy. Current instruments are very flexible and well tolerated by elderly patients. Minimal sedation is required here also, and the procedure can be done entirely on an outpatient basis. Flexible sigmoidoscopy can be easily applied in the office with no premedication or sedation required. With the flexible sigmoidoscope the distal 60 cm of the colon may be well seen, and biopsy specimens can be obtained, if needed. Polyps, diverticuli, neoplasms, and inflammatory lesions may all be inspected and sampled through the short sigmoidoscope. The long colonoscope may be introduced through the entire colon to the cecum, and therefore the colon may be well seen throughout its length. Preparation for this examination requires thorough bowel cleansing, but this is usually well tolerated by the elderly patient and can be administered at home beforehand.

Polypectomy with the colonoscope may be accomplished in an office or outpatient setting. Most large-bowel cancers have now been shown to arise from benign adenomatous polyps of the colon. If these polups have a sufficient stalk, they may be removed with a snare device passed through the colonoscope with the application of cautery current. The polyp is then retrieved and sent to the pathologist for examination. Large polyps with significant villous components may be completely removed with this technique. However, if cancer is present in the polyp, extending to the base of the polyp and into the stalk, then surgery will be required, to obtain adequate surgical margins.

All rectal bleeding, be it gross or microscopic, requires a thorough evaluation to establish its cause. It has been my practice to do total colonoscopy in these patients at the initial time of presentation. Barium studies of the lower colon may be complementary in some cases when the cecum cannot be reached, although this is unusual. However, many barium studies may produce false-positive findings, as possible polyps may appear on these studies as filling defects that later prove to be adherent to fecal debris. Conversely several polyps and carcinomas of the colon have been found at the time of colonoscopy in patients in whom previous barium enemas had revealed no abnormalities, even with fine double-contrast technique.

Endoscopic evaluation of the biliary and pancreatic tree may also be accomplished. The ampulla of Vater may be well visualized, and may be cannulated with the subsequent injection of dye retrograde into both the biliary and pancreatic ductal systems. In so doing pancreatic pathology as well as biliary disease may be demonstrated. Endoscopic sphincterotomy can be performed to facilitate the passage of common duct stones, and stents can be inserted into the biliary tree to relieve obstructing tumor masses if such entities are found. This may then eliminate the need for palliative surgery, and therefore quite significantly reduce morbidity and mortality from these serious illnesses.

As in all invasive procedures, but particularly in the elderly, extra care must be used during the procedure. Sedatives must be carefully adjusted in older patients to avoid excessive administration. Respiratory depression may occur if inadequate titration of sedation is used. Hypoxia, with associated cardiac dysrhythmias and cardiac events, may develop unless such care is taken. Bleeding during therapeutic application of endoscopy, such as polypectomy, may occur and must be carefully monitored. After the procedure is accomplished, the patient must be monitored either in an outpatient unit or at home to avoid any further complicating events. In general, endoscopy of both the upper and lower digestive tracts is well tolerated in the elderly.

ULCERS

With advancing age there is a progressive decline in acid production in the elderly. This occurs in both men and women but is more common in the former.

The role of end-organ decline (ie, stomach, gastric acid production) or vagal influences is unclear. Regardless of the cause, there is still a high incidence of ulcer disease in patients over 65, and recent studies have shown that one third of patients with duodenal ulcer disease are over 60 years of age. Gastric ulcers constitute approximately one third to one half of ulcers found in patients over 60 years of age, and approximately 85% of ulcers requiring surgery are in patients over age 75.

Gastric ulcer in the elderly may be subtle in its presentation. Pain may be minimal or almost absent. There may be a vague relationship to eating, and the patient may appear clinically to have a malignancy, with weight loss, anemia, and severe weakness. Major problems associated with gastrointestinal ulcers in the elderly are primarily hemorrhage and perforation.

Hemorrhage in the elderly patient may be life-threatening. Often it is brisk and may occur in the absence of prior symptoms. Prompt studies are needed to establish the diagnosis, and the recent availability of heater probes and laser therapy may avoid the need for emergency surgery. Gastric ulcers in the elderly tend frequently to rebleed, and prompt surgical therapy may then be required.

Perforation also is a serious event in the evolution of peptic ulcer disease. Perforation of a gastric ulcer is less common than with duodenal ulcer, but the mortality is higher than with a duodenal lesion. Frequently such patients have associated medical problems, such as cardiac, renal, or pulmonary disorders, that reduce their ability to sustain such a complication. In addition, diagnosis may be delayed because of these other medical conditions and the vague nature of the patient's presentation.

Some gastric ulcers that may appear to be benign may actually harbor malignancies. Therefore, careful endoscopic surveillance with biopsy and follow-up is indicated in every gastric ulcer, to demonstrate complete healing. Biopsies and cytology studies must be done serially until complete healing has been documented. In addition, surveillance is indicated in the near future to avoid recurrence of such a lesion.

The use of nonsteroidal drugs in the elderly is extremely common. Antiinflammatory drugs may produce both gastric and duodenal ulcer disease. Therefore, a careful history is needed to exclude the use of these agents, as they are frequently used and are readily available throughout our medical care system.

Duodenal ulcer disease in the elderly is similar in its presentation to gastric ulcer disease. Melena may again be the presenting symptom, but also epigastric pain is more common in the duodenal ulcer patient than in the gastric ulcer patient. As with gastric ulcers, hemorrhage and perforation are the major indications for surgery, with obstruction and intractability occurring much less frequently.

Medical therapy for peptic ulcer disease in the elderly is similar to that used for a younger population. Response to therapy, however, may be somewhat delayed. H_2-receptor antagonists are the drugs of choice for peptic disease in this age group as well as in younger patients, but they may cause central nervous system effects, such as confusion and disorientation. Discontinuation of all stomach-irritating agents must also be promptly accomplished. Avoidance of smoking and reduction of alcohol intake are mandatory. With these measures and with moderate dietary manipulation, the elderly patient may do quite well.

SUGGESTED READINGS

Dysphagia

Castell D: Dysphagia in the elderly. *J Am Geriatr Soc* 1986;34:248–249.

Crowther J, Ardran G: Dysphagia due to cervical spondylosis. *J Laryngol Otol* 1985;99:1167–1169.

Halpert R, Feczko P, Spickler E, et al: Radiological assessment of dysphagia with endoscopic correlation. *Radiology* 1985;157:599–602.

Mayberry J, Atkinson M: Swallowing problems in patients with motor neuron disease. *J Clin Gastroenterol* 1986;8:233–234.

Pelemans W, Vantrapper G: Esophageal disease in the elderly. *Clin Gastroenterol* 1985;14(4):635–656.

Jaundice

Geokas M, Conteas C, Majumdar A: The aging gastrointestinal tract, liver and pancreas. *Clin Geriatr Med* 1985;1:177–205.

Huibreatse K, Katon R, Coene P, et al: Endoscopic palliative treatment in pancreatic cancer. *Gastrointest Endosc* 1986;32:334–338.

Lieberman D, Krishnamurthy G: Intrahepatic versus extrahepatic cholestasis. *Gastroenterology* 1986;90:734–743.

Endoscopy

Jacobsohn W, Levy A: Endoscopy of upper gastrointestinal tract is feasible and safe in elderly patients. *Geriatrics* 1977;32(1):80–83.

Porro G, Lazzaroni M, Petrillo M: Gastroscopy in elderly patients. *Curr Med Res Opin* 1982;7:96–103.

Stanley T, Cocking J: Upper gastrointestinal endoscopy and radiology in the elderly. *Postgrad Med J* 1978;54:257–260.

Ulcer Disease

Jolobe O, Montgomery R: Changing clinical pattern of gastric ulcer: Are anti-inflammatory drugs involved? *Digestion* 1984;29:164–170.

Steinheber F: Aging and the stomach. *Clin Gastroenterol* 1985;657–688.

Watson R, Hooper T, Ingram G: Duodenal ulcer disease in the elderly—a retrospective study. *Age Ageing* 1985;14:225–229.

Chapter 7

Constipation and Rectal Bleeding in the Elderly

Glen Mogan

INTRODUCTION

Bowel elimination often preoccupies the older individual. Constipation increases with age and infirmity. Physicians are often called on to evaluate change in bowel habits and rectal bleeding. The ensuing discussion will focus on the pathophysiology and treatment of these problems.

CONSTIPATION

Preoccupation with bowel elimination is common in all age groups. Constipation has a different meaning unless it is objectively described. Constipation should be defined before embarking on a discussion of cause and management. Most important is a change in bowel habits. They may be reduced frequency of defecation, and hard scybalous stools with difficulty in elimination. Transit time is prolonged, and colonic motility is altered, often with an atonic, insensitive bowel. Little is understood concerning the cause of motility defects in the elderly. The range is from a hypermotile (irritable bowel type) to a hypomotile state (more common with increasing age). The problem may be one of general bowel motility dysfunction, or localized to lack of anorectal sphincteric relaxation.

Many practitioners classify constipation according to severity into three categories: constipation, fecal loading, and fecal impaction. The latter occurs in individuals with chronic constipation and is diagnosed by rectal examination revealing hard inspissated stool and a flat plate of the abdomen showing fecal matter throughout the colon.

The management of fecal impaction is initially with digital disimpaction followed by enemas, oral purgatives, mineral oil, and often lactulose. Good results have been reported with the addition of Golytely, a balanced electrolyte oral gut solution.

Fecal impaction affects a considerable proportion of elderly patients, both in and out of institutions. It is often regarded as a consequence of mental and physical decline of old age. Actual anorectal function has been studied by way of manometry in these individuals and controls. Their abnormalities are both neurologic and muscular, with diminished rectal sensation. Most of these patients have prolapsed hemorrhoids and seem to strain at stool. A high proportion give a history of chronic laxative abuse, which may contribute to myenteric plexus damage. The elderly often use narcotics and analgesics, which predispose to colonic inertia and constipation.

One cannot discuss constipation without understanding some basic colonic physiology. The colon absorbs water, electrolytes, and bile acids. It secretes bicarbonate and mucus. There are different frequencies and types of colonic propulsion and peristalsis that serve to complete fecal formation and expel fecal mass. The colon also serves as a reservoir, retaining stool until defecation occurs. Aging in the colon is characterized by thickening of the muscular and collagenous layers of the bowel wall, diverticular formation, and possible altered motility with decreased blood flow to the gut.

Constipation in the elderly is multifactorial; inadequate diet (low fiber, diminished volume of liquids), diminished motor function on a muscular and vascular basis, abnormal anorectal motility, overall physical inactivity, depression, and longstanding laxative abuse with neural damage. Much of the neuromuscular initiation of fecal elimination is poorly understood.

A recent study in institutionalized elderly patients demonstrated a beneficial effect on constipation by dietary alteration. By supplying a minimum of 25 g of daily dietary fiber with 1,500 mL of fluid intake a day, constipation complaints and laxative abuse were eliminated. Furthermore there were no adverse nutritional consequences.

Laxative usage and abuse are intertwined with constipation. Usage increases with age, is often covert, and is seldom medically indicated. Prevention of the constipation averts the need for laxatives. Commonly used laxative preparations include senna (Senekot), lactulose, danthron, mineral oil, dioctyl sodium sulfosuccinate, anthraquinone purgatives, phenolphthalein, and castor oil. Major complications of regular laxative use include colonic inertia with degeneration of the neuromuscular plexus, perforation, fecal incontinence, and aspiration pneumonia.

More significant than laxative abuse in the elderly is a pattern established in adulthood, leading to habituation in old age. Perhaps increased intake of high-fiber bran-type products could avert this problem. Burkitt demonstrated the direct relationship between fiber intake and stool weight, and the inverse relationship with transit time. Most studies to date demonstrate a salutory effect of oral bulk on preventing constipation and laxative abuse.

When evaluating constipation one must check for a mechanical obstruction (cancer, diverticulitis, stricture, sigmoid volvulus, and fecal impaction). After recording a detailed history and an abdominal and a digital rectal examination, an abdominal plain film is taken. If stool is seen throughout the colon and rectal examination reveals hard, impacted stool, digital disimpaction is required. It is essential to recognize nonobstructed megacolon (idiopathic), which can predispose to a surgical emergency such as a sigmoid volvulus. Occasionally idiopathic megacolon (motility disorder) is so severe that a colectomy or decompressive colostomy is required. It is imperative to search for reversible causes, such as medications that cause fecal stasis (especially antidepressants in the elderly), metabolic disorders, and generalized systemic disease (collagen vascular, circulatory, and neuromuscular disease). Most commonly no cause is discovered.

Sigmoid volvulus is an abdominal catastrophe with significant mortality. If there is no peritonitis, an endoscopic or radiographic attempt at decompression is warranted, with placement of a rectal tube. If this is successful, the patient should have an elective sigmoid resection. If this is not done, there is an extremely high recurrence rate with mortality.

In nongastrointestinal disorders, bowel habits show no real significant change with age. Exceptions include altered diet, physical activity, and medications. Milne and Williamson studied a random sample of 215 males and 272 females aged 72 to 90. They found no statistical difference as far as bowel habit was concerned between the young and the old.

Laxative usage, however, appears to increase with age. This seems to occur regardless of normal bowel movements. Many people think that regular evacuation is necessary and beneficial. Early-20th-century physicians believed that bowel stasis could lead to other medical disorders. We now understand that there are many normal patterns of bowel elimination, and one does not have to have a bowel movement daily. A reasonably good set of bowels goes a long way to patient happiness.

RECTAL BLEEDING

Most patients come to the doctor's office in fear of the worst: they've seen some blood in the toilet bowl, on the toilet paper, or in the stool itself and are convinced that they have colorectal cancer. Others are embarrassed to admit that they've been passing blood for 2 months . . . or 2 years.

Neither group of patients needs to panic, although the second group should certainly have called as soon as the symptoms appeared. Rectal bleeding is a common occurrence with numerous causes, which can be identified by a thorough radiographic or endoscopic examination of the large intestine.

Among people younger than 40, the usual causes are hemorrhoids, anal fissures (simple tears in the lowermost lining of the rectal canal), infections, and inflammatory colitis—all of which can be treated medically. On occasion the cause turns out to be familial polyp syndrome; very rarely, in this age group, is it malignancy.

Even after age 40, these problems or another medically treatable condition, diverticulosis, can cause rectal bleeding. However, this is also the age at which colorectal polyps—exuberant or excessive growths of the lining of the lower intestine—can arise.

More than 95% of all polyps are benign, yet it is imperative that they be removed immediately, for one simple reason: most colorectal cancers begin as polyps. Removing them while they are benign eliminates the possibility of malignancy.

Today polyps can even be discovered before they start to bleed, which they do in only 30% to 50% of all cases. The American Cancer Society recommends an annual Hemoccult stool test for everyone over 40. If such blood loss is discovered, sigmoidoscopy with barium enema, or colonoscopy is warranted.

About one third of all polyps lie within the 2-foot reach of the sigmoidoscope, and can be removed under local anesthesia without a surgical incision. If the source of bleeding is not within this area, then the remainder of the intestine is explored with either a carefully performed barium enema or colonoscopy. In addition, because the presence of polyps in the lower intestine increases by tenfold the chance that there are additional ones farther up, it is prudent to follow sigmoidoscopy with colonoscopy on an annual basis.

All polyps should be removed entirely and examined by a pathologist. In the relatively rare case—less than 5%—of malignancy, the surgical excision of an appropriate length of intestine prevents its spread.

It may also help to realize that early diagnosis and treatment of colorectal polyps allows us to practice preventive medicine in its purest form: removal represents cure. The incidence of a disease that claims 100,000 lives every year can be drastically reduced with readily available home tests, prompt medical consultations, accurate diagnostic tests, and effective therapy.

Colorectal cancer predominantly occurs in the older age groups and represents a major health problem for the geriatric patient. Early detection is vital and should be aimed at the proper patient population. This refers to the individual over 40, women with a history of breast and genital neoplasia, and people with a positive family history, previous polyps, and previous inflammatory bowel disease. Surgical resection remains the major treatment modality for this cancer. Age is not a contraindication to surgery and is less of a factor than physiologic status. Survival appears to be related to the stage of the neoplasm, and not to the age of the patient. The distribution of the lesion is changing, with movement of the cancer from the left to the right colon.

About 5% to 10% of the population over 40 will have one or more adenomas, and the risk rises with increasing age. It usually takes 10 to 15 years for adenomas to develop into carcinomas.

Previously mentioned groups (ie, longstanding inflammatory bowel disease, etc) are definitely at high risk for cancer transformation. More controversial is the risk of right colon neoplasia after cholecystectomy. A study from Sweden demonstrated a higher incidence of colonic cancer in both sexes, especially females, in a group of patients between ages 70 and 75 whose gallbladders had been previously removed. A possible mechanism is an alteration in the types and quantity of bile acids bathing the colon.

Clinical presentation of colon cancer differs between the elderly patient and the middle-aged patient. Anorexia, constipation, and findings correlating with anemia are more common in the geriatric population. One should never make a new diagnosis of irritable bowel syndrome beyond the age of 40 without thorough evaluation to exclude an organic intestinal disease.

Evaluation consists of a sigmoidoscopy and either barium enema or colonoscopy. The entire colon must be visualized. The choice of procedures is based on the patient's condition and physician capabilities. Preoperative serum carcinogenic embryonic antigen and radiographic visualization of the liver are done. If there is metastatic disease, one should operate only if there is bowel obstruction or massive hemorrhage. The only method of curative treatment is surgical extirpation. Adjuvant radiotherapy is reserved for rectal cancers.

Because the outcome of therapy of colorectal cancer depends on the stage of diagnosis, careful population screening is essential. In this way colon cancer can be diagnosed at an earlier stage. The entire geriatric population requires stool Hemoccults, digital rectal examinations, and sigmoidoscopy. Whether one uses flexible or rigid sigmoidoscopy depends on the local expertise. If any of these examinations is positive, full colon evaluation is warranted.

Diverticular disease is often recognized as a cause of rectal bleeding and constipation. It appears to represent an aging process of the colon. Most cases are asymptomatic, although they can be a source of bleeding, perforation, obstruction, and inflammation (diverticulitis, etc). Parks reported the presence of diverticuli in 60% of the population over 60 years old. The rectum is always spared, and the sigmoid colon is invariably involved. Epidemiologic studies argue for a major dietary role in the cause of diverticular disease. The disease is uncommon in areas of the world in which there is high fiber intake throughout life.

The complications of diverticular disease are inflammatory and hemorrhagic in nature. If a diverticulum becomes plugged by feces or a foreign body, pus builds up in a diverticular sac and abscess formation and rupture can ensue.

Diverticulitis can present with abdominal colicky pain and a mass, fever, alteration of bowel habits, and, less often, free perforation or vesical, small bowel, or vaginal fistulization. Large- and small-bowel obstruction can occur. Uncomplicated diverticulitis can be managed during the acute phase with intravenous antibiotics, antispasmodics, and low-fiber diet. Surgery is necessary if fistula, obstruction, or free perforation is present.

The other major category of complications is rectal hemorrhage. This occurs in 15% of patients and can be massive. Most bleeding is self-limited and does not require surgery. If bleeding does not cease, either subtotal colectomy or interventional angiography is required. One must exclude bleeding angiodysplasias, cancer, polyps, and other potential colonic lesions. This is done with colonoscopy, nuclear bleeding scans, and, possibly, angiography.

A major colonic disease presenting with abdominal pain and rectal bleeding is acute mesenteric ischemic bowel disease. It is most common in the elderly. Its incidence is rising, and the most common cause is low mesenteric blood flow rather than thrombosis or embolus.

The patient's complaints of severe abdominal pain associated with loose, bloody bowel movements are out of proportion to the minimal physical findings. However, if the ischemic event is not diagnosed and no intervention transpires, gangrene and shock ensue. Many cases have atypical signs and symptoms, and a high index of suspicion must be kept.

Pending definitive diagnosis and treatment, intravenous fluid and antibiotics should be instituted. A flat plate, CBC, serum amylase, lipase, and other routine laboratory studies should be obtained. Once basic resuscitation of the patient is performed, exploratory laparotomy should be performed. This offers the only proven chance of success. The role of angiographic pharmacologic intervention is controversial.

More common is the abdominal equivalent of angina pectoris. This represents chronic arterial obstruction or insufficiency with abdominal pain in response to a meal. The patient can present with malabsorption and fear of eating (sitophagia), with weight loss and postprandial abdominal pain. One must exclude peptic ulcer disease, upper gastrointestinal cancer, gallstones, esophageal pain, and myocardial or pulmonary sources of pain. Because there are no proven pharmacologic means of ameliorating the problem, vascular reconstructive surgery may be warranted.

A recent development is the recognition of colonic angiodysplasia as a major cause of rectal bleeding over the age of 50. Its recognition parallels the advent of colonoscopy. Many cases of rectal hemorrhage attributed to diverticular disease are, in reality, secondary to bleeding right colonic angiodysplasias. It can occur at any age and is much more common with increasing age, valvular heart disease, and uremia. These ectasias are not seen on barium radiographs, not felt or seen by a surgeon, and only recognized by endoscopy or angiography. The cause of these lesions is unknown. They can massively bleed, or be a source of occult blood loss. They have also been described in the upper gastrointestinal tract. They can be treated by endoscopic coagulation, laser, or, in cases of massive hemorrhage with many telangiectasias, right hemicolectomy. Recently estrogen therapy has been tried.

Rectal bleeding can be massive or in small quantity. Often, because of age, the patient has to be hospitalized. After resuscitation, CBC, coagulation parameters, and a careful history should be obtained to record all medications ingested, previous medical problems, and the type of bleeding. Melanotic stools usually indicate an upper gastrointestinal source proximal to the ligament of Treitz. This should be investigated by upper gastrointestinal endoscopy. If there is maroon or bright red blood, sigmoidoscopy is performed. If the bleeding is not massive and no obvious source is seen on sigmoidoscopy, then colonoscopy is done. In more active hemorrhage the scheme shown in Figure 7-1 is suggested.

It is my impression that andiodysplasias, diverticuli, colitis, polyps, and cancer are the leading causes of rectal bleeding over the age of 60. Most bleeding is self-limited and does not require surgery. If bleeding does not cease and interventional endoscopy or angiography has failed, then a subtotal colectomy for diverticular bleeding or a right hemicolectomy for angiodysplasia is appropriate.

As the elderly population rises and the incidence of Crohn's disease rises, the pattern of the disease in the elderly must be recognized. It is uncommon but not rare. Goligher reports an 8% incidence of a large series of intestinal disorders. Distal colonic disease, especially in areas of diverticular involvement, seems to characterize the elderly patient with Crohn's disease. Those patients uncommonly require surgery as opposed to ileal involvement in the younger group. One major difficulty in my experience is to separate the patient with active granulomatous colitis from one with a concomitant diverticular abscess. Steroids are often required in the former state and contraindicated in the latter. Rarely colon cancer

---

NUCLEAR BLEEDING SCAN

(+) → Angiogram

(−) → Colonoscopy
When less bleeding

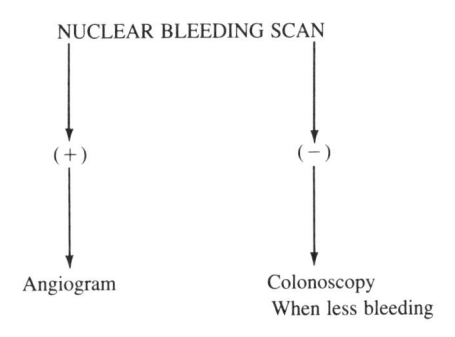

Figure 7-1 Therapy either by way of angiogram, with colonoscope, or supportive, depending on pathology.

can mimic colonic granulomatous (Crohn's) disease. There is a much better prognosis in the elderly patient with Crohn's disease compared with that of the younger, and this variant is a less aggressive form of the disease.

Crohn's disease is becoming more prevalent in the elderly. New onset can occur in the seventh and eighth decades. Differentiation must be made between diverticulitis, ulcerative colitis, cancer, infection, and ischemic bowel disease. The older patient with Crohn's disease has less ileal involvement and tends to have more left-sided disease. All the above pathologic conditions can present with diarrhea, rectal bleeding, pain, an abdominal mass, and fistulae. One should think of Crohn's disease (granulomatous ileocolitis) when perineal involvement is noted and vaginal or vesical fistulae are present, or if there are extraintestinal manifestations such as finger clubbing, pyoderma gangrenosum, erythema nodosum, gallstones or kidney stones, uveitis, sacroiliitis, and arthritis. Certain radiologic and endoscopic findings are highly suggestive, and endoscopic intestinal biopsies are often diagnostic.

Although most patients' expected survival is normal, some studies suggest a higher death rate. These are related to small- or large-bowel cancer development, chronic steroid usage with its complications, secondary amyloid, and bowel perforation. Cause is unknown, and therapy is identical to that in the young. This includes the use of an elemental diet or total parenteral nutrition during an acute exacerbation of the disease, sulfasalazine or metronidazole for colonic disease, steroids for ileal involvement and locally for anorectal disease, and immunosuppressants if the aforementioned medications fail and surgery is contemplated. Although there is a significant recurrence rate, surgery should not be withheld when indicated.

Just as Crohn's disease may present late in life, so may ulcerative colitis. There appears to be a bimodal occurrence (20 to 30 years and 60 to 70 years). The presentation in young and old is similar. There are occasional acute fulminant cases. One of the major concerns is a geriatric patient who has had longstanding chronic ulcerative colitis. There is a known risk of dysplasia and colon cancer in any individual who has had ulcerative colitis more than 7 years. The risk increases with each subsequent decade of the disease by about 20% per decade. This applies to disease that at least involves the left colon and does not appear to be related to activity of disease. This entire group requires surveillance that includes either yearly colonoscopy with biopsies or sigmoidoscopy with barium enema. I favor the former. In evaluating a new patient with possible ulcerative colitis, cultures and toxin assays must be obtained to exclude infectious etiology and antibiotic-associated colitis, including pseudomembranous colitis (*Clostridium difficile* toxin). Medical and surgical management is identical at all ages.

NUTRITION

Older individuals' nutritional needs are similar to those of younger people when healthy. A major issue is whether the elderly are, in fact, ingesting the required nutrients. Many factors decrease the ability to eat. These include oropharyngeal disorders, cancer, ability to obtain food, restricted food selection in institutions. A careful, thorough dietary history should be included in any geriatric medical evaluation. This should be corroborated by a physical examination and laboratory evaluation. Table 7-1 indicates the essential measurements. Abnormalities must not be corrected without searching for the cause. Iron deficiency is seldom dietary, and a source of gastrointestinal blood loss must be located. Fat-soluble vitamin deficiency is due to fat malabsorption and requires a small-bowel, hepatic, and pancreatic evaluation. The fat-soluble vitamins are A, D, E, and K.

Major causes of death in the elderly include cardiovascular disease, stroke, and cancer. The role of diet in these pathogeneses is controversial. However, recommending moderate fiber with bulk and lower intake of saturated fats appears prudent. One must individualize these diets to the patient's activity level, weight, and gastrointestinal tract status.

Nutrition in disease and health is receiving increasing attention. Much is unknown about the role of dietary management in major gastrointestinal illnesses. Caloric, vitamin, and trace element requirements change in the elderly, as does the need for fiber. The gut is the site of digestion and absorption of nutrients. Diseases that affect any portion of the gastrointestinal tract can be expected to alter the nutritional requirements of any patient.

Some gut disorders can be ameliorated by specific nutritional recommendations. (See Table 7-2.) These include (a) use of a high-fiber diet in nonmechanical constipation; (b) supplemented liquid or elemental diets in severe inflammatory bowel disease, acute gastroenteritis, and advanced neoplasia; (c) use of medium chain triglycerides for pancreatic and small-bowel fat malabsorption syndrome; (d) lactose exclusion in lactase deficiency or after an acute small-bowel enteritis; (e) avoidance diets in food allergies or in gluten-enteropathy; and (f) low-protein diets in advanced liver disease.

Nutritional requirements in the geriatric population are linked to subtle changes in body composition that occur with aging. There is an increase in body fat, constant body weight, and diminution of lean body mass (protein). Physical activity decreases with age, as does the basal metabolic rate. (See Figure 7-2.)

Of particular interest is the role of calcium intake in preventing osteoporosis. It is known that calcium absorption declines with age. The minimum intake should be increased to 1,000 mg. Hormonal supplementation may be required.

Brief mention will be made of correction of severe malnutrition. The same principles apply in the young and the elderly. Ideally the enteron should be used; if

---

Table 7-1 Laboratory Measurements to Assess Nutritional Status

Weight	Total lymphocyte count	TIBC
Height	Serum albumin	Transferrin level
	Serum ferritin	Hemoglobin

Table 7-2 Current Recommended Daily Intake for Elderly People in the United Kingdom (1979)

	Men		Women	
	65-74	75	55-74	75
Energy (kcal)	2400	2150	1900	1680
(MJ)	10.0	9.10	8.0	7.0
Protein (g)	60	54	47	42
Thiamine (mg)	1.0	0.9	0.8	0.7
Riboflavin (mg)	1.6	1.6	1.3	1.3
Nicotinic acid equivalent (mg)	18	18	15	15
Total folate (μg)	300	300	300	300
Ascorbic acid (mg)	30	30	30	30
Vitamin A (retinol equivalent)	750	750	750	750
Vitamin D (cholecalciferol)	*	*	*	*
Calcium (mg)	500	500	500	500
Iron (mg)	10	10	10	10

*Adults sufficiently exposed to sunlight generally need no dietary sources of vitamin D. However, adults with inadequate exposure to sunlight (eg, housebound elderly) may need a supplement of 10 μg daily.

Source: *Report on Health and Social Subjects,* No 15, pp 6–7, Department of Health and Human Services, 1979.

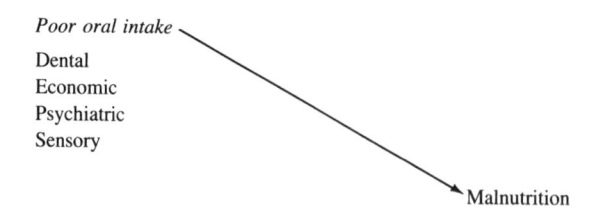

Poor oral intake
Dental
Economic
Psychiatric
Sensory

→ Malnutrition

Malabsorption
Sprue
Lactose intolerance
Bacterial overgrowth
Blind loop
Postgastrectomy
Drugs
Alcohol
Liver-pancreatic disease

Figure 7-2 Pathways Leading to Malnutrition

not feasible, then parenteral routes are utilized. Vitamin and mineral (trace element) supplements are necessary.

The role of diet in colonic carcinoma appears to be important. High cholesterol intake and low fiber are probably potentially carcinogenic. This combination results in prolonged intestinal transit time and increased contact exposure to potential carcinogens.

Serum cholesterol seems to rise with age. However, it appears that dietary manipulation must occur earlier in life to decrease cardiovascular morbidity and mortality. Low-fat diets in the elderly are seldom protective. Salt restriction is useful with significant hypertension and congestive heart failure.

One of the major problems in geriatric medicine is the multitude of medicines a person ingests. There are multiple drug–food interactions. The metabolism and elimination of drugs change with age and can affect the nutritional state of the elderly. Furthermore some medicines cause anorexia, nausea, vomiting, and, consequently, malnutrition. Others affect vitamin absorption and production. Examples include laxatives—vitamin antagonism; antibiotics—vitamin K synthesis; luminal binders (eg, cholestyramine, sucralfate)—malabsorption of nutrients and endogenous bile acids; antacids—phosphate depletion; and steroids—calcium inhibition. The physician who prescribes for the elderly must give the minimum medication in proper dosage for age and body mass.

Nutritional status appears to have a profound effect on susceptibility to infectious disease and immunologic response. Influenza, pneumonia, urosepsis, and herpetic disease often attack malnourished elderly individuals and are a significant cause of morbidity and mortality. Infection itself increases body requirements by causing increased catabolism of protein mass, and deficiency of trace elements such as zinc, phosphorus, and magnesium. The malnourished marginal geriatric patient has altered immune function. Normal aging appears to decrease the immune response. Leukocyte and cilia function may be diminished. Immunoglobulin deficiency has been noted with aging. Overall immune incompetence and malnutrition predispose to overwhelming infection and possibly neoplasia and autoimmune diseases.

Much of the population over 65 are in different types of institutions. Even the noninstitutionalized often have physical impairments. They all are at high risk for nutritional deficits. By the year 2000 the elderly population may exceed 35 million. Therefore, the problem of providing appropriate care and nutrition for these elderly will increase.

REFERENCES AND SUGGESTED READINGS

Bader TF. Colorectal cancer in patients older than 75 years of age. *Dis Colon Rectum* 1986;29:728–732.

Bedford PD, Wollner L. Occult intestinal bleeding as a cause of anemia in elderly people. *Lancet* 1958;1:114.

Boley SF, Sammartano R, et al. On the nature and etiology of vascular ectasias of the colon. *Gastroenterology* 1977;72:650–660.

Brocklehurst JC. Colonic disease in the elderly. *Clin Gastroenterol* 1985;14:725–744.

Burkitt DP, Walker A, Painter NS. Effect of dietary fiber on stools and the transit time and its role in the causation of disease. *Lancet* 1972;3:1408.

Cooke WT, Mallass E, Prior P, et al. Crohn's disease—course, treatment and long term prognosis. *Q J Med* 1980;49:363–384.

Department of Health and Human Services. Recommended daily amount of food energy and nutrients for groups of people in the United Kingdom. Report on Health and Social Subjects. No 15, 1979, pp 6–7.

Evans JG, Acheson ED. An epidemiological study of ulcerative colitis and regional enteritis in the Oxford area. *Gut* 1965;6:311–324.

Geokas MC, Conteas CN, Majumdar APN. The aging gastrointestinal tract, liver, and pancreas. *Clin Geriatr Med* 1985;1:177–198.

Lightdale CJ, Winawer SJ. Polyps and tumors of the large intestine, in Hellemans J, VanTrappen G (eds): *Gastrointestinal Tract Disorders in the Elderly*. Edinburgh, Churchill Livingstone, 1984, pp 174–184.

Milne JS, Williamson J. Bowel habit in older people. *Gerontol Clin* 1972;14:55–60.

Moore-Gillon V. Constipation: What does the patient mean? *J R Soc Med* 1984;77:108–110.

Sherlock P, Winawer SJ. Are there markers for the risk of colorectal cancer? *N Engl J Med* 1984;311:118–119.

Slack J, Noble N, Meade TW, et al. Lipid and lipoprotein concentrations in 1604 men and women in working populations in north west London. *Br Med J* 1977;2:353–356.

Spitz MR, Russell NC, et al. Questionable relationship between cholecystectomy and colon cancer. *J Surg Oncol* 1985;30:6–9.

Chapter 8

Infectious Diseases of the Aged

Leon G. Smith, Leon G. Smith, Jr., and Paul R. Summers

INTRODUCTION

Gynecological infectious diseases of the aged is a new field of scientific study only fully appreciated as our population grows older. The purpose of this chapter is to review all the known data on host defenses; changing vaginal flora; the changing pattern of infections in the vagina, vulva and uterus as compared to younger women; and proper use of antimicrobial therapy in the aged.

Under ideal conditions the human species can live up to 115 years of age, in comparison with other mammals, such as elephants (70 years), horses (46 years), cats (28 years), and dogs (20 years).[1] Shock's[2] promising work confirms folklore that aging is produced by physiological deterioration. The female genital organ system is also altered by one's life style, especially declining sexual activity. With age, the major body composition change is muscle mass. Lean body mass declines with age primarily because of loss of muscle mass,[3,4] whereby atrophy rather than hypoplasia occurs. Secondary to estrogen loss, bone mass declines with age, especially after menopause.[5] A life style of nutrition, physical activity, and hormonal replacement can modify this bone mass loss.[6] Fat mass usually increases until age 65 and then decreases considerably thereafter.[7] In summary, these physiological changes, including decreased endocrine activity, produce the milieus for age-associated diseases of the female genital tract.[8] To illustrate these age-specific diseases, we shall compare the effects of premenopause and postmenopause on various infectious diseases, antimicrobial usage, and host factors.

HOST DEFENSE

The elderly person gradually develops a number of host defense abnormalities. A delayed immune response has been demonstrated by reduced skin reactivity to dinitrochlorobenzene, *Monilia*, tuberculin, mumps, and *Trichophyton*.[9-11] Lymphocyte mitogen stimulation also decreases with aging. Phair and colleagues[12,13] also reported decreased opsonization of *Escherichia coli* and *Staphylococcus aureus* in some people over age 70.[14] The data on B cell deficiencies of humoral antibody in the aged are less clear. Three explanations of a diminished immune response are given: (1) Trace metal and vitamin deficiencies often cited in the elderly patient may reduce the cell-mediated response. (2) Blockage and subsequent stagnation of bodily fluids (eg, bladder dysfunction) will lead to colonization of organisms. (3) Nosocomial infections with resistant organisms can potentially overwhelm an otherwise normal immune system.

VAGINAL FLORA

The normal vaginal flora changes gradually with age owing to numerous factors, such as pH elevation; decreased estrogen, progesterone, and glycogen; atrophied cells; and other well-understood factors.[15] In general, the postmenopausal vagina has more Gram-positive bacteria, including *S aureus*, *Staphylococcus epidermidis*, and various streptococcal species, especially groups B, C, D, and G, than Gram-negative bacteria. *E coli*, *Proteus mirabilis*, *Proteus morgani*, *Klebsiella* sp, and *Citrobacter* sp. *Candida albicans* increases from 9.7% to 16.7% with age. The anaerobic bacterial density, which includes all *Bacteroides* sp, increases with age. Thus more potential pathogens are observed in the postmenopausal woman.

GARDNERELLA VAGINALIS, TRICHOMONAS, AND OTHER VAGINITIS

Gardnerella vaginalis infection is primarily a disease of the sexually active younger woman. However, a study from England revealed that women aged 56 to 75 had a 7% incidence by culture, whereas those aged 76 to 86 had a 15% rate.[16,17] *G vaginalis* not only can colonize the elderly vagina, but also can be associated with symptomatic vaginitis. There was no correlation between sexual practices and previous infections. *Trichomonas vaginalis* was much rarer in the elderly. Anaerobe and *C albicans* vaginal colonization increases markedly with aging but rarely produces symptoms. Elderly diabetic patients frequently acquire symptomatic candidal vaginitis. Pseudohyphae should be seen on a KOH smear, and cultures may be appropriate in recurrent cases.

A small enterovaginal fistula that develops as a complication of colitis or after pelvic surgery or irradiation may initially be confused with vaginitis. Such patients generally complain of vaginal discharge, which the gynecologist may at first erroneously attribute to atrophic vaginitis. The fistula may be difficult to identify on pelvic examination but may be demonstrated by barium enema or endoscopy. Microbiological findings of many coliform bacteria in the vaginal discharge would lead to the suspicion of an enterovaginal fistula.

Vulvitis resulting from estrogen deficiency may also be confused with vaginitis. It is important to ask the patient to identify the site of irritation and to specify her symptoms. It is also important to remember to biopsy any white or ulcerated vulvar lesion to exclude neoplasm. For atrophic conditions of the vulva, either a steroid cream or a testosterone cream may be helpful. Estrogen cream reverses vaginal atrophy but does not relieve symptoms of vulvar atrophy. Many steroid creams contain paraben preservatives, which can be highly irritating and should be avoided in the postmenopausal patient with atrophic vulvar tissues.

Urinary incontinence in the elderly woman may result in vaginal or vulvar symptoms that are similar to typical vulvitis or vaginitis. Once the mediating factor of excessive local moisture is eliminated, such symptoms may be expected to resolve.

GONOCOCCAL INFECTION

Disseminated, or even local, genital gonorrhea is not a well-appreciated entity in the elderly. This venereal disease occurs, as is expected, in people in their 20s. Based on the epidemiology of Geelhoed-Duyvestijn and colleagues'[18] cases, it would appear that a postmenopausal woman may carry the gonococcus for an extraordinarily long period after sexual contact. Harboring of gonococcus may occur even before local or systemic manifestations of arthritis, tenosynovitis, and skin lesions develop. None of these patients had an underlying disease or immunological defects.[18] With increasing promiscuous sexual activity by our elderly population, we can expect to see more of this sexually transmitted disease.

The gonococcus is generally restricted to endocervical columnar epithelium. Following the process of squamous metaplasia, generally only atrophic squamous epithelium would be expected on the typical postmenopausal cervix. Experience from the pediatric population has shown that atrophic vaginal and vulvar squamous epithelium is susceptible to gonococcal colonization, especially if these tissues are moist. Thus what would typically present as an asymptomatic endocervical gonococcal infection in the reproductive years may present as a true symptomatic vulvovaginitis in some patients with atrophic tissues.

BACTERIOLOGIC SEPSIS FROM INAPPARENT ATROPHIED GYNECOLOGIC SITE

Gynecologic sepsis (inapparent) as a cause of covert infection in the elderly is a recently appreciated phenomenon called to our attention by Horan and coworkers.[19] This English group described three women over 80 years of age with sepsis, which was detected only after a careful bimanual examination of the atrophied uteri with profuse pus from the vagina containing *E coli* and *Clostridium welchii*. Primary endometritis is an unusual infection in the reproductive years, presumably owing to many factors, including pH, estrogen stimulation, and cyclic shedding of the endometrium. The absence of pyrexia and leukocytosis in old age can make this diagnosis difficult. In essence, a careful pelvic examination must be done based on one's clinical acumen, namely, whenever there is a change from the status quo to a deteriorating status. For example, one of the patients in Horan's series appeared to have developed a stroke but actually had sepsis. She recovered with intravenous antibiotic therapy.

POSTMENOPAUSAL TUBO-OVARIAN ABSCESS

Postmenopausal tubo-ovarian abscess (TOA) is generally perceived as a disease of women in their childbearing years. Over a 5-year period, on a busy city hospital service, Heaton and Ledger[20] reported 12 postmenopausal women with TOA. They ranged in age from 46 to 71 years. Nine patients had a previous history of salpingitis. Three patients had a history of previous adnexal surgery without salpingitis.

Uterine bleeding was the most prominent symptom; pain, fever, and change in bowel habits were less prominent. A pelvic mass was the major consistent physical finding. Only 50% were TOA in the preoperative differential. Bilateral TOA were present in more than 60% of the cases. *E coli*, *Klebsiella*, *Aerobacter*, and *Pseudomonas* sp were the most common pathogens. *Actinomyces* should be suspected if the TOA is unilateral, especially in the ovulating premenopausal patient after bowel surgery. *Bacteroides* sp was present in the blood of two patients and was probably present in the abscess as well, even though *Bacteroides* sp (anaerobes) were not cultured.

In other, older series (approximately 11 centers, including Charity Hospital in New Orleans, which had the largest series of TOA)[21] ruptured TOA without surgical intervention has a mortality rate approaching 100%, especially in older patients. The use of modern antibiotics, especially those effective against anaerobes, currently results in a somewhat lower mortality rate after rupture of a TOA.

The antibiotics of choice must cover *S aureus*, coliforms, and anaerobes. Clindamycin and gentamicin remain the most commonly used, but newer combinations, or even single drugs, may prove equally effective and less nephrotoxic. Some authorities would recommend including either clindamycin or metronidazole in the regimen if an abscess is present because of evidence of greater activity of these agents on abscess fluid in comparison with penicillin, cephalosporins, or aminoglycosides.[22]

If the patient's symptoms resolve on antibiotic therapy, and surgery is not required, it is important to follow the patient's pelvic examination to exclude persistence of an adnexal mass. Rarely salpingitis may be the presenting finding in a patient with an ovarian or tubal malignancy. Any persistent pelvic mass in this setting necessitates exploratory surgery.

PYOMYOMA

Leiomyomas seldom undergo suppuration, and pyomyoma is extremely rare.[23,24] Only 75 cases have been reported. Although acute inflammation, chronic inflammation, and calcification develop in leiomyomas, suppurative complication develops in cysts, tuberculation, obstructed cervix, and liquefaction of tumor are major predisposing features. These findings are more commonly seen in subserosal leiomyomas, whereby an accompanying symptom is a large accumulation of fluid with associated abdominal pain. Although bacteremia is often absent, fever is usually present because of various pathogens, such as *S aureus*, coliform bacilli, *Clostridium perfringens*, and various species of streptococci. The incidence of pyomyoma rises in pregnancy and the postmenopausal period, when degeneration is more likely to develop. In the postmenopausal woman a ruptured viscera, especially diverticulitis, is an important, predisposing factor.

PESSARY INFECTION

Elderly patients with medical problems that prohibit operations for stress incontinence or massive procidentia will need a Gellhorn or disk-type plastic vaginal pessary.[25] Like intrauterine devices in the young, and other foreign bodies, they must be periodically checked and, with pessaries, must be removed and cleaned monthly. Vaginal ulceration at pressure sites in the vagina is not an uncommon finding. *S aureus*, *S epidermidis*, and other bacteria can attach to the pessary surface and be a source of bacteremia. If bacteria or local purulence should be present, removal of the pessary is imperative.

UNUSUAL INFECTIONS OF THE FEMALE GENITAL TRACT

Xanthogranulomatous pseudotumors, malakoplakia, and Whipple's disease can produce vaginal lesions that look and feel like tumors.[26] Only with proper electron microscopy, cultures, and staining are these conditions detectable. All of these conditions are caused by low-grade, chronic bacterial infections that respond to proper antibiotic therapy. These rare entities should be looked for if the biopsy has suggestive eosinophilic cytoplasmic granules on hematoxylin and eosin stains. These entities are thought to be due to incomplete clearance of bacteria by phagocytosis.

GENITAL ELEPHANTIASIS (LYMPHEDEMA)

In the United States elephantiasis of the male and female genitalia is extremely rare.[27,28] Except for selected pockets of filariasis, most lymphedema of the vulva is secondary to carcinoma, chronic streptococcal disease, tuberculosis, sarcoidosis, lymphoma, chronic impetigo, and chronic suppurative hidradenitis. Lymphogranuloma venereum also may eventually result in vulvar edema.

The workup of genital lymphedema must include all of the above as well as filariasis serology, streptozyme, biopsy, and lymphangiography studies. Repeat biopsies are often needed, especially in cases of carcinoma.

POSTMENOPAUSAL PELVIC TUBERCULOSIS

Postmenopausal pelvic tuberculosis is a rare entity in the United States and yet should always be searched for in patients with postmenopausal bleeding.[29] The incidence of pulmonary tuberculosis has declined considerably, but the incidence of extrapulmonary tuberculosis remains unchanged. Extrapulmonary tuberculosis rarely has an active pulmonary focus, which is generally not appreciated. Fifty percent of pelvic tuberculosis patients will have classic tuberculosis in the endometrial scrapings. On exploration the others will have a positive biopsy and culture in other pelvic organs. The tuberculin skin test is usually positive but can be negative, especially if peritonitis is present. Table 8-1 compares premenopausal and postmenopausal tuberculous symptoms.

Pelvic tuberculosis responds readily to isoniazid and rifampin therapy. Too often the diagnosis is made *after* hysterectomy or other surgery, rather than before surgery. If tuberculosis is diagnosed and treated early enough, surgery can be avoided. If after 6 months of therapy the symptoms still prevail, then surgery would be instituted. Towers, on the other hand, favors extensive ablation for those beyond the childbearing age, "since there is no need to conserve these organs."[29]

Table 8-1 Comparison of Symptoms in Premenopausal and Postmenopausal Tuberculous Endometritis

Premenopausal	Postmenopausal
Infertility	Majority of patients have had children
Menstrual disturbance not significant	Postmenopausal bleeding is significant
Amenorrhea may rarely precede discovery of disease	Amenorrhea associated with menopause
Tubes almost always involved and can frequently be palpated	Tubes not always palpable; may be involved
Onset early in life, usually in puberty	Onset usually immediately before or after climacteric
Pelvic disease limited to tuberculous process	Other lesions besides tuberculosis frequently present

Source: Reprinted with permission from *American Journal of Obstetrics and Gynecology* (1972;112[5]:681–687), Copyright © 1972, The CV Mosby Company.

PRESSURE ULCERS

Pressure ulcers in the elderly, including of the female genital tract, can develop in up to 7% of those hospitalized and in 20% of nursing home patients.[30] Up to 3 million persons have these ulcers at any one moment. Recent data demonstrate that these ulcers can be prevented if pressure can be reduced below 30 mm. Stage I and stage II lesions of blanching or hyperemia can be treated by choosing the proper low-pressure mattress. Stage III and stage IV eschar and ulcer formation require aggressive infectious and surgical control. Ulcers are always more extensive than they appear. Local iodides are contraindicated, since they are toxic to tissue. Hydrogen peroxide used as an irrigant may be absorbed systemically, resulting in life-threatening oxygen embolism.[31] Pressure saline irrigation helps to free the tissue of necrotic material and transiently lowers the bacteria count.

GENITAL FISTULAS

Genital fistulas in the elderly female that involve the vagina or vulva must be taken seriously. Fistula formation often occurs in previously diagnosed chronic illnesses. Proper studies must be taken to trace the fistula to the point of origin: carcinoma of bowel or bladder, diverticulitis, Crohn's disease, local carcinoma burrowing deeply, foreign bodies, or decubitus ulcers.[32–36] Such fistulas should be carefully studied. Often genital fistulas appear like chronic suppurative adenitis or unusual ecthyma lesions. A careful bowel study, biopsy, and fistulography will provide the proper diagnosis of these lesions.

MYIASIS IN THE GENITAL TRACT

There is evidence of myiasis in the ordinary house fly. Larvae are laid accidentally and hatch. Maggots in the vagina is thereby increasing in nursing homes.[37–39] Pneumaturia may be the first sign of such larval activity. Carcinoma may be present, but usually the patient is a victim simply because of immobilization and poor hygiene. Myiasis is most commonly seen in tropical climates, and travelers to and from these areas are more susceptible. The warble fly and the botfly produce a large boil-like lesion. *Dermatobia hominis* is seen only in states near Mexico and in South America. It produces an irregular, circular 1-mm lesion that can be necrotoxic, such as that caused by the *Loxosceles* spider bite. Most often *D hominis* looks like molluscum contagiosum, herpes simplex, streptococcal cellulitis, larva migrans, and mite infestation.

The most important aspect of maggot control is fly control. Maggots are no longer used to clean up infected ulcers.

PYODERMA GANGRENOSUM OF THE GENITALIA

Female genitalia can be the site of pyoderma gangrenosum, especially in the elderly female.[40,41] Such ulcers are often misdiagnosed as infiltrating carcinoma or pressure ulcers. Pyoderma gangrenosum is often associated with systemic illness, toward which the workup should be directed. The lesion starts as a pustule posttrauma followed by progressive painful tissue destruction and blue ulceration with advancing erythema. Secondary satellite pustules can also be seen. Regional nodes do not usually become involved, however. Patients who require iodine therapy may have aggravated lesions. Associated diseases are inflammatory bowel diseases, biliary cirrhosis, diabetes mellitus, malignancies, myeloma, sarcoidosis, and thyroid and arthritic diseases. Steroid and immunosuppressive therapy is empirical and unpredictable.

Differential diagnoses are vasculitis, Sweet's disease (acute febrile neutrophilic dermatosis), dermatitis artefacta, malignancy, chronic fungal disease, and Meleney's synergistic gangrene.

INTERSTITIAL CYSTITIS WITH VAGINITIS

Interstitial cystitis is primarily a woman's disease characterized by disabling dysuria, frequency, and pelvic pain.[42–50] Although the peak incidence is from 30 to 50 years of age (most patients are postmenopausal), interstitial cystitis can occur in the elderly. This entity was first described by Hunner in 1915 as a bladder ulcer disease. Since then the disease has been expanded to include bladder ulcers or petechiae to normal mucosa. On biopsy there is a marked increase in plasma, especially mast cells. More than 20 mast cells per square millimeter of muscle tissue is 95% diagnostic-specific. Recently we have seen a small number of patients, some elderly, who had profound culture-negative, painful vaginitis, and who also had classic mast cells on bladder biopsy. The leukorrhea amount and cell content were highly variable but always unresponsive to therapy. The myriads of therapeutic medical and surgical approaches are unrewarding. Prozazan, to block the neurogenic fibers that cause pain, and dimethyl sulfoxide, instilled directly into the bladder, are the current favorite modes of therapy. Sodium cromoglycate has been effective in clinical trials.

ACTINOMYCOSIS OF THE PELVIC ORGANS

Actinomycosis of the pelvic organs can simulate a malignancy because of its firmness and slow growth.[51,52] Often the source of this anaerobe is a ruptured viscus, especially the appendix. Adherence to pelvic organs, oviducts, and bladder with compression symptoms are the main presentations. Only by biopsy and by culturing anaerobically with proper staining can this entity that responds to long-term penicillin be diagnosed. Pelvic actinomycosis in the premenopausal patient typically presents as an oophoritis, the corpus luteum acting as the initial site of infection at the time of ovulation. Thus the majority of cases of actinomycosis salpingo-oophoritis reported in the literature have been in premenopausal women.[53]

With advancing age the increased risk of bowel disease necessitating surgery increases the opportunity for pelvic peritoneal seeding with *Actinomyces* from the bowel flora. Any female who develops pelvic peritonitis after bowel surgery, or in association with colitis, should be suspected of having a possible pelvic *Actinomyces* infection.

PINWORMS

Pinworms are primarily a disease of younger school-age children. Elderly patients, on rare occasion in nursing homes with poor hygiene, can develop anal and vaginal pruritus, appendicitis, and localized peritonitis.[54] A search for the pinworms by anal cellophane tape smears can readily make the diagnosis.

VIRUS OF THE GENITAL TRACT

The following viruses have been demonstrated from the female genital tract: herpes simplex virus, molluscum contagiosum, Epstein-Barr virus, papovavirus, cytomegalovirus, and adenovirus.[55-59] All of these viruses tend to remain in the genital tract area forever after their primary infection in the young woman. Papillomavirus evidence toward carcinoma of the cervix is impressive. The other viruses may be tumorigenic, but their role is less clear. Special electronic microscopic techniques and DNA hybridization are needed to demonstrate the carrier state. Adenovirus can be associated with bladder symptoms and hematuria.

TOXIC SHOCK SYNDROME

Toxic shock syndrome (TSS) was first described by Todd in 1978, but on reviewing the old literature, similar syndromes were reported before World War I.[60-62] Although TSS was initially described in children, most reported cases were associated with the use of extra absorbent tampons during menstruation. Less appreciated is the postsurgical form of the disease, such as post hysterectomy or even minor surgery.

In the postmenopausal woman the incidence of Gram-positive colonization of the vagina increases considerably, but TSS in the elderly remains a rare event. The incidence of protective antibodies also increases with age, but TSS can still affect the elderly female, especially in a postoperative situation. Any surgery of the genital tract that is colonized by a TSS toxin-producing *S aureus* can produce a syndrome characterized from hours to days after surgery by hypotension, hectic fever, generalized erythematous rash, and, later, desquamation. At the operative site, such as vaginal hysterectomy, there is no pus, only clear fluid containing toxigenic *S aureus*.

Too often TSS is mistaken for pulmonary emboli, drug reaction, or Gram-negative sepsis. Rapid intervention with fluids and anti–*S aureus* drugs, and clearing of the operative site with vigorous washing will produce the highest salvage rate. Culture of the *S aureus*, which is tested for toxin production, confirms the diagnosis.

ACQUIRED IMMUNODEFICIENCY SYNDROME

The acquired immunodeficiency syndrome (AIDS), caused by HTLV III/HIV retrovirus, has produced many confusing female genital lesions that are new to physicians.[63-66] These vulvovaginal lesions are atypical manifestations of various pathogens, such as molluscum contagiosum virus, tuberculosis, typical and atypical mycobacterium avium intracellular (MAI), *Cryptococcus neoformans*, herpes simplex, and, more rarely, *Nocardia* sp. It is virtually impossible to diagnose any of these lesions without a biopsy, as these pathogens in an HIV-infected individual produce atypical lesions. Lesions that look like florid molluscum contagiosum, which is seen so often in AIDS patients, can be due to *C neoformans*. *Cryptococcus* lesions, which are typically firm, nodular lesions, can appear as clusters of vesicles simulating herpes simplex. Persistent ulcers that are resistant to local care can be due to *Hemophilus influenzae* type B or group B streptococci. Hence biopsies and proper viral, bacterial, and fungal cultures are in order. Because many of the lesions, such as tuberculosis, do not reveal typical caseation granuloma, proper staining acid-fast and special culturing for atypical tuberculosis are to be used.

The incidence of AIDS in postmenopausal women is much lower than in younger, sexually active women or in those who use intravenous drugs. Thus the diagnosis can be more difficult.

The majority of postmenopausal AIDS is acquired through blood transfusions. Any unusual skin lesion in the sexually active elderly should mandate an HIV antibody screening in addition to a proper biopsy. Also, oral candidiasis (thrush) in a previously healthy elderly woman should be considered an indication for HIV screening.

ANTIBIOTICS

There are currently a bewildering number of fine antibiotics, including third-generation cephalosporins, quinolone derivatives, and monobactams.[67-71]

The Cephalosporins

Three generations of cephalosporin antibiotics are particularly attractive in treating the elderly because they are relatively safe to use and show low incidence of allergic reactions even in penicillin-allergic individuals. (See Table 8-2.) Such antibiotics are not as nephrotoxic or ototoxic as aminoglycosides. They are bactericidal, and inhibit cell wall synthesis by binding to protein binding sites. Consequently they can be used as the only drug in life-threatening infections. The incidence of penicillin allergies is higher in the elderly. Cephalosporins, therefore, can be given under observation to these patients if the penicillin reaction is the delayed allergic reaction, as the majority are. If the penicillin reaction is the immediate type of anaphylaxis, then cephalosporins can be contraindicated.

Table 8-2 Parenteral Cephalosporins Currently Available for Clinical Use in the United States

Generic Name	Proprietary Name
First Generation	
Cephalothin sodium	Keflin, Seffin
Cephapirin sodium	Cefadyl
Cephradine	Anspor, Velosef
Cefazolin sodium	Ancef, Kefzol
Second Generation	
Cefamandole nafate	Mandol
Cefuroxime sodium	Zinacef
Cefonicid sodium	Monocid
Cefoxitin sodium	Mefoxin
Cefotetan disodium	Cefotan
Third Generation	
Cefotaxime sodium	Claforan
Moxalactam disodium	Moxam
Cefoperazone sodium	Cefobid
Ceftizoxime sodium	Cefizox
Ceftazidime	Fortaz, Tazicef, Tazidime
Ceftriaxone sodium	Rocephin

Sources: *Geriatrics* (1986;41[12]:51–55), Copyright © 1986, Modern Medicine Publications Inc; *Archives of Internal Medicine* (1982;142:1267–1268), Copyright © 1982, American Medical Association.

First Generation

The first-generation cephalosporins are most effective in eradicating *S aureus*, *Streptococcus pneumoniae*, and group A streptococci, but not enterococci. Methicillin-resistant *S aureus*, so often seen in nosocomial or nursing home infections, does not respond to any cephalosporin. *S epidermidis* infections tend to elude cephalosporin therapy. Cefazolin has the longest half-life of this group and therefore provides higher blood levels for up to eight hours. Hence cefazolin is the most commonly used drug for surgical prophylaxis.

Second Generation

Second-generation cephalosporins, especially cefoxitin, are valuable drugs in female pelvic infection. Also, prophylaxis can be used, since this compound covers the *Bacteroides* sp to a high degree (75% to 85% of all strains). Cefotetan offers no benefit over cefoxitin; it is an equivalent of cefoxitin, the most commonly used cephalosporin. The other second-generation cephalosporins have little to offer in treating pelvic infection in the elderly.

Third Generation

The third-generation cephalosporins are extremely valuable as a safer alternative to aminoglycosides. To simplify their use, cefotaxime, ceftizoxime, and ceftriaxone have basically the same spectrum and can be used interchangeably, based on cost factors. Ceftriaxone has the advantage of once-a-day dosing. This subgroup generally is effective against most Gram-negative bacteria (non-anaerobes), but not *Pseudomonas* sp. On the other hand, ceftazidime and cefoperazone are frequently effective against many *Pseudomonas* strains. The third-generation group is extremely valuable in combination with other antibiotics when the bacteriology abscess, peritonitis, and sepsis in pelvis is not known. Moxalactam, however, should not be used because of bleeding side effects.

Penicillin

Penicillin is used less and less in treating female genital tract infections, with the exception of gonorrhea. The newer penicillins, such as piperacillin and mezlocillin, have an extremely broad Gram-negative spectrum, including *Pseudomonas* sp. Combined with an aminoglycoside, they are the most widely used treatment for serious *Pseudomonas* infections. Ticarcillin, when combined with a beta lactamase antagonist, has similar coverage for moderate anti–Gram-positive bacteria, such as *S aureus*. These penicillins have reasonably good anti-anaerobic coverage for pelvic infections as well. In the elderly patient, however, these doses must be regulated by renal function.

Imipenem/Cilastatin Sodium (Primaxin)

This compound of a penem antibiotic (imipenem) and a kidney enzyme inhibitor (cilastatin) has the broadest range of bacterial coverage of any known antibiotic. Its use at this time in pelvic infection is for pelvic peritonitis, infection with an unknown organism, and organisms resistant to other antibiotics. This compound is effective against most anaerobes except *Clostridium difficile*, *S aureus*, most Gram-positive bacteria, and most Gram-negative bacteria, including most *Pseudomonas* sp. Because of renal clearance of the drug and seizure possibilities, the dosage in the elderly must be carefully monitored.

Quinolones

Quinolones will replace many of the antibiotics because of their wide Gram-negative and Gram-positive spectrum. They can be given orally with excellent absorption. Quinolones act by inhibiting the DNA gyrase enzyme, which is responsible for the necessary DNA coiling. Previous quinolones, such as nalidixic acid, quickly developed resistance. These new compounds resist such a change. Their exact role in elderly pelvic infection will soon be delineated. Norfloxacillin, ofloxacin, and ciprofloxacillin shall soon appear on the market.

REFERENCES

1. Kirkwood TBL, Holliday R: The evaluation of aging and longevity. *Proc R Soc Lond [Biol]* 1979;205:531–546.

2. Shock NW: Systems integration, in Finch CE, Hayflick L (eds): *Handbook of Biology of Aging*, ed 1. New York, Van Nostrand Reinhold Co, 1977, pp 639–665.

3. Forbes GB: The adult decline in lean body mass. *Hum Biol* 1976;48:161–173.

4. Tzankoff SP, Norris AH: Effect of muscle mass decrease on age-related BMR changes. *J Appl Physiol* 1977;43:1001–1006.

5. McCarter R: Effects of age on contraction of mammalian skeletal muscle, in Kaldor G, DiBattista WI (eds): *Aging in Muscle*. New York, Raven Press, 1978, pp 1-21.

6. Exton-Smith AN: Mineral metabolism, in Finch CE, Schneider EL (eds): *Handbook of the Biology of Aging*, ed 2. New York, Van Nostrand Reinhold Co, 1985, pp 511–539.

7. Masoro EJ: Metabolism, in Finch CE, Schneider EL (eds): *Handbook of the Biology of Aging*, ed 2. New York, Van Nostrand Reinhold Co, 1985, pp 540–563.

8. Masoro EJ: Biology of aging: A current knowledge. *Ann Intern Med* 1987;147:166–169.

9. Makinodian T, Perkin EH, Chen MG: Immunologic activity of the aged. *Adv Gerontol Res* 1971;3:171.

10. Mackay IR: Aging and immunological function in man. *Gerontologica* 1972;18:285.

11. Tice RR, Schneider EL, Kram D, et al: Cytokinetic analysis of the impaired proliferative response of peripheral lymphocytes from aged humans to phytohemagglutinin. *J Exp Med* 1979;149:1029.

12. Phair JP, Kauffman CA, Bjornson A: Investigation of host defense mechanisms in the aged as determinants of nosocomial colonization and pneumonia. *J Reticuloendothel Soc* 1978;23:397.

13. Phair JP, Kauffman CA, Bjornson A, et al: Host defenses in the aged: Evaluation of components of the inflammatory and immune responses. *J Infect Dis* 1978;138:67.

14. Louria DB, Lavenhar MA, Kaminski T, et al: Staphylococcal infections in aging mice. *J Gerontol* 1986;41:718–722.

15. Blum M, Elian I: The vaginal flora after natural or surgical menopause. *J Am Geriatric Soc* 1979;27:395–397.

16. Admad FJ, Sayed SM: Vaginal infection with *Gardnerella vaginalis*. *Practitioner* 1985;229:273–277.

17. Ratnam S, Fitzgerald BL: Semiquantitative culture of *Gardnerella vaginalis* in laboratory determination of nonspecific vaginitis. *J Clin Microbiol* 1983;18:344–347.

18. Geelhoed-Duyvestijn PH, van der Meer JW, Lichtendahl-Bernards AT, et al: Disseminated gonococcal infection in elderly patients. *Arch Intern Med* 1986;146:1739–1740.

19. Horan MA, Puxty JA, Fox RA: Gynecologic sepsis as a cause of covert infection in old age. *J Am Geriatric Soc* 1983;31:213–215.

20. Heaton F, Ledger WJ: Postmenopausal tuboovarian abscess. *Obstet Gynecol* 1976;47:90–94.

21. Collins CC, Nix FG, Cerha HT: Ruptured tubo-ovarian abscess. *Am J Obstet Gynecol* 1956;72:820–829.

22. Landers DV, Sweet RL: Current trends in the diagnosis and treatment of tuboovarian abscess. *Am J Obstet Gynecol* 1985;151(8):1098–1110.

23. Scully RE, Mark EJ, McNeely BU: Case records of Massachusetts General Hospital. *N Engl J Med* 1985;312:1505–1511.

24. Weiss G, Shenker L, Gorstein F: Suppurating myoma with spontaneous drainage through abdominal wall. *NY State J Med* 1976;76:572–573.

25. Huffman JW: Gynecologic disorders in the geriatric patient. *Geriatr Gynecol* 1982; 71(1):38–51.

26. Strate SM, Taylor WE, Forney JP: Xanthogranulomatous pseudotumor of the vagina: Evidence of a local response to an unusual bacterium (mucoid *Escherichia coli*). *Am Soc Clin Pathol* 1983;79(5):636–643.

27. Chernin E: Patrick Manson (1844-1922) and the transmission of filariasis. *Am J Trop Med Hyg* 1977;26:1065.

28. Von Lichtenberg F, Lehman JS: Parasitic disease of the genitourinary system, in Harrison JH (Ed): *Campbell's Urology*, ed 4. Philadelphia, WB Saunders Company, 1978, vol 1, p 597.

29. Schaefer G, Marcus RS, Kramer EE: Postmenopausal endometrial tuberculosis. *Am J Obstet Gynecol* 1972;112(5):681–687.

30. Medical News & Perspectives: Pressure ulcers preventable, say many clinicians. *JAMA* 1987;257(5):589–593.

31. Tsai SK, Lee TY, Mok MS: Gas embolism produced by hydrogen peroxide irrigation of an anal fistula during anesthesia. *Anesthesiology* 1985;63:316–317.

32. Talbot RW, et al: Vascular complications of I.B.D. *Mayo Clinic Proc* 1986;61:140–145.

33. Mir-Madjlessi SH, et al: Clinical course and evolution of E.N. and P.G. in chronic ulcerative colitis: A study of 42 patients. *Am J Gastroenterol* 1985;80:615–620.

34. Galan E: Therapy of pyoderma gangrenosum complicating ulcerative colitis: Successful therapy with methylprednisolone pulse therapy and dapsone. *Am J Gastroenterol* 1986;8:988–989.

35. Moll JM: Inflammatory bowel disease. *Clin Rheum Dis* 1985;2:87–106.

36. Greenstein AJ, et al: The extraintestinal complications of Crohn's disease and ulcerative colitis: A study of 700 patients. *Medicine* 1976;55:401–412.

37. Hubler WR Jr, Rudolph AH, Dougherty EF: Dermal myiasis. *Arch Dermatol* 1974; 110:109–110.

38. Everett ED, DeVillez RL, Lewis CW: Cutaneous myiasis due to *Dermatobia hominis*. *Arch Dermatol* 1972;113:1122.

39. Guillozet N: Erosive myiasis. *Arch Dermatol* 1981;117:59–60.

40. Powell FC, Schroeter AL, Su WP, et al: Pyoderma gangrenosum: A review of 86 patients. *Q J Med* 1985;55:173–186.

41. Perry HO, Brunsting LA: Pyoderma gangrenosum: A clinical study of nineteen cases. *Arch Dermatol* 1957;75:380–386.

42. Parivar F, Bradbrook RA: Interstitial cystitis. *Br J Urol* 1986;58:239–244.

43. Johnston JH: Local hydrocortisone for Hunner's ulcer of the bladder. *Br Med J* 1956; 2:698–699.

44. Le Portz B, Boccon-Gibod L, Steg A: Interstitial cystitis—the arsenal of possible therapies—5 cases. *Ann Urol* 1983;17:165.

45. Messing EM, Stamey TA: Interstitial cystitis: Early diagnosis, pathology and treatment. *Urology* 1978;12:381–392.

46. Murnaghan GF, Saalfeld J, Farnsworth RH: Interstitial cystitis—treatment with Chlorpactin WCS-90. *Br J Urol* 1969;42:744.

47. Murphy DM, Zincke H, Utz D: Interstitial cystitis. *J Urol* 1982;128:606.

48. Parsons CL, Schmidt JD, Pollen JJ: Successful treatment of interstitial cystitis with sodium pentosanpolysulvate. *J Urol* 1983;130:51–53.

49. Stewart BH, Shirley SW: Further experience with intravesical DMSO in the treatment of interstitial cystitis. *J Urol* 1976;116:36–38.

50. Wishard WN, Nourse MH, Merz JH: Use of Chlorpactin WCS-90 for relief of symptoms of interstitial cystitis. *J Urol* 1957;77:420–423.

51. Meade R, et al: Primary hepatic actinomycosis. *Gastroenterology* 1980;78:355.

52. Pheil MG, et al: Abdominal actinomycosis. *Surgery* 1984;51:345.

53. Niebyl JR, Parmley TH, Spence MR, et al: Unilateral ovarian abscess associated with the intrauterine device. *Obstet Gynecol* 1978;52(2):165–168.

54. Amin OM, Mwokike FG: Prevalence of pin worms and whipworm investigation in institutionalized mental patients in Wisconsin, 1966-1976. *Wis Med J* 1980;7(3):31–32.

55. Wertheim P, Galama J, Geelen J, et al: Epidemiology of infections with cytomegalovirus (CMV) and herpes simplex virus in promiscuous women: Absence of exogenous reinfection with CMV. *Genitourin Med* 1985;61(6):383–386.

56. Posevaia TA, Kulcsar G, Horvath I, et al: Detection of the virus-specific antigens of adenoviruses and herpes simplex virus in patients with malignant genital diseases. *Vopr Virusol* 1984;29(6):727–730.

57. Kumari TV, Shanmugam J, Prabha B, et al: Prevalence of antibodies against herpes simplex and adenovirus in oral and cervical cancer patients—a preliminary report. *Indian J Med Res* 1982;75:590–592.

58. Kaufman RH, Faro S: Herpes genitalis: Clinical features and treatment. *Clin Obstet Gynecol* 1985;28(1):152–163.

59. Editorial: EBV and the uterine cervix. *Lancet* 1986;2(8516):1134–1135.

60. Thomas D, Withington PS: Toxic shock syndrome: A review of the literature. *Ann R Coll Surg Engl* 1985;67:156–158.

61. Smith CB, Jacobson JA: Toxic shock syndrome, in *Disease a Month*. Chicago, Year Book Medical Publishers, 1986, pp 78–118.

62. Editorial: Toxic shock syndrome: Back to the future. *JAMA* 1987;257(8):1094–1095.

63. Kostianovsky M, Orenstein JM, Schaff Z, et al: Cytomembranous inclusions observed in acquired immunodeficiency syndrome. *Arch Pathol Lab Med* 1987;111:218–223.

64. DeVita VT, Brodei S, Fauci AS, et al: Developmental therapeutics and the acquired immunodeficiency syndrome. *Ann Intern Med* 1987;106:568–581.

65. Fahey JL, Sarna G, Gale RP, et al: Immune interventions in disease. *Ann Intern Med* 1987;106:257–274.

66. Walkinshaw SA, Cordiner JW, Clements JB, et al: Prognosis of women with human papillomavirus DNA in normal tissue distal to invasive cervical and vulval cancer. *Lancet* 1987;1:563.

67. Gleckman RA, Bergman MM: Newer antibiotics: Their place in geriatric care. *Geriatrics* 1986;41(12):51–55.

68. Malangoni MA, Condon RE, Spiegel CA: Treatment of intra-abdominal infections is appropriate with single-agent or combination antibiotic therapy. *Surgery* 1985;98:648–655.

69. Wilson SE, Williams RA, Lewis RT, et al: Multicenter comparative study of cefotetan vs moxalactam in the treatment of intra-abdominal infections. *Infect Surg* 1985;4(April suppl):29–34.

70. Lipsky JJ: N-methyl-thio-tetrazole inhibition of the gamma carboxylation of glutamic acid: Possible mechanism for antibiotic-associated hypoprothrombinaemia. *Lancet* 1983;2:192–193.

71. Gleckman R, Gantz NM: The third-generation cephalosporins: A plea for restraint. *Arch Intern Med* 1982;142:1267–1268.

Chapter 9

Psychiatric Aspects of Aging

Hilda B. Templeton and Donald D. Scalea

INTRODUCTION

The physician's own feelings about the aging process are important as he or she approaches the geriatric patient. In examining one's own feelings it is important to keep in mind that the younger physician often feels threatened by the elderly because they may arouse concerns about the physician's own age. In addition, the elderly patient may cause the physician to need to address conflictive relationships with his or her parents. The physician may even feel that his or her efforts may be wasted on the older patient because the patient may be dying shortly. This is of particular concern given the fact that the death may stimulate within the physician conflicts regarding his or her competence. Some physicians even look on gerontologists as having a morbid preoccupation with death, and specific interest in the elderly is sometimes regarded as "sick."[1]

"The old medical school maxim to address the total patient, with attention to the interplay of the biomedical, the psychological, and the social, is perhaps more relevant with the geriatric patient than with any other."[1] It is important for the physician to convey a sense of empathy toward the patient. Empathy is to be distinguished from sympathy; the latter would unnecessarily "infantilize" the patient and convey the sense that the patient is overly dependent on the physician. Likewise, in speaking with the elderly patient, it is important to include somewhat controversial topics, such as sexuality. Including such topics conveys a sense of self-esteem to the patient and provides the physician with important details. Shaking hands with the patient may also help to give the patient a sense of importance and self-esteem. Gentle touching can be quite reassuring, and it may communicate genuine caring.[2] It may be important for the physician to greet the elderly patient by his or her last name, rather than by first name. If nothing else, such a sign of respect may be important in terms of bolstering the patient's self-esteem. If the evaluation is occurring in a hospital setting, the physician should sit in a chair near the patient, being sure to provide the patient with a comfortable amount of distance. Sitting on a patient's bed or standing next to the patient's bed may give the patient the idea that the physician has little time, and may imply a familiarity in the relationship that is inappropriate.

A complete evaluation is important in order to adequately diagnose psychiatric illnesses in the elderly. The history should include not only past illnesses, but also an assessment of ability to meet one's own activities of daily living, including meal preparation and grocery shopping. In addition, sexual dysfunction, feelings of dependence, and loneliness should be elicited. One must always be particularly aware of depression and suicidal ideation, as often the elderly patient will not immediately offer these complaints, and will voice them only if questioned directly.

After the history a complete medical and laboratory evaluation should be performed, certainly no less so than would be provided for a younger patient. Often pelvic and rectal examinations are omitted in the older population, and they certainly should be performed as they would in any younger patient. The patient's family also should be involved in the information-gathering process, as information that is important in the diagnostic process is frequently obtained from the family. In involving the family, the physician may be confronted with resistance, frustration, and anger on the part of family members. It is important that family members not be alienated, as often they have made the contact with the physician and may be the only source of support for the patient. The family should have an opportunity to ventilate their concerns.

It may be important to further evaluate the family to ensure that the patient is not being physically or emotionally abused. Perhaps the most common form of abuse is neglect. Causes of this type of abuse include alcoholism in the family member, financial stress, and long-term familial conflict. Occasionally abuse is brought to medical attention by unexplained multiple "falls," fractures, and bruises. In terms of neglect, nonambulatory patients may be left unattended for long periods.[3]

In taking the history, it is important to include an evaluation of the patient's sleep patterns. If the patient has difficulty sleeping, this may indicate an underlying treatable illness. Anxiety may be suggested by difficulty in initially falling asleep, and early-morning awakening often suggests an underlying depression. Failure to pursue a sleep disorder may be catastrophic, given the fact that suicide is common in the elderly depressed population.[1]

Cohen offers seven general rules for assessing the elderly patient for psychiatric illness: (1) Do not assume that mental changes in the elderly represent senility. (2) Do not accept systematic mental changes in older people as being within normal limits. (3) When dementia does occur, it may not be the senile type; it may be an acute organic brain syndrome. (4) Psychogenic changes later in life can masquerade as organic changes. (5) Both psychogenic and organic changes can coexist. (6) Many psychogenic and organic changes in the aged that cause mental symptoms can be treated. (7) When psychogenic and organic problems coexist, either or both may respond to proper treatment, with overall improvement in the patient's clinical state.[1]

General Diagnostic Issues

Numerous erroneous assumptions should be kept in mind by the practitioner who is assessing and potentially treating the elderly female patient. One should not assume that because an irreversible condition exists, treatment is not indicated. Even if an elderly patient suffers from a disease process that is irreversible, often much can be done to minimize the severity of the problem by providing supportive treatment. For example, treatment of hypertension may be appropriate when patients suffer from multi-infarct dementia.[4] Further, one must avoid considering decreased appetite, diminished memory, weakness, tremulousness, and other stereotypic symptoms of the aging process as merely signs of old age. Frequently such symptoms suggest an underlying psychological illness that may be treatable. Such symptoms also may represent side effects of medications. Early on in the assessment of this patient population it should be determined whether or not aphasia exists. Aphasia may be mistaken for dementia, owing to difficulty the patient has in communicating. Impaired visual or auditory acuity may be mistaken for paranoid ideation.[4] Dementia, depression, delirium, and paranoia are not part of the normal aging process. The issue of sensory deprivation must be kept in mind. Of note is that hearing loss occurs in approximately 30% of elderly patients and is potentially quite problematic. In severe forms paranoia may result.

As patients age, their cognition diminishes. Given the fact that impaired mental status is a symptom of many common illnesses, it is a major health issue. Given the large number of depressed patients in the elderly population, and given the high rate of suicide in the population, diagnosing and treating psychological illnesses are of paramount importance. Further, physical illnesses are exacerbated by psychological symptomatology.

General Treatment Issues

Elderly patients who are intellectually impaired should be moved to new locations as infrequently as possible, since it is difficult for marginally oriented people to cope with unfamiliar surroundings.[4] Often institutionalization is considered in the overall treatment plan of the elderly patient. "A well-known but often neglected aspect of this care system is the fact that the death rate among elderly people climbs dramatically as they move from community to institution, regardless of the nature of the institution."[5]

Analysis of cause-specific deathrates among 750 elderly psychiatric inpatients revealed a markedly increased risk of death from cardiovascular disorders during the first year of hospitalization. Although the risks of cardiovascular death are considerably less among longer-stay patients, the pneumonia risks remain high. This suggests differing preventive strategies. To help prevent cardiovascular deaths, more attention should be paid to avoiding transfer-trauma and its attendant stress. To help prevent pneumonia deaths, high priority should be given to an aggressive program of immunization, adequate nutrition, reduction of hospital overcrowding, and recognition of early pneumonia symptoms.[5]

Compliance is an issue in this population. Any obstacles that exist in the physician's office may decrease the patient's likelihood of receiving treatment. Access to the office should be ensured. Likewise, ordering numerous outpatient tests on the same day may contribute to a decrease in compliance. Compliance issues may be further complicated by the need of the elderly patient to make use of public transportation. Home visits might be considered, if at all possible. Oftentimes the elderly patient can better tolerate several short visits rather than one long one.[2]

As a final note regarding the general guidelines for assessment of the elderly female, it should be noted that "the older patient can be troubled by any of the psychiatric disorders found in younger adults. Studies indicate that the incidence of major psychiatric syndromes in old age is in the area of 18% to 25%, depending on what is included and the severity of the condition."[1]

SEXUALITY

There is a preponderance of widows and divorced females in the aged population. Because there are more women than men available, men tend to be in a "buyer's market." Widowers and single men have a greater opportunity because of traditional male freedom and mobility in society to affect social relationships with a number of women. On the other hand, widows and divorcées are much less able to find sexual partners. Fifty percent of women between the ages of 70 and 75 are widows. Between the ages of 60 and 64 more than 25% of women are widowed and only 6% of men. The death rate appears to increase in the first year after the death of a spouse. Depression is also significantly increased, and there is an apparent increase in suicidal gestures.[6]

Men continue to function at a lower level of sexual interest and at the same time develop general health problems, such as prostate difficulties, while in their 50s and 60s. A common response to any medical or surgical problem is decreased sexual interest. In the aging woman there is some chemical change that slows down vaginal lubrication and results in less vigorous contractions of the organic platform. Intensity of erotic stimulation decreases. Elderly women, though, remain capable of having multiple orgasms, whereas their male partners tend to have a higher incidence of impotence. Postmenopausal women retain their capacity for sexual desire and sexual pleasure. The capacity to reach orgasm remains intact. There may in fact be increased libidinal response after menopause. This development is usually indicative of psychological rather than physiological phenomenon, since women often feel freed of the fear of pregnancy as they also find that they are still desirable love objects.[6]

A consequence of the aging process that results in lessened availability of estrogens and progesterones may render sexual intercourse painful to the aging female. Adequate steroid replacement retards these changes and helps to prevent vaginismus and secondary dyspareunia. However, regular sexual activity during the menopausal and postmenopausal years tends to retard the development of involutional changes in the female genitalia. With regular intercourse, women can retain the capacity for orgasm and sexual gratification well into their later years. The aging process itself neither physiologically nor psychologically predisposes women to decreased libido and orgasmic response.

MENOPAUSE

The impact of the menopause on women's emotional status is undergoing an enlightened reconceptualization. Past literature is rife with inaccuracies, biases, and myths about the effects of menopause. Freud and others viewed the climacteric as a time of crisis, in that many previously undisturbed women developed neuroses. "Menopausal women," Freud said, "tended to behave in a quarrelsome, obstinate, petty, and stingy manner and to exhibit sadistic and anal-erotic features which they did not show before."[7]

Deutsch, a psychoanalyst in the early 1900s, viewed the climacteric as a "stage of emotional struggle; a struggle against inevitable decline, more organically and psychologically demanding for women than the mid-life period was for men." The climacteric was regarded by Deutsch as a woman's last traumatic experience as a sexual being and the "third edition" of the infantile state (the second being menarche), during which time a woman acted out certain unconscious fantasies, such as rape or prostitution. She described changes in a woman's behavior at the time of menopause to include irritability, depression, anxiety, and giddiness, and referred to "hysteria reactions." Deutsch's views served as the basis for others who described the menopause as a rather negative, unfulfilled period in a woman's life.[6]

As the number of postmenopausal women in the general population increases, feminists and medical researchers are taking a new look at menopause. Most studies show that attitudes toward menopause relate to the sociocultural expectations in a society. In cultures where attitudes toward the elderly are more positive, menopause is less stressful. Conversely, in those societies where aging is looked on as the end of a fruitful existence, complaints and psychiatric illness during the climacteric are increased.

Symptoms attributed to the menopause are lengthy. Perhaps depression is most significant, and in previous psychiatric literature, involutional melancholia was directly attributed to endocrinologic changes that take place at the time of the menopause. Insomnia, headaches, dizzy spells, palpitations, weight changes, giddiness, lethargy, forgetfulness, and weight gain have all been associated with menopausal changes. Studies show that although the climacteric does not precipitate psychiatric illness, there is a higher morbidity of psychiatric problems at this time in a woman's life. These symptoms are not present in all women during the climacteric. In fact studies show that the number of women reporting uncomfortable symptoms in the climacteric is significantly declining in relation to the number of complaints reported by a similar population of women years ago. This change seems to coincide with more positive attitudes concerning aging and menopause. Bachman and Mijuta describe a study done in 1965 in which a majority of climacteric women sampled complained of irritability, lethargy, depression, forgetfulness, and weight gain. In contrast, they referred to a study conducted in 1984 at the University of Medicine and Dentistry of New Jersey, Rutgers Medical School, in which a minority of climacteric women voiced the same complaints.[7]

What, then, is the etiology of climacteric complaints? They appear to be multifactorial with psychological factors, sociocultural factors, and hormonal changes being primary. The majority of studies have shown that estrogens are beneficial in alleviating some of the psychiatric symptoms at the time of menopause, such as changes in mood with anxiety and depression, insomnia and irritability. It is also reported that hormonal replacement helps to improve sexual activity in terms of satisfaction and capacity for orgasm.

Psychological factors in terms of personality structure are also very much involved. Those individuals who are well able to handle changes in life as seen in adolescence or during middle life will also be expected to handle the life changes associated with the time of menopause with the same ease. Those women, though, who are so involved in their role as mother may find the adjustment to an empty nest a difficult one and develop psychiatric symptoms at this time coinciding with the end of menses. Important also is the lack of a distinct correlation between the intensity of psychiatric symptoms that may develop at this time and the degree of hormonal change. Socioeconomic factors such as race, economic status, religion, educational level, and type of work all contribute to a woman's mental health. A positive attitude toward women in their changing roles as they approach their later years reflects most significantly on their mental health. In a study by Bar,

> the most intense climacteric symptoms have been reported in women who, during the reproductive years, complained of premenstrual fatigue and tension, dysfunctional uterine bleeding, and dysmenorrhea. On the other hand, climacteric symptoms are lessened in women who are in general good health and are not totally absorbed in the mother role.[7]

The number of climacteric complaints appear to be higher in women with limited education and lower economic status. Those women who have alternative life interests to motherhood also have fewer climacteric complaints. Women who are most adversely affected by changes in menopause are those women whose primary activity in life has centered around family and children and who have limited education and few interests outside their homes. Women who are in stable marriages with extended family and friendships have decreased symptoms.

When we are talking about menopause, we are basically talking about loss. There is a fear of aging, dying, of losing one's looks, of losing health, of losing a spouse, and the loss of children as they move away and develop families of their own. If we continue to conceptualize menopause as a time of obsolescence, then resolution of all of these losses becomes quite difficult; but if we redefine this period of time as a positive one, with many good years ahead, then the resolution of these conflicts and losses will be done in a healthy way. The issue of feeling good about one's self is the key to the psychology of menopause.[7]

Psychotherapy at this time must deal with the "repair, support, and maintenance" of the patient's self-esteem. Support groups can be very helpful.

DIAGNOSTIC CATEGORIES

Depression

> The importance of depression as a psychopathologic syndrome in the elderly is stressed by the estimate that about 30% of persons over the age of 65 may be expected to experience an episode of depression severe enough to interfere with daily functioning. Depression is the chief cause of psychiatric hospitalization among the elderly, and it bares great potential for death through inanition or suicide. Loss of mastery (ability to cope) and the onset of helplessness are frequent dynamic issues in the development of depression or behavioral problems in the elderly. Geriatric stereotypes contribute directly to helplessness by reinforcing such behavior. Stereotypes also minimize the chance of appropriate response

outcomes relative to needs. Rolelessness, a partial result of stereotyping, leads to anomie, alienation, and lowered self-esteem.[8]

Social losses of the elderly that are significant issues in the development of depression include social support systems such as children, friends, and spouse. There is also loss of social roles, for example, occupational, family, sexual, and gender. There are also associated losses of housing, income, health, independence, and mobility.[8]

> Therapeutically, the redevelopment or reacquisitions of meaningful role functioning is a major goal of psychotherapy or sociotherapy with the elderly. An attempt is made in therapy to correct social losses by helping the old person to find new social outlets (for example, senior citizens or friendship groups), to find a job, or to gain satisfaction at the traditional roles of the elderly (for example, grandparenthood). Psychotherapy is frequently targeted to help the older person regain increasing mastery over the environment so that feelings of helplessness, fear and anger diminish, thus alleviating psychopathologic symptoms.[8]

The essential feature of depression is either a dysphoric mood, which is usually described as depression, or loss of interest or pleasure in usual activities. These symptoms are relatively persistent and may be associated with appetite disturbance, weight change, sleep disturbance primarily characterized by early-morning awakening (terminal insomnia), psychomotor agitation or retardation, decreased energy, feelings of worthlessness and guilt, impaired concentration, and suicidal ideation. Some patients may not be able to verbalize their depression and may instead complain of "feeling empty," "not caring anymore," "nothing makes me happy anymore." Strong isolation is also characteristic of depression in the elderly.

Difficulty concentrating, slowed thinking, and indecisiveness are frequently associated with complaints of memory loss. "Misdiagnoses of pseudo-dementia is a common cause of psychiatric hospitalization of the elderly and a major factor leading to long term institutional care."[8]

Some associated features of depression include panic anxiety attacks, phobia, somatic preoccupation and concern, tearfulness, anxiety, brooding, and depressed appearance. Patients may not be as concerned about their personal hygiene and grooming. Psychotic features may accompany a depression and may include delusions and hallucinations that are most often mood congruent. Less common are mood incongruent psychotic features.

Differential diagnosis of a major depressive episode in the elderly must be given careful consideration. The presence of disorientation, apathy, impaired concentration, and memory loss may indicate both organic and functional disorders.

Depression in the elderly is primarily reactive or situational. For example, grieving the loss of a spouse is usually time-limited, and after a brief period most individuals are able to return to a normal baseline functioning. Some people, however, are unable to do this, and their depressive symptoms linger and become severer over time. Some depressed geriatric patients may also be unable to recall a primary precipitating event for their depression. These individuals have a chemical depression or, as stated in the *Diagnostic and Statistical Manual of Mental Disorders,* third edition (DSM-III), and DSM-III-R, a major affective disorder—depressed. Nondetection of a major depression may result in significant morbidity and mortality. A significant common complication of untreated depression in the elderly is suicide. Elderly males in particular have an increased suicide rate.[9]

The elderly woman may present in a variety of ways to her primary care physician. She may present with a masked depression, that is, present with a multiplicity of nonspecific complaints for which she has seen many physicians for symptom relief. She may also complain of persistent lack of energy. A decreased activity level is another common complaint. There is often a role reversal or regression. Preoccupation with the past is often present. Malnutrition, suicidal ideation, and memory and concentration problems are also hints to the physician that a major depression may be present.

Some patients have their initial onset of major depression as they reach old age. Others may have had postpartum depression and are presenting again with a depressive disorder after menopause. It is estimated that more than 50% of individuals with a major depression will have another depressive episode some time in their lifetime. Those individuals with recurrent major depressions are at greater risk of developing a bipolar affective disorder. After successive treatment most patients with depressive disorders return to normal functioning. Only a small number of patients, between 20% and 35%, remain socially impaired and/or have considerable residual symptoms. This is more likely to occur when there are frequent recurrent episodes of depression. The disorder is estimated to be twice as common in females as in males.[10] "There is evidence that prevalence of the disorder has increased in the age cohort that came to maturity after the second World War."[11]

Most studies show that major depression is 1.5 to 3.0 times more common among first-degree biological relatives than among the general population.[11]

Available studies indicate that approximately 33% of medical inpatients report mild or moderate symptoms of depression, and that up to 25% may suffer from a depressive disorder. Depression in cancer patients is significant. A study by Bukbert et al reports that 42% of cancer patients meet modified DSM-III criteria for major depression. However, a study of women with breast tumors found that the severity of depression did not depend on whether or not the tumor was malignant.[12]

Studies have reported up to 50% of patients with significant depressive symptoms after acute stroke. The high-risk period of depression after a stroke extends for 2 years. Depression is common also in other neurologic conditions, including amyotrophic lateral sclerosis, Parkinson's disease, temporal lobe epilepsy, and multiple sclerosis. Neuroendocrine disturbances are also commonly associated with depressive syndromes. These primarily include altered pituitary-adrenal axis and thyroid axis diseases. Hypothyroidism, autoimmune thyroiditis, hyperparathyroidism, diabetes mellitus, hyperinsulinism, Cushing's disease, adrenal cortical hyperplasia, and Addison's disease have all been associated with depressive symptomatology.[12]

Patients with medical illness may present with a major depressive episode, or they may present with less severe depressive disorders. Among these is an adjustment disorder with depressed mood in which there are maladaptive reactions to some indefinable psychosocial stressor, with symptoms occurring within a 3-month period from the onset of the stress. Physical illness may be a precipitant of an adjustment disorder with depressed mood. Dysthymic disorder refers to a more chronic disturbance of mood. Here depressive symptoms may be present as a major affective disorder, but they lack sufficient severity and duration to meet the criteria for a major depressive episode. Again, chronic physical illness may be a common precipitant. In organic affective syndromes, which DSM-III refers to as organic mental syndromes, the disturbance is primarily that of mood. Unspecified symptoms are present for at least a 2-week period on a daily basis, and there is evidence of a specific etiological organic factor.[9,11,12]

There may be covert or indirect manifestations of depression without prominent cognitive or affective symptoms. Patients may present with somatization, abnormal illness behavior, and pain. They may also present with dementia and pseudodementia symptoms. There may also be suicidal behavior and refusal of medical treatment. When patients refuse medical treatment in the face of serious medical illness, an underlying affective disorder must be ruled out.

Treatment of depression in the elderly is becoming an increasingly important subject, considering the rising incidence of major depression in this growing population. Somatic therapies usually include the use of tricyclic antidepressants (TCAs), monoamine oxidase (MAO) inhibitors, and electroconvulsive shock therapy (ECT). TCAs carry the risk of significant side effects in the elderly, particularly in those who are medically ill. These side effects include sedation, hypertension, atropinelike effects, and heart block or other cardiac dysrhythmia.[13]

A previous history of a TCA-responsive major depression or an ECT-responsive depression, or a family history of major depression successfully treated with ECT or TCAs all tend to increase the likelihood of a patient's responding to a TCA. Those patients who tend to have major depressions with mood congruent or mood incongruent psychotic features appear to respond better to ECT therapy rather than to TCAs.

Patients over the age of 65 who are being treated with TCAs must be approached cautiously because of the possibility of side effects. An adequate drug trial for an elderly individual must be a minimum of 4 to 6 weeks. Younger individuals may respond and receive maximal benefit within a 3- to 4-week period. Often TCA levels are affected by age.[14]

Side effects of a TCA primarily involve the peripheral, autonomic nervous system, the central nervous system, and the cardiovascular system. Anticholinergic or atropinelike side effects result in difficulty in urination, constipation, and pupil dilatation.

In order of potency, amitriptyline is the most anticholinergic followed by imipramine, nortriptyline, and doxepin. TCAs are contraindicated in patients with narrow-angle glaucoma. The concomitant use of pilocarpine may help to overcome the atropinelike side effects of TCAs.

The central atropinelike activity of TCAs can lead to disorientation, confusion, delusions, and ataxia. Geriatric patients are primarily vulnerable to these side effects. Parenteral administration of physostigmine is the antidote for this anticholinergic central nervous system effect. TCAs affect cardiac conduction, rhythm, and contractility, and blood pressure regulation. There is QRS interval prolongation noted with most tricyclics. Tricyclics have a quinidinelike effect and may be helpful in some cardiac dysrhythmias. Studies primarily of imipramine have shown that this drug suppresses atrial and ventricular premature contractions. Orthostatic hypotension is the most common cardiovascular side effect with the routine administration of TCAs, and patients who experience dizziness in association with orthostatic change should not be continued on that particular TCA. A trial of a different TCA may prove successful.

Barbiturates frequently used to treat sleep disorders in geriatric patients are inducers of microsomal enzymes and, as a consequence, can result in decreased TCA concentrations. Tobacco smokers also develop lower plasma concentration than nonsmokers because of the stimulation of microsomal enzymes caused by tobacco use. Although most sedative-hypnotic drugs decrease TCA levels, flurazepam does not, and therefore it may be a good choice for elderly patients with depression accompanied by insomnia. Methylphenidate inhibits microsomal enzymes and can be used concurrently with TCAs to increase plasma concentration.

Other drugs with anticholinergic side effects used concurrently with TCAs may exacerbate the anticholinergic side effects of the TCAs. Some of these drugs include phenothiazines, antiparkinsonian agents, the belladonna alkaloids, and anticholinergic antispasmodics.

Diuretic agents exacerbate TCA-induced orthostatic hypertension. Guanethidine and clonidine are inhibited by TCAs. Reserpine and alpha-methyl dopa precipitate depression and should not be used in the depressed elderly. Quinidine and procainamide have properties similar to the antiarrhythmic properties of the TCAs. Coadministration of these agents along with a TCA may produce toxic effects on the cardiac tissue. The dose of antiarrhythmic agents may be decreased in patients being treated for their dysrhythmia who are also on TCAs. Anticoagulation drugs, such as bishydroxycoumarin or warfarin sodium, along with TCAs potentiate excessive bleeding in patients on concomitant treatment. Patients with pacemakers can be safely treated with TCAs. In treating patients with cardiovascular disease, the major cardiovascular side effects of the TCAs are as follows: the most anticholinergic is amitriptyline (Elavil) followed by imipramine (Tofranil), desipramine (Norpramin), and doxepin (Sinequan). The most adrenergic to the least, desipramine, imipramine, amitriptyline, and doxepin.

MAO inhibitors are also well tolerated in the elderly. Reports on the comparative efficacy and safety of MAO inhibitors versus TCAs indicate that anticholinergic side effects were more frequently reported in the TCA group. Orthostatic symptoms have been reported with similar frequency in both drug groups, and overall, both are well tolerated.[15]

Lithium is usually well tolerated, but in view of the longer elimination half-life in the elderly, patients are at greater risk for developing side effects. They also usually need lower dosage levels for effectiveness. Lithium is the drug of choice for maintenance treatment of bipolar affective disorders. Its efficacy has also been proved in the maintenance of unipolar depressive disorders. Still, antidepressants are probably the first choice in treating the acute depressive episode, with lithium treatment being used for maintenance either alone or with a TCA.

ECT is efficacious but needs to be used with caution, particularly in those over age 75 with cardiovascular disease. It is the treatment of choice in those patients who have previously responded successfully to ECT treatment, those with psychotic depressions, and those with imminent suicidal ideation with intent, unable to wait for antidepressant response.

Dementia

Dementia is a symptom complex that has many possible causes. It is multifaceted, with deficits in memory, judgment, abstract thought, and a variety of other higher cortical functions. Changes in personality and behavior also occur. The diagnosis is not made if these features are due to clouding of consciousness, as in delirium. DSM-III defines dementia on symptoms alone, and does not connote prognosis. Dementia may be progressive, static, or remitting.[9]

The most prominent symptom of dementia is memory impairment. There is intellectual deterioration that is severe enough to interfere with occupations or social performance.[9,16] Patients may need to have directions and statements repeated a number of times. Patients may forget addresses, telephone numbers, and medical directions. Dementia may progress so that memory impairment involves not only present recall but also past memory. Short-term memory deficits are usually noted early on. Long-term memory defects are also noted as the disease progresses. There may be impairment in abstract thinking and frequently in both judgment and impulse control as well. This is often manifested by neglect of personal appearance and hygiene, poor judgment, and lack of awareness of actions that may affect personal safety.

Personality change is also present in dementia. What may be seen is a change or accentuation of premorbid personality traits. According to DSM-III, a common pattern "is for normally active individuals to become increasingly apathetic and withdrawn."[9]

The range of social involvement narrows. The personality loses its sparkle, and the individual is described by others as "not herself." Another pattern of change is for a previously neat, meticulous person to become slovenly and unconcerned about appearance. On the other hand, some individuals display an accentuation of preexisting compulsive, histrionic, impulsive, or paranoid traits. Irritability and cantankerousness are also common features of dementia.

Associated features of dementia include the following: There may be significant mood disorder when a patient notices that he or she is becoming forgetful. Paranoid ideation may also be a significant finding in patients with early dementia. It is often noted that a jealous individual may accuse his or her spouse of infidelity, and numerous case reports of assault have been reported.[9]

Dementia is predominantly seen in the elderly, although it may occur at any age. The course of the illness depends on whether or not there is a clearly defined episode of neurologic disease or whether one is dealing with a primary degenerative dementia. When there is a clearly defined neurologic disease, such as cerebral hypoxia or encephalitis, dementia may be fairly sudden in onset and then relatively static for long periods. Primary degenerative dementia, on the other hand, is insidious and relentlessly progressive.

As the dementia progresses the individual becomes totally oblivious of his or her surroundings and is in need of constant care. Usually the diagnosis of dementia is first made when there is a significant enough change in intellectual functioning so that social or occupational functioning becomes impaired.

The incidence of Alzheimer's disease is highest among people in their ninth decade. As the average age of the population over 65 increases (and the age group that is older than 85 is the fastest-growing part of our population because of the considerable reductions in mortality that have occurred in the past 15 years), the prevalence of dementia among those older than 65 should increase more than that estimated in earlier studies.[16] First-degree biological relatives of people with presenile onset of this disorder are more likely to develop dementia than are members of the general population. In rare cases Alzheimer's disease is inherited as a dominant trait.[11] The most common cause of dementia is primary degenerative dementia of Alzheimer's type. Other causes may include tertiary syphilis, tuberculosis, fungal meningitis, viral encephalitis, Jakob-Creutzfeldt disease, brain trauma, toxic metabolic disturbances such as hypothyroidism, pernicious anemia, folic acid deficiency, vascular disease characterized primarily by multi-infarcted dementia, neurologic diseases, as well as postanoxic or posthypoglycemic states. Also significant in terms of causative factors is pseudodementia. In this condition patients with major depressive episodes may complain of memory impairment, impairment in thinking and concentrating, and basically significant reduction in intellectual functioning. These factors may be proved on mental status examination and by neuropsychiatric testing. In pseudodementia the mood disorder is the primary condition with cognitive deficits secondary to the disturbed affect, and cognitive symptoms resolve with adequate somatic treatment of the affective disorder.

Dementia is not synonymous with aging. It remains controversial, however, whether or not the changes in intellectual functioning that are noted in the normal process of aging are to be considered pathologic.

Primary degenerative dementia usually is of senile onset, after the age of 64. Few cases ever develop before age 49. The course of the disease is insidious with uniform and gradual progression. It is estimated that with senile onset the duration of symptoms from onset to death is approximately 5 years.

A computed tomography scan of the head shows the brain to be atrophied, with widened cortical sulci and enlarged cerebral ventricles. Histopathologic changes include senile plaques, neurofibrillar tangles, and granulovacuolar degeneration of neurons. Rarely one sees histologic features of Pick's disease, mixed vascular degenerative disease, or nonspecific pathologic changes. To date there is no definitive treatment for Alzheimer's disease.

Delirium

According to DSM-III, the diagnostic criteria for delirium include a clouding of consciousness, with a reduced capacity to shift, focus, and sustain attention to environmental stimuli. In addition, at least two of the following symptoms are necessary for diagnosis: (1) perceptual disturbance: misinterpretations, illusions, or hallucinations; (2) speech that is at times incoherent; (3) disturbance of the sleep-wakefulness cycle, with insomnia or daytime drowsiness; (4) increased or decreased psychomotor activity. In addition, disorientation and memory impairment are noted. Clinical features develop over a short period, usually hours or days, and tend to fluctuate over the course of the day. Also usually present is evidence, from the history, physical examination, or laboratory evaluation, of a specific organic factory judged to be etiologically related to the disturbance. Systemic infections, disorders of metabolism, and substance intoxication and withdrawal are all common causes of delirium. Metabolic causes include hypoxia, hypercapnia, hypoglycemia, ionic imbalances, hepatic or renal disease, and thiamine deficiency. Certain focal lesions of the right parietal lobe and inferomedian surface of the temporal lobe may present as delirium.[9]

Often a delirium is preceded by a prodrome. Symptoms of such a prodrome include restlessness, difficulty thinking clearly, hypersensitivity to auditory and visual stimuli, nocturnal insomnia, daytime hypersomnolence, vivid dreams, and nightmares.[9]

It is important to note that a diagnosis of delirium is particularly complicated when an underlying dementia exists. A diagnosis of delirium should be entertained when a mental status change suddenly occurs in an elderly patient who has no history of prior psychiatric illness.

Emotional disturbances are common in delirium. These may include depression, irritability, anger, anxiety, fear, euphoria, and apathy.[9] Hallucinations, delusions, disordered thinking, and impaired speech may also be present. However, these symptoms are random, given the fluctuating course of the delirium.

> One cannot diagnose dementia in the presence of significant delirium, because the symptoms of delirium interfere with the proper assessment of dementia. Only a definite history of pre-existing dementia allows one to decide that an individual with delirium also has dementia.[9]

"A prominent symptom may be panic or terror and sometimes this is the most important presenting complaint."[17]

Paranoid Disorders, Schizophrenia

Paranoid disorders generally occur in middle age or later in life. According to DSM-III, paranoid disorders are characterized by persistent persecutory delusions that are not caused by another mental illness. Paranoid disorders must be distinguished from major affective disorders, paranoid personality disorder, and schizophrenia. DSM-III defines paranoid disorders as lasting less than 6 months. It is rare that one's ability to function on a day-to-day basis is impaired. One's intellect and ability to function on the job usually remain intact. The character of the delusions may include delusional jealousy, conspiracy, a patient feeling as if he or she is being poisoned, or having harm done. People often become angry, and occasionally violent; grandiose delusions are common. Paranoid disorders must also be distinguished from brief reactive psychosis, in which psychotic symptomatology appears after a recognizable stressor and which is usually accompanied by incoherent thought processes, hallucinations, and grossly disorganized behavior. In addition, in a brief reactive psychosis, the psychotic symptoms last anywhere from a few hours to 2 weeks.[9]

Antipsychotic medications are quite useful in the elderly population, but the adverse side effects of this family of medications can be quite problematic. Bothersome side effects include sedation, syncope, light-headedness, anticholinergic symptoms, blurred vision, disorientation, and delirium. Also possible are akathisia and tardive dyskinesia. A given dose of antipsychotic medication may produce a higher blood level in an elderly patient than in a younger or middle-aged patient.[8] This does not explain in total the higher incidence of side effects in the elderly population. A complex interplay of pharmacodynamic factors, possibly at the receptor level, may account for this phenomenon.

Antipsychotic drugs may potentiate the plasma levels of TCAs. This is particularly important, given the fact that these medications are often used together.

When beginning a patient on antipsychotic medication, the dose should be very low, and increased gradually. The increase in the dose should be continued until the desired effect occurs, or until side effects occur. Blood pressure must be monitored, and clinical examinations performed frequently. Blood pressure should be taken, both seated and standing.

Routine medication evaluation before beginning the antipsychotic medications may include a baseline electrocardiogram, as the antipsychotic medications are known to prolong cardiac conduction time.

If at all possible, treating extrapyramidal symptoms with anticholinergic medications should be avoided, given the fact that the antipsychotic medications themselves have anticholinergic activity.

In choosing a particular medication, the specific side effects of each medication should be considered. If orthostatic hypotension is a particular problem, and if sedation is particularly worrisome, higher-potency medications should be considered. These include haloperidol and fluphenazine. If patients are particularly prone to extrapyramidal side effects, lower-potency medications should be considered. In general, in the elderly population, one of the higher-potency medications is initially the best choice. Again, the dose initially should be very low, and raised only gradually.[18]

In general clinical practice the antipsychotic medications are often used to treat confusional states and dementia, if accompanied by aggressive behavior. However, these medications should not be used in delirious states. Antipsychotic medications should be avoided in treating simple anxiety and simple depressions. Often in these latter clinical problems the medications may cause a worsening of symptoms.[18]

In the past, paraphrenia denoted schizophrenia that developed for the first time in the elderly population. According to DSM-III, schizophrenia must have its onset before age 45. DSM-III-R and other authors acknowledge that schizophrenia may have its onset later in life.[8,19] DSM-III divides schizophrenia into catonic, paranoid, residual, and undifferentiated types. Characteristics of the disorder include delusional thinking, auditory hallucinations, incoherence, a blunted, flat, or inappropriate affect, and grossly disorganized behavior.[9]

In the past, as noted earlier, paraphrenia was defined as schizophrenia that developed later in life. It was thought to occur far more often in females, particularly those who were isolated from society. Notably present were visual and auditory hallucinations and paranoid delusional thoughts. The delusional thinking was frequently sexual in nature, and behavior became at times quite bizarre. Paraphrenia was thought to be quite adequately treated with antipsychotic medication, if the medication was instituted early on in the illness.[17]

Personality Disorders

DSM-III distinguishes between personality traits and personality disorders. Personality traits are patterns of behavior that persist throughout life and that are seen as within normal limits. It is only when such traits become fixed and inflexible that a diagnosis of a personality disorder is made. Often the symptoms that suggest the diagnosis of a personality disorder are present by adolescence or early adulthood. DSM-III also notes that often the characteristics appear less notable in middle or old age. Features suggestive of the personality disorders may exist in the context of another acute psychiatric illness. A personality disorder should be diagnosed only when the symptoms are long term and characteristic of the patient's overall level of functioning.[9]

DSM-III-R groups these disorders into three clusters: (A) paranoid, schizoid and schizotypal personality disorders; (B) antisocial, borderline, narcissistic, and histrionic; (C) avoidant, dependent, obsessive-compulsive, and passive-aggressive personality disorders. Cluster A personalities often appear odd or eccentric. Cluster B individuals often appear dramatic, emotional, or erratic. Cluster C personalities appear anxious and fearful. Some individuals may have personality characteristics from each of these clusters.[11]

Individuals who suffer from paranoid personality disorder are seen by others to be hostile, defensive, rigid, and uncompromising. They seem to have a fear of intimacy, and are noted often to be egocentric and at times grandiose. They appear to be jealous of people in power or control positions. If stressed to an extreme, psychotic symptoms may be demonstrated. These individuals usually function adequately in society, given the fact that they understand that their unusual ideas are different from the general population, and therefore keep them to themselves. If the symptoms are severe, all interpersonal relationships are affected.

In the schizoid personality disorder emotional aloofness is often apparent, as well as the absence of caring feelings for other people. There is an indifference to the comments of other people, and close relationships are rare.

In the schizotypal personality disorder there is often an unusual speech pattern or unusual behavior, but an absence of loose associations and no evidence of incoherent thought. Magical thinking, as exemplified by clairvoyance, or superstition may also be present. Ideas of reference may be present, as well as social withdrawal, paranoid thought or suspiciousness, and anxiety in social situations. Illusions may also occur. It is important to note the distinction between a schizotypal personality disorder and a schizoid personality disorder, and both should be differentiated from schizophrenia.

In the histrionic personality disorder what is most often noted is a dramatic, intensely emotional presentation. These people tend to want to be the center of attention, and there may be an inner drive to pursue exciting or dramatic events. These individuals usually overreact to a given situation and become irrational or inappropriately angry at times. However, they tend to seem superficial to others and may appear overly concerned with their appearance, dependent, and manipulative. Suicidal gestures are common.

In the narcissistic personality disorder patients tend to exhibit a self-centered, grandiose sense of themselves. These individuals, perhaps out of an inner, deeper insecurity, suggest themselves as being overly powerful and overly important. Often they demonstrate exhibitionism, which may take the form of constant need for attention and reassurance. Rare reactions may occur, as well as intense feelings of insecurity and inferiority. These individuals frequently demonstrate a sense of expectation for special treatment, and may take advantage of other people in interpersonal relationships. Also, many lack the ability to empathize with others.

In the antisocial personality disorder there is often a history of truancy, suspension, or expulsion from school, or juvenile delinquency. These individuals have a history of lying, having casual sexual encounters, indulging in substance abuse, and committing crimes such as theft and vandalism. School performance is poor, and there is a frequent and persistent violation of rules, regulations, and authority. Interpersonal relationships are few and unstable, and work performance is poor. Unemployment is common, jobs are held for only brief periods, and often there is an inability of these patients to get along with their bosses. Impulsivity is common, and aggressive behavior is often noted. Multiple arrests are common. Perhaps most notable in these individuals is an inability to feel guilt and to empathize with others.

In the borderline personality disorder impulsivity and unpredictability are paramount. There are frequent self-destructive tendencies, which may result in self-laceration, frequent suicide attempts, promiscuous sexual activity, substance abuse, overeating, or the commission of petty crimes. Interpersonal relationships are characteristically unstable, and manipulative behavior toward other people is central. There is a marked disturbance of identity, which may surface in the area of sexual identity or gender identity. These people have a marked inability or serious difficulty in being alone, and may appear quite desperate at times. There is an inner sense of a void, and overwhelming emptiness.

In the avoidant personality disorder a hypersensitivity to rejection is noted. What may seem like an insignificant remark to other people will seem like a direct insult to these individuals. Interpersonal relationships tend to be unusual, and these people enter into a relationship only if given strong reassurance that they will not be rejected. There is an overwhelming desire for acceptance, a markedly impaired sense of self-esteem, and social isolation.

In the dependent personality disorder a marked passivity is noted. These people find it difficult to accept responsibility and find it almost impossible to function on their own. Personal needs are placed secondary to the needs of others, so long as other people will see to it that the dependent personality individual is cared for.

In the compulsive personality disorder there is a difficulty in expressing tender feelings toward other people. These people may appear rigid, rude, and insensitive to others. Often there is a overwhelming drive for perfection, and preoccupation with small or minute details. There is a lack of understanding for any other person's method of doing things, and insensitivity to other people. These individuals often immerse themselves in work, to the exclusion of warm interpersonal relationships. Ambivalence and difficulty in making decisions are noted, and often these people are overly preoccupied with money, and seem stingy when compared with other people.

In the passive-aggressive personality disorder what is central is the individual's resistance to performing in both social and interpersonal arenas. However, the resistance is not demonstrated in a direct fashion, and occurs through methods such as tardiness, intentional poor performance, and stubbornness. Given the individual's overwhelming need to resist in a passive fashion, interpersonal relationships are poor and job performance is impaired.

Adjustment Disorders

In the adjustment disorder of adulthood the significant factor is a maladaptive or inappropriate reaction to psychosocial stress. According to DSM-III-R, the reaction must occur within 3 months of the particular stress. The maladaptive aspect of the reaction is notable in terms of poor social functioning or poor work performance. However, the reaction also may refer to responses that themselves would be within normal limits, but given the severity of the responses, they become inappropriate. Once the stressor is removed, the symptoms subside. If the stress remains, the patient is able to eventually adapt in an appropriate fashion, and the maladaptive response no longer exists. Stresses may include separation from a loved one, either by divorce or death, difficult business situations, bankruptcy, the onset of an acute or chronic illness, family discord, loss of a job, or a natural occurrence such as an earthquake or a hurricane. The adjustment disorder may occur in any age group, although, as noted earlier, it must occur within 3 months of the identified stress.

DSM-III-R divides adjustment disorders into the following subtypes: adjustment disorder with depressed mood, adjustment disorder with anxious mood, adjustment disorder with mixed emotional features, adjustment disorder with disturbance of conduct, adjustment disorder with mixed disturbance of emotions and conduct, adjustment disorder with work inhibition, adjustment disorder with withdrawal, and adjustment disorder with atypical features.[11]

Uncomplicated Bereavement

Among the most frequently encountered psychiatric occurrences seen by the gynecologist in the care of the aged female is uncomplicated bereavement. This is when the focus of attention or treatment is a normal reaction to the death of a loved one.[9,11]

Symptoms associated with uncomplicated bereavement are depression, loss of appetite, and sleep disturbance. The individual usually perceives these symptoms as being normal for some period of time after the death. The duration of normal bereavement varies considerably with different cultural groups.

Rarely does uncomplicated bereavement develop into a major depression that requires psychopharmacologic intervention. If this should develop, there is frequently preoccupation with worthlessness, prolonged and marked functional impairment, and often marked psychomotor retardation. The reaction to a loss usually occurs immediately afterward. Rarely does this phenomenon occur after 2 or 3 months.

Somatoform Disorders

Conversion Disorders

Conversion disorders usually have their onset in adolescence but may occur in middle age or in the later decades of life. Essential for the diagnosis is a loss or alteration in physical functioning that suggests a physical disorder. Such a change generally affects the sensory motor system without defined underlying pathologic findings. Symptoms are often symbolic of underlying psychological conflicts. Patients may experience episodes of these symptoms through the years, and the site and nature of the symptoms may vary. Symptoms may develop in clear response to psychological stress, and onset may be sudden. The phenomenon of "la belle indifférence," the total indifference to the conversion symptom, may be present. The symptoms expressed in a conversion disorder are not under voluntary control.[11]

Somatoform Pain Disorder

There are a significant number of patients in whom the only primary complaint is that of pain. In both somatization disorder and conversion disorder pain may also be a factor, but it is not the primary or only complaint. In the case of psychogenic pain disorder the pain is usually described as severe and prolonged, and may be inconsistent with anatomical possibility. In most instances patients undergo significant medical workup without any significant organic pathology being found. Psychological factors are the primary ideology for this disorder. Frequently a temporal relationship between the onset of pain symptoms and a significant environmental stress that is perceived by the patient as being noxious is noted. There may be some secondary gain in the unconscious development of this symptom. Treatment of patients with somatoform pain disorder is difficult because there is often a lack of psychological mindedness, and patients are often resistant to insightful psychotherapy. A close, supportive, and trusted relationship with a primary physician is often one of the ways in which a patient may be able to give up her pain.

Hypochondriasis

Hypochondriasis may first appear at any age, from early childhood on, but the peak incidence in females is in the fifth decade. The essential feature is physical complaints without demonstrable organ pathology. Women often go from physician to physician seeking relief but receive none from either negative workup or physician reassurance. There is a resulting impairment in social and occupational functioning owing to this unrealistic fear or belief of having a disease. Hypochondriasis is notoriously refractory to treatment. Supportive physician relationships may be helpful.

Anxiety Disorders

DSM-III-R divides anxiety disorders into generalized anxiety disorder, obsessive-compulsive disorders, post-traumatic stress disorders, agoraphobia, social phobias, simple phobias, and panic disorders.[11]

The generalized anxiety disorder is diagnosed when there is evidence of generalized muscle tension, autonomic hyperactivity, apprehensive expectation, and vigilance and scanning. Motor tension includes symptoms such as generalized tremulousness, muscle discomfort, and difficulty relaxing. Signs of autonomic hyperactivity include excessive sweating, rapid heart rate, gastrointestinal distress, the sensation of a lump in one's throat, dry mouth, and increased respiration rate. DSM-III-R defines apprehensive expectation as a sense of foreboding. Vigilance and scanning are described by DSM-III-R as an extreme sense of foreboding, to the point that people become irritable, have difficulty concentrating, difficulty sleeping, and fatigue owing to impaired sleep.[11]

Obsessive-compulsive disorder is noted by DSM-III-R to consist of obsessions or compulsions that provide a significant amount of anxiety to the patient. Obsessions are recurrent thoughts or ideas that are inconsistent with the individual's normal thought process, and the patient often attempts to put them out of her mind. Compulsions are repetitive acts that occur in a stereotypic fashion. Such acts assist the patient in diminishing the amount of anxiety that she feels. At the same time the patient is aware of the purposeless aspect of her behavior and attempts to minimize or, at times, discontinue it. An example is the repeated handwashing that is often observed in patients who may be attempting to minimize the amount of guilt that they feel regarding a sexual encounter.[9,11]

In the posttraumatic stress disorder there exists a particular stressor that the patient has experienced, which would prompt a significant amount of stress. In addition, the patient reexperiences the emotion that she may have experienced at the time of the stress. This may include recurrent memories of the event, recurrent dreams in which the patient reexperiences the event, and an acute sense that the event may be happening again, as a result of a thought that may be associated with the event. Also included in the posttraumatic stress disorder may be a diminished response to the individual's environment, which may surface as withdrawal, restrictive affect, or a sense of detachment from other people. There may be associated sleep disturbance, feelings of guilt, poor memory, impaired concentration, and hyperalertness.[9,11]

Agoraphobia is diagnosed when the patient has a fear of being alone or a fear of being in enclosed places. At times this fear may be overwhelming, and may result in the individual's restriction of her daily life. This disorder is most frequently diagnosed in women.[9,11]

In social phobias there is an overwhelming fear of contact with other people. Oftentimes the individual has a sense that he or she may be ridiculed or embarrassed in certain situations. Individuals afflicted with this illness are intellectually aware that their fears are of inappropriate degree, yet they are unable to control them.[9,11]

In the simple phobia individuals experience irrational fear of certain objects or situations. There is an overwhelming need to avoid these objects. Examples of simple phobias are fears of heights or of particular animals, such as snakes. As in the social phobias, individuals afflicted with this disorder are aware that their fears are of inappropriate degrees.[9,11]

According to DSM-III-R, panic disorders are diagnosed when individuals experience more than four panic attacks in a 4-week period. These attacks are not associated with any particular object or situation, but seem to occur on their own. Panic attacks consist of times of overwhelming fear and may be accompanied by shortness of breath, rapid heartbeat, chest pain, dizziness, numbness and tingling in the extremities, sweating, faintness, and an overwhelming sense of doom. Panic disorders are diagnosed far more often in women than in men.[11] Mitral valve prolapse may be an associated condition but does not preclude diagnosis of panic disorder.[11]

The drug of choice for individuals suffering from agoraphobia and obsessive-compulsive disorder is imipramine. In the elderly population a starting dose of 25 to 50 mg may be used. This dose should be given on a once-daily basis and is most often given at bedtime. The dose may be increased up to 250 mg per day, if the individual is able to tolerate the side effects. However, in the elderly population, anticholinergic symptoms are common, and daily doses of 75 to 100 mg are often sufficient. Also of use in agoraphobia is alprazolam. Starting doses are 0.25 to 0.50 mg twice daily. Caution should be used in prescribing this drug, as the possibility for dependence exists. In addition, side effects of benzodiazepines include dizziness, confusion, and sedation. These are of particular concern in the elderly population, as falls may be complicated by fractures. Other benzodiazepines that may be helpful in the treatment of anxiety in the elderly population include lorazepam and buspirone. Anxiety disorders in the elderly population are often amenable to a regimen of psychotherapy.[20]

Substance Abuse

It is perhaps difficult for some clinicians to imagine elderly people addicted to alcohol or other drugs. However, the problem is far more widespread than most people believe. "When elderly patients present with repeated falls, alcohol abuse must be considered in their differential diagnosis."[21] Presenting symptoms of alcohol abuse in the elderly include repeated falls, confusion, and self-neglect.[21] Such patients rarely complain of alcohol abuse or difficulties regarding alcohol to the clinician. The issue of denial, as being perhaps the primary dynamic issue in the disease, deserves some mention.

It is difficult for some people to understand the degree to which denial affects the substance abuser. It is not unusual to speak with a flagrantly intoxicated person and have that person deny that she uses alcohol. Denial is a family phenomenon, and often it is not only the person doing the drinking who denies the severity of her problem. Oftentimes the spouse or child of an alcoholic is unconsciously invested in the alcoholic continuing her drinking, for a variety of dynamic reasons. It is due to this denial, which again can occur in anyone associated with the alcoholic, that makes diagnosis of the disease so difficult.

DSM-III makes a distinction between alcohol abuse and alcohol dependence. In order to make a diagnosis of alcohol abuse, three situations must exist. First, a pattern of pathologic alcohol use must be present. Second, impairment in social or occupational functioning owing to the alcohol use must be noted. Third, the duration of the abuse must be for at least 1 month. The pattern of pathologic alcohol use may become apparent when noting a need for daily use of alcohol, when noting an inability to decrease the amount of alcohol used or to stop drinking completely, and when noting binge-drinking and black-out episodes. The latter are periods of amnesia for events that occurred during the time the patient was intoxicated. Another pattern of pathologic use that is seen is a patient who continues to drink despite the serious physical or medical harm it is causing her. A number of possible impairments in social or occupational functioning are listed in DSM-III. They include violence during the intoxicated episode, absence from work owing to either intoxication or "hangovers," losses of employment, legal difficulties that can include arrests for driving while intoxicated, and arguments or difficulties with family relationships owing to the excessive use of alcohol.[9]

In order to make a diagnosis of alcohol dependence, DSM-III states that the patient must exhibit the following: either a pattern of pathologic alcohol abuse or impairment in social or occupational functioning owing to alcohol abuse, and either tolerance to or withdrawal from alcohol. DSM-III defines tolerance as a need for markedly increasing amounts of alcohol to achieve the necessary or desired effect. It also notes that the patient may experience a decreased effect given regular use of the same amount of alcohol. Withdrawal is defined as the development of a withdrawal syndrome and malaise that are relieved by ingestion of alcohol. A withdrawal syndrome may occur not only after discontinuing the alcohol consumption but also after a decrease in amount used.[9]

Another category mentioned in DSM-III is alcohol intoxication. In order to make such a diagnosis there must be a recent history of consumption of alcohol, evidence of maladaptive behavior after such an ingestion, and at least one of the following physiological indicators: (1) slurred speech, (2) incoordination, (3) unsteady gait, (4) nystagmus, (5) flushed face. In addition, at least one of the following psychological signs must exist: (1) mood change, (2) irritability, (3) loquacity, (4) impaired attention. Maladaptive behavior may include aggressiveness and impaired judgment. In addition, the individual's normal behavior may be accentuated or altered. Someone who is usually paranoid may experience an increase in the paranoid ideation and therefore in the demonstrable paranoid behavior. Another individual who is usually quiet and withdrawn may experience an increase in social interactions when under the influence of alcohol.[9]

DSM-III also mentions that despite the fact that alcohol is a central nervous system depressant, initially as one becomes intoxicated, the behavioral effects that are demonstrated may be otherwise. Therefore, an individual may appear uncommonly animated, and even hyperactive. She may feel unusually intelligent and experience a rare sense of well-being. As the blood alcohol level increases, however, the individual may experience mental slowing, depression, withdrawal, and dullness and eventually even lose consciousness. Intoxication usually occurs with blood alcohol levels between 100 and 200 mg/dL. Death can occur with levels above 400 mg/dL. The latter occurs either by directly depressing the individual's respiration, or by aspiration of vomitus.[9]

DSM-III mentions that at least half of all highway fatalities involve either a driver or a pedestrian who has ingested alcohol. It also mentions that more than half of all murderers and their victims are thought to have been intoxicated at the time the act occurred. Many individuals who commit suicide are intoxicated at the time of their death.

As mentioned earlier, the elderly individual often comes to medical attention with given symptoms of neglect. Not mentioned earlier were sunburn and frostbite. In addition, the possibility of depression of the immune system has been entertained, and it is thought that infections may be more prevalent in individuals who abuse alcohol.[9]

There is a great variability in the blood levels of alcohol at which a patient becomes intoxicated. DSM-III notes that some individuals become intoxicated with blood levels as low as 30 mg/dL, whereas other individuals appear unintoxicated at levels of 150 mg/dL. In part, and at times, this may be due to the phenomenon of tolerance, mentioned earlier. An individual who has developed tolerance may not appear intoxicated after having consumed alcohol over the course of many hours. In addition, the severity of the episode varies, depending on how quickly the alcohol was consumed, whether it was consumed in the presence of food, and the type of alcoholic beverage ingested.

According to DSM-III, a diagnosis of alcohol idiosyncratic intoxication is made in individuals who demonstrate a marked behavioral change secondary to a recent ingestion of alcohol, although the amount of alcohol would be insufficient to cause similar changes in other individuals.

The alcohol withdrawal syndrome is described in numerous textbooks of medicine, and will not be pursued in depth here. According to DSM-III, a withdrawal syndrome is diagnosed when there is a cessation or decrease in the amount of alcohol consumed and when tremors of the hands, tongue, and eyelids are noticed. It is accompanied by nausea and vomiting, malaise, and autonomic hyperactivity, as demonstrated by tachycardia, diaphoresis, elevated blood pressure, anxiety, depressed mood, irritability, and orthostatic hypotension. Patients may suffer from gastritis, impaired sleep, and hallucinations—visual, auditory, and tactile. The withdrawal syndrome may be complicated by epilepsy. Most clinicians, therefore, may medicate patients who have a history of seizure disorder to prevent the occurrence of seizures. Patients may also exhibit malnourishment, depression, fatigue, and other physical illnesses. According to DSM-III, a differential diagnosis should include barbiturate or sedative withdrawal, hypoglycemia, diabetic ketoacidosis, and essential tremor.[9]

The authors in DSM-III consider alcohol withdrawal delirium as a separate diagnostic entity. It should be diagnosed in the presence of a delirium that occurs within 1 week of the decrease or cessation of alcohol use. This disorder is accompanied by autonomic hyperactivity. In the past it has been called delirium tremens.[2] According to DSM-III, alcohol withdrawal delirium usually occurs after approximately 5 to 15 years of heavy alcohol ingestion and is therefore most often first diagnosed in patients between the ages of 30 and 50 years.

Another diagnostic category in DSM-III is alcohol hallucinosis. This is diagnosed in the presence of organic hallucinosis, with the presence of auditory hallucinations, which develop shortly after the decrease or cessation of heavy alcohol use, in the patient who is dependent on alcohol. It usually develops within 48 hours of the decrease in use. No clouding of consciousness is present.

Intoxication can occur with substances other than alcohol. Barbiturates and sedative-hypnotics cause intoxication similar to alcohol intoxication. Likewise, the withdrawal syndromes are similar, as are withdrawal deliriums. Also described in DSM-III is a barbiturate or sedative-hypnotic amnestic disorder.

In the amnestic syndrome the essential feature is impairment in the short- and long-term memory, which occurs without a clouding of consciousness. This diagnostic entity should be distinguished from a delirium or dementia, which have both been described earlier.[9]

REFERENCES

1. Cohen GD: Approach to the geriatric patient, Symposium on Psychiatry in Internal Medicine. *Med Clin North Am* 1977;61:855–866.

2. Goodstein RK: The diagnosis and treatment of elderly patients: Some practical guidelines. *Hosp Community Psychiatry* 1980;31:19–21.

3. Steuer J, Austin E: Family abuse of the elderly. *J Am Geriatr Soc* 1980;28:372–375.

4. Task Force Sponsored by the National Institute on Aging: Senility reconsidered. *JAMA* 1980;244:261–262.

5. Craig TJ, Lin SP: Mortality among elderly psychiatric patients: Basis for preventive intervention. *J Am Geriatr Soc* 1981;29:181.

6. Reed DM, Sadock BJ, Kaplan HI, et al (eds): *The Sexual Experience*. Baltimore, Williams & Wilkins, 1976.

7. Bachman GA, Mijuta JJ: The emotional impact of the menopause. *Postgrad Obstet Gynecol* 1985;5:1–5.

8. Solomon K: The depressed patient: Social antecedents of psychopathological changes in the elderly. *J Am Geriatr Soc* 1981;29:14–18.

9. Grossberg GT, Nakra BRS: Treatment of depression in the elderly. *Compr Ther* 1986;12(10):16–22.

10. American Psychiatric Association: *Diagnostic and Statistical Manual of Mental Disorders,* ed 3. Washington, DC, American Psychiatric Association, 1980, pp 101–203.

11. American Psychiatric Association: *Diagnostic and Statistical Manual of Mental Disorders,* ed 3—rev. Washington, DC, American Psychiatric Association, 1987.

12. Rodin G, Voshart K: Depression in the medically ill: An overview. *Am J Psychiatry* 1986;143:696.

13. Askinazi C, Weintraub RJ, Karamouz N: Elderly depressed females as a possible subgroup of patients responsive to methylphenidate. *J Clin Psychiatry* 1986;47:467–469.

14. Kantor SJ, Glassman AH: *Psychopharmacology of Aging: The Use of Tricyclic Antidepressant Drugs in Geriatric Patients.* Spectrum Publications, 1980, pp 99–117.

15. Georgotas A, McCue RE, Hapworth W, et al: Comparative efficacy and safety of MAOIs versus TCAs in treating depression in the elderly. *Biol Psychiatry* 1986;21:1155–1166.

16. Katzman R: Alzheimer's disease. *N Engl J Med* 1986;314:964–970.

17. Louden DM, Wray SR, Melville GN: Common psychological illness in the elderly. *West Indian Med J* 1985;34:148–153.

18. Raskind MA, Risse SC: Adverse effects of antipsychotic drugs in the elderly. *J Clin Psychiatry* 1985;46:17–22.

19. Volavka J: Late-onset schizophrenia: A review. *Compr Psychiatry* 1985;2:148–156.

20. Turnbull JM, Turnbull SK: Management of specific anxiety disorders in the elderly. *Geriatrics* 1985;40:75–81.

21. Wattis JP: Alcohol problems in the elderly. *J Am Geriatr Soc* 1981;29:131–134.

Chapter 10

Musculoskeletal Problems

Sheldon D. Solomon

INTRODUCTION

The aged woman may present to her gynecologist with any of the 100 conditions that constitute a textbook of rheumatology.[1] However, knowledge of a much smaller number of common entities will enable the gynecologist to diagnose about 95% of patients, leading to adequate management.

CLASSIFICATION OF MUSCULOSKELETAL PROBLEMS

These conditions may be divided pathogenetically, as seen in Table 10-1. It behooves the physician to appropriate the patient's musculoskeletal (M-S) syndrome into the correct category, since the prognosis and management programs among these categories vary widely. For example, the patient whose neck and shoulder pain is caused by polymyalgia rheumatica (PMR) will be managed entirely different than if her pain is secondary to degenerative, cervical arthritis.

DIFFERENTIAL DIAGNOSIS

In the differential diagnosis of these conditions, the basic history and physical examination are the most important tools. In most cases the clinical evaluation allows for grouping of the patient in one of the categories in Table 10-1. Then further testing with laboratory or x-ray may be needed to pinpoint the exact diagnosis. It is also helpful to attempt to determine the anatomical site of the patient's pain (Table 10-2). Often it is easy, even for the untrained physician, to differentiate an axial syndrome as osteoarthritis of the lumbar spine from rheumatoid arthritis (RA) affecting the hands and feet. More difficult may be the

Table 10-1 Pathogenetic Classification of Rheumatic Disorders

1. Degenerative or "wear-and-tear" disorders
   a. Osteoarthritis
   b. Low-back syndrome
   c. Bursitis, tendinitis
2. Metabolic
   a. Osteoporosis
   b. Paget's disease
3. Inflammatory
   a. Polymyalgia rheumatica
   b. Crystal deposition diseases
      (1) Gout
      (2) Pseudogout
   c. Rheumatoid arthritis
   d. Systemic lupus erythematosus
4. Neoplastic
   a. Bone tumors
      (1) Multiple myeloma
      (2) Metastasis from breast, lung, etc
   b. Peripheral effects of breast or pelvic malignancy
      (1) Dermatomyositis
5. Neuropsychiatric
   a. Fibromyalgia

---

distinction between a cervical radiculopathy and a carpal tunnel syndrome: both cause similar symptoms (ie, numbness and paresthesias in the hand), yet both require very different management.

Interview

The most critical tool in arriving at an appropriate diagnosis is the interview. Sir William Osler once said, "Listen to the patient; they will reveal their diagnosis." In evaluation of musculoskeletal pain this is particularly true. All too often the clinician is misled by a laboratory or radiographic abnormality that may have little to do with the patient's complaints. For example, the patient with PMR will often have radiographs of the cervical spine that demonstrate osteoarthritis simply because of the patient's advanced age; yet the pain syndrome has nothing to do with these radiographic abnormalities.

In evaluating the pain, first determine whether it is unifocal or multifocal. Often this is not simple, since unifocal pain syndrome may refer pain to other areas, hence mimicking a multifocal problem. An example of this would be a trigger point secondary to fibromyalgia that could cause pain in the scapula, shoulder, axilla, arm, and anterior chest wall. Next one needs to evaluate the *quality* of the pain. A dull, achy pain across the knuckles aggravated by motion suggests

Table 10-2 Anatomical Site of Rheumatic Disorders

1. Axial
   a. Cervical
   b. Thoracic
   c. Lumbosacral
2. Peripheral
   a. Articular
   b. Nonarticular
      (1) Tendon
      (2) Ligament
      (3) Bursa
      (4) Myofascial
      (5) Nerve compression

---

inflammation of the joints, whereas a burning, tingling in the hand, sometimes worse at night while sleeping, suggests a nerve compression syndrome. Is the pain made better with rest? Most degenerative and metabolic problems such as osteoporosis would certainly be better with rest. However, the M-S pain of malignancy is not helped with rest and actually is worsened. Is there associated stiffness with the M-S complaint? Although almost all types of rheumatism have some degree of stiffness, inflammatory conditions such as RA are characterized as being associated with prolonged stiffness after a period of inactivity. In the morning this stiffness generally lasts for longer than one hour, whereas the stiffness of "gelling" that is associated with a degenerative disorder or osteoarthritis usually lasts for five to ten minutes in the morning. Another associated symptom to evaluate in the interview is fatigue. With most degenerative or wear-and-tear disorders, such as bursitis and low-back pain, there are no associated systemic symptoms such as fatigue. However, in inflammatory conditions such as RA, PMR, and systemic lupus erythematosus (SLE), fatigue is usually an integral part of the patient's complaints, and usually comes on a few hours after arising in the morning. This is in contrast to the fatigue that is associated with neuropsychiatric musculoskeletal pain such as in fibromyalgia. Here the patient often awakens fatigued and stays tired the entire day. In all patients with M-S pain the information above must be obtained. Occasionally the history has to be expanded, depending on the clinical situation. For example, if PMR is suspected, the physician should inquire whether the patient has temporal headaches or blurred vision; these complaints may suggest temporal arteritis, which is seen in about 10% to 20% of PMR. If malignancy is suspected, inquiry about weight loss, anorexia, or fever may also be important.

Physical Examination

At this point, after taking a history, the gynecologist should have a strong suspicion about the patient's problem. If the patient is complaining about a painful peripheral joint, examine it for swelling, increased heat, erythema, or loss of mobility (LOM). In inflammatory conditions (RA) the joint will be boggy or spongy to palpation, whereas in degenerative arthritis the joint will demonstrate hard, bony swelling. A classic example is the Heberden's nodes involving the distal interphalangeal (DIP) joints, representing degenerative arthritis or osteoarthritis. Evaluate whether the patient's pain is emanating from the joint or from a neighboring soft tissue structure (ie, tendon or bursa). As far as axial complaints are concerned, the physical examination helps more in excluding problems that refer or mimic back pain. A patient with an abdominal aneurysm causing back pain may have unequal femoral pulses or a bounding, pulsatile abdominal mass. A patient with midthoracic or right scapular pain may have tenderness to deep palpation in the right upper quadrant, making the clinician suspicious of gallbladder disease as the cause.

SPECIFIC RHEUMATIC DISEASES OF THE ELDERLY WOMAN

Degenerative Arthritis or Osteoarthritis

Osteoarthritis (OA) is the most common type of arthritis in the elderly and is almost inevitable as the aging process proceeds. Obesity, wear and tear, and injuries influence the location, frequency, and severity. Even genetic factors are important, as demonstrated by familial patterns.[2]

Clinical Course

The patient will usually complain of insidious, dull, aching pain aggravated by exercise, eased with rest, associated with transient stiffness in the morning (gelling) that is relieved by motion or a hot shower in 10 to 20 minutes. These symptoms may occur in one, a few, or several areas of the body. The most common areas are listed in Table 10-3. Other areas, if affected by OA, usually have had preexisting injury or another preexisting rheumatic disease. Examination will reveal crepitus and pain on range of motion (ROM). There may be mild heat and erythema, since inflammation does play a small but important role in the development of OA.[3] Bony swelling is noted secondary to joint space narrowing and subsequent bony proliferation. This swelling is most classically seen in the DIP and proximal interphalangeal (PIP) joints of the hands, where it is called Heberden's and Bouchard's nodes, respectively. Although severe gait disorders may occur secondary to OA of the hip, knee, or spine, no real systemic or constitutional symptoms should occur. Laboratory tests should be normal, including a complete blood count (CBC) and biochemical evaluation. Most important, the erythrocyte sedimentation rate (ESR) should be in the normal range. The ESR

Table 10-3 Common Sites of Osteoarthritis

1. Spine
   a. Lumbar
   b. Cervical
2. Hand
   a. Distal interphalangeal joint
   b. Proximal interphalangeal joint
   c. First carpal–metacarpal joint—thumb
3. Hip
4. Knee
5. First metatarsophalangeal

---

is a valuable tool to exclude significant disease processes such as RA, PMR, and malignancy. However, the ESR does rise in healthy individuals as they age.[4] Radiographs will usually reveal the characteristic joint space narrowing, sclerosis, and osteophyte formation. OA can be quite disabling when it involves the base of the thumb (first carpal–metacarpal joint), the hip, the knee, or the spine. In the neck the proximity of the cervical nerve roots to the joints of Luschka makes them vulnerable to compression secondary to degenerative changes.[5] The patient may exhibit pain, paresthesias, and weakness in her upper extremity. Occasionally impingement on the cord can lead to a myelopathy, resulting in a severe gait disorder with little pain. If an elderly woman complains of difficulty walking and has evidence of hyperflexia and a positive Babinski's sign, cervical OA would be the most common cause, even in the absence of severe neck pain.

Treatment Program

Although the management of OA does not produce dramatic responses, the results can be quite rewarding to both patient and physician. First, realistic goals must be established. Frustration occurs when the patient expects a "cure." Goals that must be established include (a) decreasing pain, (b) improving function, and (c) preventing further joint destruction by joint protection. Pharmacologic management is discussed in the last section of this chapter. Proper rest is obviously important, particularly with weight-bearing joints such as low back, hip, or knee. The patient's daily activities must be reviewed and modifications suggested so as to minimize step walking or prolonged walking, for example, moving the washer and dryer from the basement to the first floor to avoid carrying heavy loads up steps. Also, an hour or two of rest in the afternoon should be introduced into the patient's program. A non–weight-bearing exercise program is also essential in management. Such a program is usually initiated by a physiotherapist, who can teach the patient nonstressful ROM and isometric muscle strengthening to prevent muscle atrophy, a common sequela of a painful joint. The therapist will also instruct the patient in proper use of local heat to be used to help "loosen up" during exercises. Joint protection is obviously helped by rest, but specific measures should also be suggested. Proper use of a cane will protect an osteoarthritic knee or hip, whereas using a wide-bodied pen will protect an osteoarthritic thumb joint. In order to obtain compliance, the patient should be educated in the above by not only the physician, but also a physiotherapist. Weight reduction must be stressed, particularly in obese patients with OA of the back or knee. Although these patients claim that they cannot lose weight because of lack of exercise, an aquatic program on a regular basis will usually *not* aggravate the joint and will help to expend calories. In a patient with significant pain unresponsive to conservative measures, reconstructive joint surgery, including total knee and hip prostheses, can reverse the pain and immobility.

The portions of the spine usually affected by OA include the neck and low back. In the neck the nerve roots exiting the intervertebral foramina are often compressed by spurs or degenerative disks, leading to pain radiating down the arm associated with paresthesias and weakness. This author has found immobilization with a soft cervical collar, in conjunction with intermittent cervical traction and other physiotherapy modalities, to be extremely effective in improving this condition. Most patients respond to these conservative measures, and surgery is almost never required. Low-back pain involving the lumbar spine probably reflects degenerative change involving disks, the facet joints, paraspinal ligaments, and muscles. Nerve root compression usually occurs at L4-L5 or L5-S1 in 95% of patients and, once again, responds to conservative measures such as bed rest, traction, mild exercise, and bracing. Spinal stenosis, a variant of the above, usually arises from proliferative spurring of the intervertebral joints, producing a pseudoclaudication syndrome. Patients complain of pain and numbness on standing, relieved by rest. This syndrome does not respond well to conservative measures and often requires a surgical approach.

Osteoporosis

The clinical state of osteoporosis is best defined as that in which skeletal bone is normal in nature but deficient in amount or mass. The principal site of morbidity is the thoracolumbar spine, where vertebral compression fractures occur in 25% of white females over age 65.[6] Other sites with a propensity to fracture include the hip, distal head of the radius, and ribs. Is osteoporosis a disease, or merely an expression of age? Because 80% of white women over age 65 have radiographic bone demineralization, it is difficult to define it as a disease. This figure will probably be found to be higher as the newer, more sensitive studies, such as dual photon absorptiometry, begin to be used clinically.

Pathogenesis

Bone is a dynamic organ system that undergoes a lifelong process of remodeling. Osteoblasts that form bone are tightly coupled with osteoclast-mediated matrix resorption and mineral release. Bone resorption is known to be enhanced by the aging process and estrogen withdrawal, whereas dietary intake of calcium and intestinal absorption decrease with age.[7]

Differential Diagnosis and Laboratory Testing

In the vast majority of white, postmenopausal females a spontaneous fracture of the vertebral body will be secondary to idiopathic, senile, or postmenopausal osteoporosis. Probably a few, simple laboratory studies should be done, particularly in a black female, to screen for rare causes of radiographic bone demineralization (osteopenia). A biochemical profile will help to rule out the rare case of hyperparathyroidism, in which case calcium and alkaline phosphatase levels would be elevated. The presence of anemia coupled with a very elevated Westergren ESR should make the clinician suspicious of multiple myeloma in a patient with bone pain. As mentioned earlier, most patients will have no other etiology except age and status postmenopausal. In a patient with a radiographic fracture it is almost impossible to determine the age without a bone scan. The scan will show increased uptake or activity only during the early stages of the fracture. A history of chronic steroid use may be a contributing factor in the pathogenesis.

Clinical Picture

Vertebral compression or crush fractures are the most disabling feature of osteoporosis. These often occur with mild activities, such as bending down to pick up a light object. Microfractures may occur chronically, resulting in a "dowager hump" accompanied by a loss of height. Actual nerve compression is rare. Spontaneous resolution of symptoms occurs gradually with fracture healing in 2 or 3 months. If symptoms persist or a bone scan remains "hot," then entities such as myeloma or other malignancies must be considered. In the osteoporotic patient femoral neck fractures may occur with mild trauma, such as sitting down on a hard chair or a minor collision.

Management

If a patient develops a vertebral fracture, care is directed toward control of pain. It is unusual to see cord compression with these types of fractures, but bed rest is mandated by the degree of pain. Sometimes hospitalization for complete rest, pelvic traction, and narcotic administration is necessary for patients with severe pain. Although bed rest increases bone resorption, this author has found that healing of the fracture, which is the immediate problem, occurs much faster with complete rest. As healing begins after 1 to 2 weeks, a program of supervised exercises under a physiotherapist is begun. In most cases bracing is not required.

Once the acute fracture has healed, the focus of management becomes the prevention of new fractures. A recent study[8] revealed that a combination of calcium, sodium fluoride, and estrogen therapy dramatically reduced the recurrent fracture rate as compared with a control group. Vitamin D in large doses did not seem to help; because it may cause hypercalcemia or hypercalciuria, it is not recommended by this author.

In the postmenopausal, asymptomatic geriatric woman, what program should be instituted? Although good epidemiologic data is lacking, a reasonable estimate is that a 60-year-old American white woman has a 25% to 50% risk of sustaining one or more fractures in her remaining years. Table 10-4 lists the factors that increase the patient's risks.

To begin, every patient should be instructed to become less sedentary. A daily walk or exercise program is essential. Calcium has been well documented to increase bone mass, decrease fracture rate, and produce positive calcium balance.[9] Each geriatric patient should receive an oral calcium supplement of at least 1.0 g of elemental calcium daily. Calcium in the form of calcium carbonate (40% calcium) is probably the most convenient form of therapy, since fewer tablets are needed (four tablets, 0.5 g each). In patients with multiple risk factors, three or four tablets are needed. Another convenient form of calcium is antacid tablets (Tums), which are also calcium carbonate. Vitamin D should not be given, since it may cause hypercalciuria. It may be used in small doses, 400 IU (international units), for nutritional balance.

Hormones. The role of estrogens for the asymptomatic geriatric woman is still controversial. The risk of endometrial carcinoma is greatly reduced by addition of progestogen to the estrogen therapy. Which patients should receive just calcium or a combination of calcium plus hormones currently has to be individualized, depending on each patient's number of risk factors. For example, an active, heavy-boned black woman probably requires only calcium supplementation.

Table 10-4 Risk Factors for Osteoporotic Fractures

- Slender build
- Early natural or surgically induced menopause
- Excessive alcohol consumption
- Sedentary life style
- Low calcium intake
- Exogenous steroid therapy or Cushing's disease
- Rheumatoid arthritis or other disabling types of arthritis
- Thyrotoxicosis

However, a slender patient who consumes alcohol heavily, has rheumatoid arthritis, and is on steroids should, no doubt, be on calcium plus hormones.

Fluoride Treatment. Doses of 40 to 60 mg daily of sodium fluoride has definitely been shown to decrease fracture rate.[8] However, large double-blind studies have not yet been completed. Also, side effects such as nausea and bone pain in a significant number of patients should temper our enthusiasm for its use in asymptomatic patients.

Is radiographic osteoporosis without fracture a cause of chronic back pain? The fact that some of these patients seem to respond to osteoporotic therapy suggests that there is a connection. Therefore, it is worth a trial of calcium supplementation, hormonal therapy, and, possibly, sodium fluoride.

Paget's Disease

Although Paget's disease is seen more commonly in men, its incidence is 3% in patients over 60, so that gynecologists should be aware of this entity. This bone abnormality results from coupling of excessive bone resorption with the rapid and disorganized deposition of fibrous connective tissue and trabecular bone, which is larger, softer, more deformable, and more easily fractured than normal bone.

Clinical Picture

An important consideration is that *80%* of people with radiographic abnormalities of Paget's disease are asymptomatic and have no clinical complaints or findings.[10] This is critical, since many patients presenting with low-back pain secondary to OA may be thought to have a more significant clinical problem if the radiographs reveal Paget's. Paget's disease as the sole cause of back pain appears to be rare. The diagnosis is secured by the radiographic abnormalities coupled with an elevated serum alkaline phosphatase. A bone scan will reveal increased uptake in pagetoid bone.

Other areas of pagetoid bone, as in hip or knee joint, may be painful secondary to the degenerative arthritis that may accompany Paget's. These patients can be managed with acetylsalicylic acid (ASA) or other nonsteroidal anti-inflammatory agents (NSAIDs). Although there is specific treatment for the disease process, this is usually withheld in most patients. Drugs such as diphosphonates, calcitonin, and mithramycin should be reserved for patients with severe complications of the disease, such as spinal involvement with paraplegias, severe skull involvement with platybasia, severe deformities, and hearing loss (Paget's of the petrous ridge). At this point the gynecologist should obtain either rheumatologic or orthopedic consultation, since these drugs are potent and have the potential to produce a number of side effects.

Once again, it must be stressed that all too often a patient presents with a minor M-S problem (ie, bursitis)—if x-rays are obtained, Paget's may be reported. Therapy here should be directed to the bursitis. If the patient improves, then she has asymptomatic Paget's disease, which would require *no* specific therapy.

Polymyalgia Rheumatica

PMR is probably the most common type of *inflammatory* rheumatism seen in the geriatric female population. In addition, it is easily treated and its prognosis is very good; so all gynecologists who care for elderly women should be able to recognize and diagnose it.

Clinical Picture

These patients have a characteristic clinical profile. The interview reveals that PMR begins in most patients rather abruptly with diffuse aching in the proximal muscles, particularly the neck, shoulders, upper arms, low back, buttocks, hips, and thighs. Stiffness, particularly with inactivity, is particularly severe. Often the patient becomes almost totally incapacitated. Although patients attribute their functional limitation to weakness, it is usually due to muscle pain. These patients also have systemic complaints consisting of fatigue, anorexia, and weight loss. In contrast, the physical examination reveals little. Once again, these patients appear weak, but it is really due to muscle soreness that they display difficulty getting out of a chair, lifting their legs into the stirrups, or raising their arms over their head. Although this is a *non*articular form of rheumatism, occasionally these patients do reveal synovitis of wrists and knees.[11]

Diagnosis

The diagnosis is made clinically. The laboratory is used to exclude other entities that can mimick PMR. Laboratory studies will reveal *normal* muscle enzymes such as serum glutamic oxaloacetic transaminase and creatine phosphokinase, normal thyroid studies, negative antinuclear antibodies, and normal biochemical profiles. The only abnormal test, and one that, for all intents and purposes, is required for confirmation, is elevation of the Westergren ESR. Usually this is greater than 60 mm/hour, but levels greater than 100 mm/hour are not unusual. The triad of the clinical picture of nonarticular rheumatism in a woman over age 60 with an ESR greater than 60 mm/hour is most consistent with a diagnosis of PMR.

Therapy

A therapeutic trial is warranted if the clinical picture described above exists. An initial dose of 15 mg of prednisone should produce a dramatic response, usually within a couple of days. If improvement does not occur, then the diagnosis of PMR must be questioned and further diagnostic workup and consultation are required. This author usually begins to lower the dose after ten days to doses under 10 mg/day. An attempt is made to use the minimal amount of steroid possible (ie, 3 or 4 mg daily). Usually the ESR will drop precipitously (ie, from 120 mm/hour down to 60 mm/hour); however, no attempt to "treat the sed rate" should be made, since often the patient feels fine even though the ESR does not come down to "normal levels."

Prognosis

Generally the prognosis is good. Patients require very low dose prednisone for 1 to 5 years, and then this can be discontinued and the patient remains asymptomatic.

It is important to keep in mind that less than 10% of these patients may have underlying temporal arteritis (TA).[12] Local manifestations secondary to inflammation of the temporal artery and its branches may include unilateral blindness and severe unilateral headache. Often TA may produce a dramatic systemic picture of fever of unknown origin, severe anemia, and/or weight loss. If this entity is suspected, appropriate emergency consultation with ophthalmologist, neurologist, or rheumatologist is necessitated. These patients require high-dose prednisone (greater than 60 mg daily) and usually develop many of the severe side effects of steroids, such as diabetes mellitus, vertebral collapse, and increased susceptibility to infection.

Rheumatoid Arthritis

It is important for the gynecologist to be aware of the early manifestations of RA. Often the gynecologist is the first physician to examine these patients. It is imperative to diagnose RA early so that the inflammatory response leading to joint destruction, deformity, and functional limitations may be diminished. In one clinic 34% of the patients with RA were over age 60.[13]

Clinical Picture

The onset is usually gradual but may occur acutely, involving many small and large joints in a symmetrical fashion. The most common presentation involves the hands. Here it is important to differentiate RA from OA. RA is usually a proximal distribution involving the wrist, metacarpal phalangeal (MCP), and PIPs, whereas OA usually is more distal, involving the DIPs and occasionally the PIPs. OA does not affect the wrist, but does involve, as mentioned earlier, the first carpal–metacarpal, causing pain at the radial aspect of the wrist (at the base of the thumb).

The inflammatory process produces boggy, warm, swollen joints, whereas OA produces the hard, bony abnormalities discussed previously (Heberden's nodes). Patients with RA normally complain of prolonged morning stiffness (usually at least one hour) as compared with the transient stiffness of OA.

The laboratory cannot definitely make a diagnosis of RA. The rheumatoid factor (RF) determined by the latex fixation test may be positive in up to 35% of patients who do not have rheumatic diseases.[14] Not only is this method not specific, but it is also a poor screening device. In early cases under one year the study is usually negative in greater than 60%. A more important study, although nonspecific, is the ESR, as alluded to earlier. If the physician is suspicious clinically of RA, an elevated ESR would strengthen the diagnosis.

Treatment

At this point basic management consisting of rest, exercises, and medication could be instituted. The patient must be instructed in the importance of proper daily rest periods. Ten to 12 hours of bed rest are essential. A proper exercise program must also be performed daily to prevent the muscle atrophy and flexion contractures that are so common in this disease. This can easily be taught to patients by a physiotherapist. Water exercise therapy (WET) is an excellent method to exercise inflamed joints without damaging them. This is particularly true if weight-bearing joints are involved, as the knees. Pharmacologic therapy with proper doses of ASA or NSAIDs is also indicated. More than 50% of patients will respond to this regimen. If the disease progresses, then rheumatologic referral is indicated for consideration for more potent therapies, such as intra-articular steroid injections and gold or methotrexate therapy. Finally, pamphlets and information about support groups and other aides for these patients can be obtained by contacting the local chapter of the Arthritis Foundation.

Systemic Lupus Erythematosus

SLE is another inflammatory disease characterized by the production of autoantibodies that participate in immunologic tissue damage. Multiple organ systems may be involved, particularly the joints, skin, kidneys, microcirculation, nervous system, and serous membranes. Women are affected nine times more frequently than males. Although the highest incidence is between the second and fourth decades, it can be seen at any age (I have cared for one woman whose onset was at age 84).

The clinical findings are protean. The most common manifestations involve the joints and skin. In more than 90% of lupus patients one of these two organ systems is involved. The arthritis differs from RA in that the most common presentation is really arthralgias and myalgias. To a lesser degree, patients present with a mild synovitis. Rarely do patients have deforming arthritis as in RA. Systemic complaints are prevalent, including extreme fatigue, often chronic fevers, and weight loss. The classic finding is an erythematous rash in a butterfly distribution over the nose and cheeks. Another common dermatologic manifestation is a maculopapular erythematous rash in exposed areas, such as the face, chest, and arms. About 25% of patients give a history of precipitation of either rash or systemic symptoms after sun exposure. This information is helpful in establishing the diagnosis. Because of the many organ systems that may be involved, the gynecologist should refer these patients to a rheumatologist if he or she is suspicious of SLE.

Regional Syndromes

Regional syndromes or nonsystemic M-S problems are common in the elderly female. The most common sites are listed in Table 10-5.

Clinical Course

All of these entities share pain as their common denominator. Patients may present in a very acute stage in severe pain or with a chronic mild discomfort. None of these patients should have any accompanying systemic complaints, such as weight loss, fever, or fatigue. Usually the pain is aggravated by exercising the afflicted area and made better by rest. For example, a patient presenting with a bicipital tendinitis will relate how painful it is to attempt to comb her hair, but if she keeps her arm down, the pain is minimal. Some knowledge of M-S anatomy is required so that during the physical examination, the gynecologist can reproduce the pain by palpating over the anatomical structure.

Management

Generally the management of all of these entities is similar. If it is an acute situation, then local application of ice often dulls the pain. For more chronic cases, wet heat, such as a bath or wet heating pad, is useful. The area involved must be rested. For example, if a weight-bearing structure such as the trochanteric bursa is involved, then the patient should be instructed to walk as little as possible, particularly steps. The only exception to this is pathology involving the shoulder.

Table 10-5 Common Sites of Regional Syndromes in Geriatric Women

1. Shoulder
   a. Subdeltoid bursitis
   b. Bicipital tendinitis
2. Elbow
   a. Lateral epicondylitis
   b. Medial epicondylitis
   c. Olecranon bursitis
3. Hand and wrist
   a. de Quervain's tenosynovitis
   b. Flexor tendinitis (trigger finger)
   c. Carpal tunnel syndrome
4. Hip
   a. Trochanteric bursitis
   b. Iliopsoas bursitis
5. Knee
   a. Anserina bursitis
6. Foot and ankle
   a. Achilles tendinitis
   b. Plantar fasciitis
   c. Mechanical metatarsalgia

Here, too much rest will lead to a periarthritis (frozen shoulder). To prevent this the patient should be instructed in simple pendulum exercises, performed by allowing the arm to rotate in a circle hanging down with the body flexed at the waist. Pharmacologic management includes NSAIDs and analgesics. If the condition does not improve, the patient should receive a series of injections of deposteroid into the involved structures concomitantly with physiotherapy. The majority of these patients do well, and it behooves the gynecologist to have patience and *primum non nocere*.

Crystal Deposition Diseases

Gout

It is important for the gynecologist to realize the following: (a) Gout, although rare in a menstruating woman, in the postmenopausal woman begins to be seen as commonly as in men the same age. (b) Gout, by definition, is the inflammatory response incited by the deposition of crystals within the joint space. It is not an M-S pain associated with a high uric acid.

About 50% will present with an acute severe inflammatory arthritis affecting the big toe (podagra) or dorsum of foot. The attack is often monoarticular, but occasionally a few joints are involved. The pain is excruciating. Examination reveals a tense, hot, swollen, painful joint. To make a definitive diagnosis, aspiration of the joint and identification of sodium urate crystals under a first order-compensated polarizing microscope is needed. In the absence of joint fluid or the polarizing microscope, the gynecologist may try an NSAID such as indomethacin (Indocin), 100 to 150 mg/day, for a few days. Remember that in the differential diagnosis of an acute monoarticular arthritis is a septic joint, so that if there is any suspicion for this (ie, leukocytosis, fever greater than 100 °F, staphylococcal infection elsewhere in the body), joint aspiration and synovial fluid studies are mandatory. If the patient has repeated attacks, once the acute process quiets down, a regimen consisting of one tablet of colchicine, 0.6 mg daily, plus allopurinol, 300 to 600 mg daily, is instituted. The colchicine is discontinued when the serum uric acid is stabilized at a low level.

Pseudogout

This entity may either mimic gout or be entirely asymptomatic. Once again, the acute attack is treated with an NSAID such as Indocin. During the intercritical period there is no treatment, since there is no known drug to bring down the calcium pyrophosphate level in pseudogout like allopurinol lowers the uric acid level in gout.[15]

MANAGEMENT OF THE ELDERLY FEMALE WITH PHARMACOLOGIC THERAPY

Analgesics

Simple analgesics, such as acetaminophen, low-dose aspirin (six to eight a day), and propoxyphene are helpful for the patient with mild, intermittent pain. Propoxyphene seems to work better with acetaminophen in chronic arthritic pain, although propoxyphene in other studies has been shown to be no better than a placebo.[16] Also, the elderly should be warned about using alcohol with propoxyphene, since serious respiratory depression has been reported.[16] Low-dose NSAIDs such as ibuprofen, fenoprofen, naproxen sodium, and diflunisal have been approved by the Food and Drug Administration (FDA) for analgesic therapy not only in musculoskeletal problems, but also for all pain syndromes.

Steroids

The gynecologist should rarely have to prescribe steroids. The only disease mentioned in the text above for which patients should receive systemic steroids is

PMR. Steroids may be given in crystalline form occasionally into the joint or a surrounding soft tissue problem; otherwise, there is little place for them in the gynecologist's armamentarium.

Nonsteroidal Anti-inflammatory Drugs

NSAIDs are valuable agents in the treatment of most of the rheumatic conditions discussed above. The goal in their use is to reduce inflammation, hence relieving pain and improving function. This is critical in the elderly female, particularly if she is attempting to live alone and remain independent. These agents seem to work by decreasing the body's supply of prostaglandins, which are active mediators in the inflammatory response (probably the reason ibuprofen works so effectively in menstrual cramps). However, prostaglandins are also needed by the body for other functions. For example, with aging, there is a decrease in the renal plasma flow probably secondary to renal arterionephrosclerosis. Prostaglandin E_2 acts as a compensatory mechanism in these patients, increasing renal blood supply. Hence the gynecologist would have to be cautious in giving an elderly woman an NSAID because it will decrease not only prostaglandins that decrease the inflammatory response, but also those that are needed as a compensatory good effect on the kidney.

At least 15 NSAIDs are available (aspirin is included here), and several are waiting in the wings (see Table 10-6). Not listed are benoxaprofen (Oraflex), zomepirac (Zomax), phenylbutazone (Butazolidin, Azolid), and oxyphenbutazone (Tanderil, Oxalid). All of these latter drugs are currently not allowed by the FDA except phenylbutazone, which is allowed but probably has no place in a gynecologic practice.

The gynecologist, in using these drugs in the elderly, must keep the following points in mind.

- Aging produces physiological changes that may affect drug disposition (ie, the renal blood flow mentioned earlier). There is also a reduced hepatic blood flow as well as decreased hepatic enzyme activity, leading to a greater accumulation of drug, possibly to toxic levels.
- In the United States, most clinical drug trials do not allow elderly patients in the protocol; hence when reading the product literature, this is not useful for very elderly women (over age 70).
- Also, these protocols usually exclude patients with mild renal or hepatic insufficiency as seen in the elderly.

Table 10-6 Nonsteroidal Anti-inflammatory Drugs

Generic Name	Trade Name
Salicylates	
aspirin	—
aspirin with buffering agent	Bufferin, Ascriptin
magnesium salicylate	Magan
salsalate	Disalcid
choline magnesium trisalicylate	Trilisate
diflunisal	Dolobid
Proprionic Acids	
ibuprofen	Advil, Nuprin, Motrin, Rufen
fenoprofen calcium	Nalfon
naproxen	Naprosyn
naproxen sodium	Anaprox
Indoleacetic Acids	
indomethacin	Indocin
tolmetin sodium	Tolectin
sulindac	Clinoril
Anthranilic Acid	
meclofenamate	Meclomen
Oxicam	
piroxicam	Feldene

Use of Specific Agents

Salicylates, which generally, in high doses, are the treatment of choice for inflammatory conditions, are more limited in the elderly. The major reason for this is that tinnitus, which is used as a guide to tell us when therapeutic levels of salicylate concentration have been reached, often does not occur in the elderly with underlying hearing loss.[17] Also, the elderly seem to develop more central nervous system manifestations such as confusion and vertigo.

This author favors drugs with twice-a-day dosing in elderly patients because such patients are usually not compliant with three times-a-day or four times-a-day drugs. Once-a-day programs, as with piroxicam, are more dangerous, since the patient may not realize she has taken her medication that day and take an extra one. This will lead to toxic levels in a short time. NSAIDs that are taken twice a day include Trilisate, Disalcid, and Dolobid (salicylates), Naprosyn, and Clinoril.

All of these NSAIDs may cause gastrointestinal upset, so they must be taken with food (ie, breakfast and dinner). This is another good reason to use twice-a-day drugs, since rarely will the elderly woman eat three or four times a day. All of the NSAIDs may cause edema and congestive heart failure, so the physician must instruct the patient not to use an excessive amount of salt. Table 10-7 gives the gynecologist some guidelines as to which drugs to use in the specific M-S condition with which the patient presents. Keep in mind that these guidelines are based on my bias, since good clinical trials comparing "apples to apples" are lacking. As shown in Table 10-7, NSAIDs' effects vary widely in different diseases; hence one of the reasons to make an appropriate diagnosis. For example, Indocin is tremendously effective in gout and certain types of OA, but is minimally effective in the majority of patients with RA.

Dosage

Here we must remember that the dosage recommended in the *Physician's Desk Reference* is the dose range tested in clinical trials with patients who are generally healthier and certainly younger. It is important to know the minimum–maximum daily dose of each drug. The physician should begin at the low end of the scale and then increase the dose accordingly. A generalization with most of these drugs is that the higher the dose, not only the more effective it is, but also the more toxic the drug becomes. For example, if an elderly patient complains of a chronic bad back, I may give her a prescription for Dolobid with the following directions: take 250 mg at breakfast and dinner for 1 week; then 500 mg at breakfast and 250 mg at dinner for 1 week; then 500 mg at breakfast and dinner. If the patient is frail, I probably will not go up to the maximum allowable dose of 1,500 mg. If the problem is acute, one may not have the luxury of time. For example, a woman presenting with acute podagra may receive the following prescription: take 50 mg of Indocin with breakfast, lunch, and dinner on the first day, 50 mg with breakfast

Table 10-7 NSAIDs in Specific M-S Problems

	Trilisate, Disalcid	Dolobid	Naprosyn	Clinoril	Indocin
OA	+	+	+	+	+ +
RA	+ +	+ +	+ +	+	0
Gout	0	+	+	+	+ +
Bursitis	+	+	+ +	+ +	+ +

+ + Very effective
+ Moderately effective
0 Mildly effective

and dinner the second and third days, and then 50 mg on the fourth day. Here higher doses were recommended initially and rapidly reduced.

Drug Interactions

Patients on warfarin sodium (Coumadin)-type compounds should not take any form of aspirin. Other salicylates and other NSAIDs could be used (except phenylbutazone), but there may be some mild synergistic effect. For this reason more frequent prothrombin times should be acquired until a new steady state is reached. Indocin has recently been reported to interfere with the antihypertensive effect of beta blocking agents.[18] An important point for gynecologists to remember is that little is known about the interaction of two or more NSAIDs. For example, if a patient is already taking Indocin for OA of the neck, the addition of Dolobid for knee pain would probably add nothing and in fact be dangerous.

Generalizations

- The gynecologist should use NSAIDs if simple analgesics such as acetaminophen are ineffective in M-S disease.
- Aspirin in high doses is cheaper but causes more GI side effects and has poorer compliance than most of the twice-a-day NSAIDs.
- The NSAIDs should not be changed rapidly. As mentioned earlier, start with a lower dose and increase slowly, allowing at least 2 to 3 weeks to determine efficacy. If drug A is ineffective, drug B may do very well and so on.
- True allergic reactions are not uncommon. The risk of cross reaction is high with another agent also.
- All the NSAIDs are anti-inflammatory, antipyretic, and analgesic.
- If patients are going to remain on these drugs, periodic monitoring of CBC, liver function tests (SGOT, alkaline phosphatase), and kidney function studies (BUN, urinalysis, serum creatinine) is mandatory.[19]

CASE DISCUSSIONS

Case #1

A 64-year-old obese woman complains of pain in her low back while you are performing a pelvic examination. After the examination she tells you that her back has been painful for about 2 years. Over-the-counter drugs have not been helpful.

She has about ten minutes of stiffness in the low back on arising but otherwise feels fine without constitutional symptoms. Examination reveals only some mild tenderness to deep palpation over the lower lumbar spine. A CBC, ESR, and biochemical profile are normal. Radiographs reveal evidence of osteoarthritis of the lumbar spine. You proceed to instruct the patient on the need for weight reduction. You then give her a prescription for a physiotherapist to teach back exercises and back protection. A prescription for an NSAID is given. Six months later the patient returns, 20 lb lighter, and states that she has almost no pain. You check her CBC and liver and kidney function studies, and maintain her on the NSAID.

Case #2

A 69-year-old woman comes in for a routine checkup. While you are taking her blood pressure she winces because of shoulder pain. In further questioning you determine that over the past 3 months she has had pain in both hands, shoulders, knees, and feet associated with morning stiffness of at least one hour, and generalized fatigue. Your examination reveals boggy PIP joints, wrists, and knees, and limitation of motion of the shoulders. Laboratory studies reveal an ESR of 72 mm/h and a positive rheumatoid factor. Radiographs are negative. You make a presumptive diagnosis of RA. You instruct the patient in a proper rest program of 12 hours a day, give her a prescription to see a physiotherapist for a proper daily exercise program, and start her on an NSAID. At her next visit she reports much less pain and stiffness and more ability to take care of herself. Examination reveals less swelling. You maintain her on this regimen.

Case #3

A 62-year-old woman informs you that she thinks she has bursitis in her left shoulder. She has pain constantly that is not necessarily worsened by use and, in fact, can even awaken her from sleep. She is anorectic and has lost 20 lb since her last visit. You recommend rest, pendulum exercises, and an NSAID. However, 1 week later she calls you, stating that the pain is no better and, in fact, worse. You refer her for rheumatologic consultation. The rheumatologist, on physical examination, finds a Horner's syndrome and orders a chest x-ray, which reveals a Pancoast's tumor of the lung, causing her shoulder pain. The patient is now receiving palliative radiation therapy.

Case #4

While interviewing a 61-year-old woman who presents for a routine physical, you notice an erythematous malar rash. She then admits to mild joint pains, low-grade fevers, and a generalized sense of malaise. Laboratory tests reveal an ESR of 81 mm/hr, hemoglobin level of 10.2 g/dL, and proteinuria (3+) with many red blood cells (RBCs) and RBC casts. You refer her to a specialist, who confirms the diagnosis of lupus with nephritis. After a 6-month course of high-dose prednisone, she is entirely well and in remission.

Case #5

A 72-year-old female, 20 years postmenopausal, presents with rather abrupt midback pain, better with rest, worse with weight bearing. She is frail, eats poorly, and avoids dairy products because of a lactase deficiency. Laboratory tests are normal, but radiographs reveal moderate osteopenia with collapse of T-7 and T-10 vertebrae. You recommend complete bed rest for ten days, wet heat, and Tylenol with codeine. In 2 weeks the patient informs you that the pain is much improved. You then instruct her in a regimen of calcium carbonate, 1,500 mg/day; sodium fluoride, 50 mg/day; and cyclical estrogen and progesterone. Two months later she is actually engaged in walking daily and swimming twice weekly.

SUMMARY

On a daily basis the gynecologist will come in contact with patients with M-S complaints. Determining the cause of their complaints through a short interview and examination, coupled with some basic laboratory tests, can then lead to a proper management program. In those patients suspected of having more serious rheumatic conditions, appropriate consultation can then be accomplished.

REFERENCES

1. McCarty DJ: *Arthritis and Allied Conditions*, ed 9. Philadelphia, Lea & Febiger, 1979.

2. Kellgren JH, Lawrence JS, Bier FL: Genetic factors in generalized osteoarthritis. *Ann Rheum Dis* 1963;22:237.

3. Pegron J: Inflammation in osteoarthritis: Review of its role in the clinical picture, disease progress, subjects and pathophysiology. *Semin Arthritis Rheum* 1981;11:115.

4. Gilbertsen EF: Laboratory medicine, ESR rates in older patients. *Postgrad Med* 1965;38:A44–A52.

5. Goldin RH, McAdam L, Lous JS, et al: Clinical and radiological survey of the incidence of osteoarthritis among obese patients. *Ann Rheum Dis* 1976;35:349.

6. Smith RW, Eyler WR, Melinger RL: On the incidence of osteoporosis. *Ann Intern Med* 1960;52:773–781.

7. Avioli LV, McDonald JE, Lee SW: The influence of age on the intestinal absorption of 47 Ca in women and its relation to 47 Ca absorption in postmenopausal osteoporosis. *J Clin Invest* 1965; 44:1960.

8. Riggs LB, Seeman E, Hodgsen SF, et al: Effect of the fluoride/calcium regimen on vertebral fracture occurrence in postmenopausal osteoporosis. *N Engl J Med* 1982;306:446.

9. Marcus R: The relationship of dietary calcium to the maintenance of skeletal integrity in man—an interface of endocrinology and nutrition. *Metabolism* 1982;31:93–102.

10. Barry HC: *Paget's Disease of Bone*. Edinburgh, E & S Livingstone, 1969.

11. Healy LA: Longterm follow up of polymyalgia rheumatica. Evidence of synovitis. *Semin Arthritis Rheum* 1984;13:322–328.

12. Huston KA, Hunder GG, Lie JT, et al: Temporal arteritis—a 25-year epidemiological, clinical and pathologic study. *Ann Intern Med* 1978;88:162–167.

13. Terkeltaub R, Esdaile J, Decary F, et al: A clinical study of older age RA with comparison to a younger onset group. *J Rheum* 1983;10:418.

14. Heimer R, Levin EM, Rudd E: Globulin resembling rheumatoid factor in serum of the aged. *Am J Med* 1963;35:175–181.

15. McCarty DJ, Solomon SD, Warnock ML, Paloyan E: Inorganic pyrophosphate concentrations in the synovial fluid of arthritic patients. *J Lab Clin Med* 1971;78:216–229.

16. McBay AJ, Hudson P: Propoxyphene overdose deaths. *JAMA* 1975;233:1287.

17. Morgan E, Kelly P, Nils K, et al: Tinnitus as an implication of therapeutic serum salicylate levels. *JAMA* 1973;226:142.

18. Durao V, Prata MM, Goncalves LMP: Modification of anti-hypertensive effect of β-adrenoceph-blocking agents by inhibition of endogenous prostaglandins synthesis. *Lancet* 1977;2:1005.

19. Solomon SD: Nonsteroidal, anti-inflammatory drugs. *J Med Soc NJ* 1985;82:143–145.

Part III

Selected Surgical and Gynecological Problems of the Older Woman

Chapter 11

Urinary Incontinence in the Elderly: A Clinician's Viewpoint

George L. Sexton Jr.*

INTRODUCTION

This chapter provides an overview of the modalities available to the clinician for the effective assessment and management of geriatric urinary incontinence. It focuses on the variables found in the elderly that may affect the successful therapeutic outcome.

The data discussed in this chapter are mainly gathered from the author's experience with 151 community-dwelling women over 65 years of age who had adequate cognitive and physical ability to seek medical help in an office setting. The methods of managing those individuals who were incontinent because of severe cognitive impairment and mobility limitations are not included in this chapter.

CLASSIFICATIONS OF INCONTINENCE

The Standardization Committee of the International Continence Society (ICS) defines urinary incontinence as a condition in which involuntary loss of urine is a social or hygienic problem and is objectively demonstrable. The ICS describes four major types of incontinence, each caused by the disruption of some aspect of the complex cycle of urine storage and micturition.[1]

---

*Acknowledgments:
 Phyllis A. Brace, RN, Health Care Professional, Women's Clinic, Ltd, for her aid in data retrieval and follow-up.
 Holter Hausner International, 3rd & Mill Streets, Bridgeport, PA 19405 USA, for their aid in the development of the synthetic alternatives described in this chapter.
 John R. Bolles, 34 Buckwalter Road, Royersford, PA 19468 USA, for his invaluable assistance in the preparation of the manuscript.

1. Genuine stress incontinence—the involuntary loss of urine when the intravesical pressure exceeds the maximum intraurethral pressure in the absence of detrusor activity
2. Urge incontinence—the involuntary loss of urine associated with a strong desire to void. Urge incontinence is subdivided into two categories: unstable bladder, which is associated with uninhibited detrusor contractions, and irritable bladder, which is not due to uninhibited detrusor contractions, but is the result of strong sensory input from the bladder and urethral sensory receptors.
3. Overflow incontinence—the involuntary loss of urine when the intravesical pressure exceeds the maximum intraurethral pressure owing to an elevation of intravesical pressure associated with bladder distention, but in the absence of detrusor activity
4. Reflex incontinence—the involuntary loss of urine caused by abnormal activity of the spinal cord in the absence of sensation usually associated with the desire to void

In this author's experience a number of women presented with the findings of both genuine stress incontinence and urge incontinence and, therefore, were evaluated as a fifth distinguishing type, "mixed."

FACTORS THAT PREDISPOSE TO TYPES OF GERIATRIC INCONTINENCE

From the clinician's point of view, it can be useful to consider each patient with geriatric incontinence as falling into one of two broad categories. The first is that patient with an acute incontinence of sudden onset, usually associated with an acute medical or surgical condition. The second type is the patient with a chronic incontinence of increasing severity that is usually without a clear precipitating medical or surgical cause.

Acute Incontinence

Acute incontinence will most often resolve spontaneously after the acute medical or surgical condition has subsided. In this author's experience the most common causes of acute incontinence were acute cystitis, restricted mobility after orthopedic surgery, medications, and fecal impaction.

Acute cystitis, which might ordinarily cause symptoms of frequency and urgency, is capable of producing incontinence in an elderly patient. Treatment of the acute inflammation may quickly restore continence.

The patient with restricted mobility may continue to be aware of the need to void but may be unable to reach the toilet. To compensate, the patient may voluntarily retain urine, and this action, when continued, can result in overflow incontinence.

Diuretics, especially the rapid-acting loop diuretics, can cause a sudden polyuria and precipitate acute overflow incontinence. Anticholinergic drugs may produce urinary retention and overflow incontinence by relaxing the detrusor muscle. Narcotics, sedatives, and antipsychotics may diminish awareness and mobility needed to void.

Fecal impactions should be considered in all acutely ill geriatric patients. Once the external pressure applied to the bladder neck has been alleviated, continence should be restored.

Chronic Incontinence

The five classifications of chronic urinary incontinence can be divided into two groups; disorders of storage, which include stress, urge, and mixed incontinence, and disorders of evacuation, which include overflow and reflex incontinence.

Disorders of Storage

In a four-year study of 151 patients whose average age was 73, stress incontinence was the second most prevalent type of chronic incontinence (Table 11-1). This type seemed to be much more prevalent in a group of 150 patients who were under 65 (average age 47) (Table 11-2). In the geriatric group three predisposing factors contributed to urethral incompetence (Table 11-3).

Anatomical weakness that causes stress incontinence is most commonly associated with genital prolapse. If the urethra is involved with the genital prolapse, it in turn responds inadequately to unequally transmitted intra-abdominal pressure, so that the intravesical pressure exceeds the intraurethral pressure.[2]

Table 11-1 Types of Geriatric Incontinence

Incontinence Type	No. of Patients
Stress	38
Urge	
Unstable bladder	25
Irritable bladder	47
Mixed	16
Overflow	12
Reflex	13
Total	151

Table 11-2 Types of Incontinence of Patients under 65

Incontinence Type	No. of Patients
Stress	91
Urge	
Unstable bladder	12
Irritable bladder	33
Mixed	8
Overflow	4
Reflex	2
Total	150

Physiologic causes of lowered intraurethral pressure are primarily based on hormonal effects. Many patients experience the onset of incontinence during the menopause owing to hypoestrogenism. This causes decreased periurethral vascularity, mucosal atrophy, and a loss of muscle tone in the estrogen-dependent urethra and trigone. These changes are intensified in the elderly.[3]

Pharmacologically induced weakness was found infrequently in the study. Adrenergic blockers may cause a hypotonia of the urethral smooth muscle, which results in urinary incontinence.[4]

In the geriatric group urge incontinence was the most frequently seen chronic disorder (Table 11-1). In most cases the cause of the unstable bladder was unknown (Table 11-4). In other cases upper motor neuron disease owing to cerebrovascular disease, internal hydrocephalus, multiple sclerosis, and Parkinson's disease was present. Irritable bladder was the more common of the two types of urge incontinence. The main predisposing factor in these cases was atrophic urethritis. Other factors included cystitis, pressure from extrinsic mass, pressure from genital prolapse, bladder calculus, bladder tumor, and urethral diverticulum. The elderly patient, because of diminished corticoregulatory response and compromised mobility, may not be able to sustain the inhibition of the detrusor reflex. Elderly women tend to be sensitive to caffeine, and chronic use or abuse may aggravate the irritable bladder.

Table 11-3 Predisposing Factors in Stress Incontinence

Factor	No. of Patients
Anatomical weakness	30
Physiologic atrophy	5
Pharmacologic (alpha-adrenergic blockers)	3
Total	38

Table 11-4 Predisposing Factors in Urge Incontinence

Factor	No. of Patients
Unstable bladder	
Idiopathic	19
Upper motor neuron disease	
CVA—stroke	3
Internal hydrocephalus	1
Multiple sclerosis	1
Parkinson's disease	1
Total	25
Irritable bladder	
Atrophic urethritis	25
Cystitis	8
Extrinsic mass	6
Genital prolapse	5
Bladder calculus	1
Bladder tumor	1
Urethral diverticulum	1
Total	47
Total unstable and irritable bladder	72

Some patients may have a combination of stress incontinence and urge incontinence. In this group of patients urethral incompetence was more often associated with an idiopathic unstable bladder than with an irritable bladder (Table 11-5). Predisposing factors were in keeping with those described earlier in the respective categories.

Disorders of Evacuation

Overflow incontinence may occur secondary to lower motor neuron disease.[5,6] In the geriatric group studied predisposing factors such as diabetes mellitus, chronic overdistention from genital prolapse, Guillain-Barré syndrome, polyneuritis, and meningioma resulted in peripheral neuropathy (Table 11-6). Other

Table 11-5 Chronic Geriatric Mixed Incontinence

Type	No. of Patients
Unstable and incompetent urethra	9
Irritable and incompetent urethra	7
Total	16

Table 11-6 Predisposing Factors in Overflow Incontinence

Factor	No. of Patients
Lower motor neuron disease	
Diabetic neuropathy	6
Chronic overdistention (genital prolapse)	2
Guillain-Barré syndrome	2
Polyneuritis	1
Meningioma	1
Total	12

causes of peripheral neuropathy not found in the series are tabes dorsalis and the denervation effect of radical pelvic surgery.

Reflex incontinence may occur secondary to upper motor neuron disease and is most commonly caused by cerebrovascular disease.[5,6] Other diseases, including metastasis to the central nervous system, spinal cord injury, and multiple sclerosis, were also found in the study (Table 11-7).

DIAGNOSTIC EVALUATION OF GERIATRIC INCONTINENCE

Elderly women who admit to urinary incontinence have usually lived with their symptoms for many years. It is most difficult for them to submit to an examination, so the clinician should request that the patient be accompanied by a friend or family member. Every effort should be made to assure the physical well-being of the patient during evaluation. It must be remembered that many patients will have physical limitations; the presence of a support system to provide comfort and reassurance may be the deciding factor in carrying out an adequate evaluation.

Table 11-7 Predisposing Factors in Reflex Incontinence

Factor	No. of Patients
Upper motor neuron disease	
Cerebrovascular	10
CNS metastasis	1
Spinal cord injury	1
Multiple sclerosis	1
Total	13

Medical History

Adequate time must be left on the schedule for a careful interview and for precise history taking. Communicating in understandable terminology in a face-to-face, unpressured setting is important.

In addition to direct discussion, the questionnaire proposed by Hodgkinson is an excellent aid in documenting urinary incontinence.[7] The questionnaire is so arranged that affirmative responses in group 1 indicate intrinsic urinary tract disease, in group 2 indicate neuromuscular dysfunction, and in group 3 indicate the physical factors that cause stress incontinence.

Details of the history should emphasize general medical and surgical conditions and the orthopedic status of the patient, as well as medications that have been prescribed for these conditions. The clinician must consider the role that these factors might play.

Neurologic disorders that cause upper motor neuron disease and lower motor neuron disease are common in the elderly. A history of loss of sensation, poor bladder control, and no awareness of incontinence will alert the clinician to the presence of these disorders. Diabetics may have not only the atonic bladder associated with lower motor neuron disease, but also polyuria owing to poorly controlled sugars, resulting in incontinence. Patients with congestive heart failure and venous insufficiency may increase urine production when they assume the horizontal position, resulting in nocturia and urge incontinence at night.

In addition to the medical history, the genitourinary history—particularly a history of recurrent urinary tract infection, pelvic irradiation, and bladder calculi—may provide clues to the cause of chronic incontinence.

Elderly women commonly have stress incontinence, that is, a history of losing small amounts of urine with increases in intra-abdominal pressure. However, most symptomatic urine leakage in the elderly is urge incontinence. It is important to remember that urge incontinence associated with a strong desire to void may not always be an irritable bladder, but may be associated with detrusor instability such as is seen in the unstable bladder. Although usually idiopathic, the unstable bladder may be an early manifestation of upper motor neuron disease.

Physical Examination

When evaluating the elderly patient, the clinician must be particularly aware of the patient's cognitive and physical status. The patient should be observed for these faculties during the history-taking interview and while being positioned on the examining table. Ability to reach the toilet in time without assistance is an important observation. Independent personality types may insist on performing toilet function without assistance, but doing so can result in an incontinence episode. This in turn may lead to depression and may lessen the patient's motivation to try again.

The abdomen should be examined for the presence of a mass, ascites, or a distended bladder. The pelvic examination must be done with a good deal of reassurance. In addition to observing for vulvar and vaginal lesions, inspecting for uterogenital prolapse is to be emphasized. Genital prolapse may be associated with outlet obstruction and high residuals, resulting in overflow incontinence. Stress incontinence may be suspected if there is hypermobility of the vesical neck, a positive Bonney test, and a positive Q-Tip test. These clinically observed tests, although limited in their predictive value, often indicate the need for further testing.

Neurology

The clinician should perform a simple screening neurologic examination. Its purpose is not only to document findings compatible with a neurologic history, but also to help identify unrecognized neurologic disorders that may better explain the type of incontinence present.

Changes brought about by lower motor neuron disease may explain a loss of bladder sensation and overflow incontinence. This may be checked by testing for perianal and perineal sensation, sphincter tone, and the simple ability of the patient to evacuate the contents of the bladder on command.

Upper motor neuron disease may be evaluated by the gait of the patient, deep tendon reflexes, bulbo-cavernous reflex, and lower-extremity sensations. These findings may explain a loss of bladder sensation and reflex incontinence.

Residuals

High residual urine volumes may be seen with both reflex and overflow incontinence. This finding, in association with the presence of signs of either lower or upper motor neuron disease, supports such a diagnosis. If residual urine is absent and the sensory system is intact, stress or urge incontinence is likely.

Although the postvoid residual determination is an important component of the diagnostic evaluation, it may be difficult to obtain in the geriatric patient. Many patients have an inhibition of spontaneous voiding because of nervous tension. (Again, reassurance of a health-care professional is supportive.) A psychological cause of urinary retention may bias the postvoid residual determination. Also, elderly patients frequently empty the bladder with delay in uroflow, and require a Valsalva maneuver or Credé maneuver to achieve evacuation. Such patients should be encouraged to "take their time" and perform whatever maneuvers they usually rely on to achieve evacuation.

Patients with high residual urine who have significant uterogenital prolapse should have repeat testing after the insertion of a Gellhorn or folding pessary to alleviate the obstruction.

Laboratory Studies

A catheterized urine specimen for urinalysis and urine cultures, in addition to a urethral culture, should be obtained on all incontinent patients. The clinician should do a urinary sediment examination and observe for the presence of pyuria and hematuria.

It must be remembered that urethritis may not be associated with positive catheterized urine specimen findings. Tenderness elicited on palpation of the urethra and trigone may indicate urethritis as accurately as urethral culture findings.

Persistent urinary tract infection, with or without hematuria, is an indication for a complete urologic evaluation to rule out upper tract disease and intrinsic bladder disease.

Because of the high incidence of diabetes and renal disease in the elderly, blood glucose, creatinine, and blood urea nitrogen levels should be obtained on all patients.

Urodynamic Investigation

With the diagnostic assessment methods described earlier, most cases of geriatric incontinence can be identified as either disorders of storage (ie, stress and urge incontinence) or disorders of evacuation (ie, overflow and reflex incontinence). Whether or not further study, in the form of urodynamic investigation, is necessary should be decided at this point. Many patients with disorders of storage can be treated by nonsurgical methods without further investigation. Patients who have persistent symptoms of urinary incontinence, or patients with disorders of evacuation warrant further evaluation.

Adequate urodynamic testing of the elderly requires that the geriatric patient have the cognitive ability and physical mobility to, first, sit comfortably on a uroflometry chair and, second, lie in the lithotomy position with the thighs in abduction to allow cystometry and endoscopy. There is a certain amount of discomfort associated with these tests, and for many frail and elderly patients this becomes a burden that they are not willing to accept. Again, care and support from health professionals can make the difference.

Cystometry

Cystometry is a method used to determine the relationship between bladder pressure and volume. A normal cystometry result is generally characterized by a bladder capacity of 300 to 500 mL, with a rise in intravesical pressure of less than 10 cm H_2O, and normal sensation that enables the patient to appreciate bladder filling. The first desire to void is usually noted in the middle range of the functional bladder capacity, and this feeling is usually suppressed until the bladder is approximately three fourths full, at which point a more urgent desire to void occurs.[8]

The ability of the patient to suppress the detrusor reflex must be carefully evaluated in the elderly because of the discomfort and anxiety produced by this invasive study. In general, the unstable bladder is associated with an idiopathic detrusor instability. The patient with this type of urge incontinence is unable to suppress the detrusor contraction.

In the elderly patient the presence of bladder instability associated with the urge to void during filling should be viewed as an indication for further neurologic evaluation. The presence of such bladder activity with apparently normal sensation may be an early manifestation of central nervous system disease. Upper motor neuron disease associated with uninhibited detrusor contractions is usually accompanied by an absence of normal bladder filling sensation.

Uroflometry

Uroflometry is a noninvasive procedure that provides a graphic record of voiding.[9,10] The volume of urine voided and the length of time of voiding are recorded. The average flow rate is then found by dividing the volume of urine voided by the time. The normal female completes voiding in less than 20 seconds with a flow rate greater than 20 mL/s. A flow rate of less than 15 mL/s indicates abnormal voiding.

Ideally a neurologic abnormality that affects the bladder will manifest itself in either poorly sustained or totally absent bladder contraction. With decompensation of the bladder from chronic overdistention, the patient is noted to strain, or must apply a Credé maneuver to void. In the elderly, uroflometry may be unsuccessful because of discomfort, with a resulting inhibition to void.

Cystourethroscopy

The possibility of intrinsic urethral or bladder disease must be considered. The finding of tumor, stone, diverticula, or radiation or interstitial cystitis will require specific modalities of treatment. The clinician can obtain sufficient diagnostic information by dynamic urethroscopic testing.

Carbon dioxide is used to insufflate and monitor the urethra and bladder. The patient is asked to perform maneuvers—such as holding urine and bearing down—in order to stimulate the detrusor contraction. The urethroscope permits observation of the bladder neck during filling, as well as evaluation of the patient's ability to suppress the detrusor contraction.[11,12]

TREATMENT MODALITIES FOR GERIATRIC INCONTINENCE

Urinary incontinence in the elderly population is not an inevitable consequence of aging and can usually be treated effectively. Several types of treatment modalities are available and are, to a large extent, similar to those applied to the younger age group. Which treatment is the most appropriate depends on the type of incontinence.

Behavioral Therapy

For those elderly incontinent patients who are capable of learning self-managing procedures, both bladder habit training and simple environmental changes, such as toileting modifications, may be most rewarding. The principle of this treatment is based on the benefits of reducing the time it takes for the patient physically to reach the toilet. We have found this particularly helpful for patients with urge incontinence who have diminished cortico-regulatory response to the storage of urine and, to a lesser degree, for those with a loss of sensation, as seen with overflow and reflex incontinence.

Toilet location problems can be obvious. With proper adjustment in toilet access, many older people can eliminate their voiding delay and remain continent.

Bladder habit training has been most helpful with patients who have disorders of storage. Effectively, this is done by establishing a voiding routine, usually every one to two hours whether or not a sensation to void is present. Frequently the interval between voidings may be lengthened as the patient gains confidence and learns to "say no" to the detrusor reflex. Patients who have disorders of evacuation may lessen residuals by shortening the interval between voidings (ie, "double-voiding").

Drug Therapy

The postmenopausal patient with urinary incontinence who demonstrates vaginal and urethral atrophy may benefit from the topical application of estrogenic cream to the vagina. Local estrogen stimulates and supports urethral and trigonal smooth musculature and epithelium, thereby improving physiologic function of these structures. The mechanism by which estrogen replacement may improve the symptoms of incontinence may be related to one of the several factors that contribute to the maintenance of intraurethral pressure, such as urethral smooth-muscle tone or blood flow in the urethra. Estrogen receptors in the human female lower urinary tract have been demonstrated, further supporting the rationale for estrogen replacement in incontinent patients with atrophic genitourinary findings.[13] One study demonstrated a significant increase in maximum intraurethral pressure and urethral length at rest in women after treatment with estrogen.[14]

This author's current approach to the treatment of both stress and urge geriatric incontinence includes estrogen vaginal cream whether or not other treatment modalities are indicated. Either the synthetic estrogen (dienestrol) or the conjugated estrogen creams are effective in doses of 0.3 to 0.6 mg, inserted intravaginally at bedtime two or three times a week. In treating geriatric incontinence I have not found oral estrogen to have any advantage over topical vaginal estrogen. At these doses systemic effects have not been noted.

Bladder Relaxants

A wide variety of drugs have bladder relaxant properties. It has been useful to involve a family member to help monitor the treatment cycles of drugs that have bladder relaxant properties. The patients may experience troublesome side effects, including constipation, blurry vision, tachycardia, esophageal reflux, and dry mouth. (If dryness of the mouth is a persistent problem, then guaifenesin 200-mg tablets three times a day may increase the salivary secretions and lessen the dryness of the mucous membranes.) These agents can also precipitate urinary retention, which can be managed in some patients while maintaining continence between intermittent catheterizations. Some patients become confused and unsteady while taking these medications. A fall with resulting fracture is a potential risk and complication of the use of these medications. The importance of a family member's involvement in monitoring the patient on such medications cannot be overemphasized.

Anticholinergic and antispasmodic agents are most commonly used for urge incontinence and reflex incontinence. Several of these drugs—Bentyl (dicyclomine), Urispas (flavoxate), Ditropan (oxybutynin), and Daricon (oxyphencyclimine)—are reported to have a direct relaxant effect on bladder muscle in addition to their anticholinergic activity.[15] Tofranil (imipramine) has both alpha-adrenergic and central effects in addition to its anticholinergic properties (Tables 11-8 and 11-9).[16,17]

The pharmacologic effects of these drugs are thought to be due to the inhibition of acetylcholine-mediated bladder contractions. Although this effect may promote

Table 11-8 Drugs Used to Treat Urge and Reflex Incontinence

Drug	Dosage	Potential Side Effects
Anticholinergic/ antispasmodic		
Dicyclomine	10–20 mg tid	Dry mouth
Oxyphencyclimine	10 mg tid	Constipation
Flavoxate	300–800 mg/day in divided doses	Blurred vision Elevated intraocular pressure
Oxybutynin	2.5–5.0 mg tid	Postural hypotension
Propantheline	15–30 mg tid	
Anticholinergic/ alpha-adrenergic		
Imipramine	1–2 mg/kg/day in divided doses bid	All of above plus cardiovascular toxicity

symptomatic improvement in many patients, the improvement is difficult to predict. This may be explained in part by the phenomenon of atropine resistance. Although atropine will completely inhibit the bladder smooth-muscle response to exogenously administered acetylcholine, it will only partially antagonize the bladder's response to pelvic nerve stimulation, suggesting that a component of this response is mediated by neurotransmitters other than acetylcholine.[15]

In this author's experience imipramine has been the single most effective bladder relaxant for geriatric incontinence. The usual therapeutic dose schedule for imipramine found to be effective has been from 1 to 2 mg/kg/d, not to exceed 4 mg/kg/d. The dose tolerance will vary from patient to patient, and the effective dose also varies considerably. This is due, in part, to the metabolism of imipramine, which primarily occurs in the liver by hydroxylation followed by glucuronide conjugation.[18] Enzymes in the liver control hydroxylation and are

Table 11-9 Drugs Used to Treat Stress Incontinence

Drug	Dosage	Potential Side Effects
Alpha-adrenergic		
Pseudoephedrine	15–30 mg tid	Headache Tachycardia
Phenylpropanolamine	75 mg bid	Elevated blood pressure
Anticholinergic/ alpha-adrenergic		
Imipramine	See Table 11-8	See Table 11-8

stimulated by barbiturates, alcohol, and smoking. Drugs such as haloperidol and some narcotics may prolong imipramine toxicity by interfering with hydroxylation. Because of these factors the mean half-life in both therapeutic dose and overdose is extremely variable, ranging from 10 to 81 hours. It is essential that the clinician be assured of an accurate accounting of the dose schedule so that cardiovascular toxicity does not occur. A potentially lethal dose occurs at 15 to 20 mg/kg.[18]

Occasionally combined low doses of two agents with complementary actions—such as oxybutynin and imipramine—will maximize the benefits and minimize the side effects. If incontinence occurs at predictable times, such as at night, one should not hesitate to prescribe a rapidly acting drug, such as oxybutynin. As with all anticholinergics, caution should be exercised when using these medications in patients with glaucoma.

In this author's experience 13 of 25 patients with the unstable bladder and 25 of 31 patients with the irritable bladder reported a good result with drug treatment. Nine of 13 patients with reflex incontinence reported a poor result; the other 4 reported only a fair result with bladder relaxant treatment.

Alpha-Agonists

The rationale of drug therapy with alpha-agonists is based on the effect of alpha-adrenergic stimulation to increase intraurethral pressure.[17,19] Both imipramine and phenylpropanolamine have been used effectively in treating stress incontinence.

Many patients with geriatric incontinence will have hypertension and will not be good candidates for the alpha-adrenergic agonists. Imipramine at therapeutic doses has had a lesser hypertensive effect on the cardiovascular system and is well tolerated.

Pessaries

Vaginal pessaries have been widely used in female patients to alleviate symptoms of pelvic relaxation and occasional urinary incontinence. The types of pessaries that have been effective have been the Gellhorn pessary and the folding pessary. The Smith-Hodge pessary is helpful in evaluating patients with stress incontinence resulting from genital prolapse.

One author reports a high degree of success with the pessary test as a simple diagnostic and prognostic tool when used during urodynamic evaluation.[20] A suitable size Smith-Hodge pessary may be placed and the patient tested in the erect position with a full bladder. The patient should be observed for urine loss during or after coughing. Uroflometry can be more effectively obtained after pessary correction of an obstructive prolapse.

Pessaries are reserved for those patients who are not suitable for corrective surgery on the genital tract. Of 38 patients with stress incontinence, 30 were medically and surgically treated; the remaining 8 either refused or were not medically suited for surgery and so were treated with pessary. Of those eight, four were successfully treated; the other four were unhappy with their pessaries and requested removal. Of 12 patients with overflow incontinence, 2 were treated effectively with pessary and intermittent catheterization for correction of outlet obstruction.

Proper pessary care entails a commitment on the part of not only the patient, but also a family member or home health aide to monitor its use. A pessary must be frequently removed during the first 6 to 8 weeks after its insertion to observe for abrasion, vaginal laceration, and infection. An estrogen cream should always be prescribed, and a cleansing saline douche should be administered on a weekly basis. If ulceration and abrasion of the vaginal wall occur, the pessary should be changed to a smaller size. If a pessary is forgotten and becomes entrapped, further vaginal ulceration with resulting bladder and/or rectal fistula may occur. It is wise for the clinician to have an informed consent on the patient's chart with documentation of the proper follow-up care.

In general, this author favors correction of uterogenital prolapse and stress incontinence by the surgical approach rather than by use of a pessary. All too often pessaries are inserted for "medical reasons," only to find later that the patient has successfully undergone urgent or emergency surgery for some intra-abdominal pathology without any particular morbidity. In addition, the pessary inserted in the geriatric patient may become a difficult nursing problem in later years, when surgery is no longer feasible.

Surgery

Several surgical options for elevating the bladder neck and removing a urethral obstruction are available to the clinician. Although these options are generally known, certain considerations in treating the geriatric patient surgically merit special attention.

Preliminary Considerations

Positioning for Surgery. The patient should be positioned on the operating table so that the hips are at the level of the two stirrups. Elastic stockings are used to provide venous compression. The ankles are suspended from the stirrups in such a fashion that acute angulation of the leg will be avoided, thus maintaining unobstructed venous return.

The full lithotomy position is ideal for colporrhaphy. However, if flexion of the thighs is limited, the patient may be operated in the semilithotomy position. This position is preferred for retropubic surgery, as it will permit vaginal palpation during the procedure.

Suture Material. In the surgical correction of geriatric incontinence the suture material used should allow for sufficient wound healing time before absorption takes place.

Plain catgut is of limited usefulness in vaginal surgery because it is more irritating, causes greater tissue reaction, and is absorbed more rapidly than chromatized catgut. Chromatized catgut provides greater resistance to absorption than plain catgut but is unpredictable in the duration of its tensile strength.

Absorbable sutures made of polyglycolic acid or polyglactin offer minimal tissue reaction and a delay in absorption. Both these sutures are available as braided stitches and provide continued tensile strength for 2 to 3 weeks.[21-23]

Polydioxanone (PDS) and polyglycolic acid–trimethyl carbonate (Maxon) offer the longest delay in absorption and duration of tensile strength. These sutures provide 55% of their tensile strength for 4 to 6 weeks.

Knot Tying. Studies of knot-tying techniques (particularly of the sliding knots frequently used by gynecologic surgeons) have indicated that nonidentical and parallel knots differed little with respect to reliability.[24] When monofilament sutures were used, five-throw knots were generally stronger than three-throw knots. Braided sutures were found to be just as strong with three-throw knots as with five-throw knots; therefore, a square knot followed by a third knot will afford maximum strength.

The gynecologist will compromise knot strength by using less than five throws with monofilament suture, whether absorbable or nonabsorbable.

Hemostasis. The local infiltration of the vaginal wall with a solution of adrenalin (1% lidocaine with 1:200,000 adrenalin up to 30 mL total) for hemostasis is well tolerated in the geriatric patient, provided it is compatible with the general anesthetic being administered. In the presence of genital atrophy the solution aids in the dissection by elevating the vaginal wall from both the vesicovaginal space and the rectovaginal space.

In the geriatric patient the vaginal wall is thin and the blood supply reduced. Consequently bipolar coagulating current is often adequate for providing rapid and complete hemostatis.

If serious intraoperative hemorrhaging should occur during retropubic surgery, the bleeding can be controlled by simultaneously applying manual pressure intravaginally and by way of the space of Retzius. Once the bleeding point has been precisely identified, a hemoclip or suture can be placed.

Technical Considerations

If geriatric incontinence is surgically treated using standard materials and methods, recurrence will be common. In view of the atrophic tissues and stress factors frequently encountered in the elderly patient, materials and methods must be modified to help ensure an improved result.

Anterior Colporrhaphy. The colpotomy incision is made into the avascular vesicovaginal space from the vesical neck to the anterior wall of the cul-de-sac. Because of tissue atrophy, denuding the vaginal wall to create two layers may not be beneficial.

The bladder should be treated as a hernia and fully mobilized from the adjacent vaginal wall and peritoneum of the anterior cul-de-sac. Redundant peritoneum, if present, should be excised at this point. After mobilization of the bladder, the bladder itself and any available endopelvic fascia are reinforced by a purse-string stitch using a #0 or #2-0 delayed absorbable suture. This stitch will reduce the protruding cystocele.

To succeed in correcting stress incontinence, the dissection must be extended laterally to the pubic rami, permitting access to the pubourethral ligaments, before the first layer of plication sutures can be placed. These ligamentous condensations of vaginal fascia that insert on the pubic ramus must be approximated at the level of the vesicourethral neck with delayed absorbable #0 suture material. If insufficient fascia is present, then plication sutures using #2-0 nonabsorbable monofilament or braided polyester sutures should be placed. The remaining first-layer plication sutures of the anterior vaginal wall are usually accomplished using delayed absorbable sutures; in geriatric surgery, however, this layer should be reinforced with #2-0 nonabsorbable monofilament or braided sutures. The most inferior plicating stitch should incorporate the prepared peritoneum of the anterior cul-de-sac to reinforce the plication.

After excess tissue from the anterior vaginal wall has been excised, the remaining tissue is approximated by interrupted #0 delayed absorbable plicating suture.

The urethra itself should not be included in plication. Plication of the urethra may result in scarring and rigidity, which can inhibit the mechanisms responsible for maintaining intraurethral pressure.

Retropubic Operations. In treating cases of severe stress incontinence in the elderly, a retropubic procedure should be considered as the operation of choice.

Whether performing a urethropexy or a colposuspension, precise identification of the bladder neck is critical to ensure proper suture placement. Shortening of the urethra and funneling of the bladder neck—both seen frequently in the elderly—will obscure the exact location of the vesicourethral angle, even in the presence of an indwelling Foley catheter bulb. Cystotomy is always indicated to determine the location of the bladder neck, particularly in cases of recurrent stress incontinence after previous retropubic surgery.

The author prefers #2-0 nonabsorbable braided polyester suture in these procedures. If periosteum of the symphysis pubis is not adequate for a urethropexy, the periurethral sutures may be fixed to the condensation of fascia formed by the aponeurosis of the internal oblique and transverse abdominis, just lateral or medial to the pubic tubercle. This same anatomical structure is also preferred over an atrophic Cooper's ligament in colposuspension.

Vaginal Colpopexy. Because incontinence can be associated with significant uterogenital prolapse, conventional corrective procedures should be augmented by vaginal colpopexy in the geriatric patient, to prevent recurrence. The vagina may be effectively fixed to the sacrospinous ligament, the round ligaments, and the properly prepared peritoneum of the cul-de-sac. When antomically feasible, all three sites should be used, to maximize effectiveness in the geriatric patient. The #2-0 nonabsorbable braided polyester sutures have been most effective.

Synthetic Alternatives

Great strides have been made in the development and application of medical-grade synthetic polymers. Nearly every surgical specialty has been augmented by implantable devices or materials to replace weakened or worn-out tissues.[25]

Many types of geriatric incontinence are caused by damaged or weakened tissues. Unfortunately the same inherent poor tissue quality in these patients can make the outcome of conventional surgical techniques uncertain. Stress factors such as chronic cough and obesity further limit the potential for success. In such difficult cases synthetic tissue supports can provide strength the natural tissues no longer possess.

Modifications of stress incontinence procedures using such materials as Mersilene and Marlex as substitutes for homologous tissues have been developed. The ready availability of these synthetics and their ability to provide instantaneous support produce early results that appear promising. However, tissue reaction to these materials has been significant (10% to 23%), necessitating removal of the material, which results in recurrence of the anatomical defect.[26-28] Moreover, removal of the mesh is made difficult by ingrowth of the adjacent tissues.

More than 30 years after its first implant application, silicone elastomer remains one of the most widely used of the synthetic polymers. It can be compounded in a variety of hardnesses, can be formed to practically any shape, and can be attached to or remain free of the living tissue, as required. In its solid, smooth, molded elastomeric form, silicone causes minimal tissue reaction; does not absorb, necrose, or change chemically; and is not metabolized.[25,29,30] These characteristics make silicone particularly well suited to incontinence surgery.

In an attempt to improve the outcome of stress incontinence surgery, the author has developed a colposuspension using a Dacron-reinforced silicone elastomer Hunter tendon rod.[31,33]

The epiurethral suprapubic vaginal suspension (ESVS) utilizes the lamina propria of the vagina and the conjoined tendon, structures that afford adequate strength for the implant in all patients, young or old. After the space of Retzius has been opened, the implant is inserted through the full thickness of the vagina on each side of the urethra. The implant is placed at the level of the vesicourethral angle, lateral enough to the urethra to prevent abrasion injury. The implant is placed over the urethra, not beneath it. The conjoined tendon adjacent to the lacunate ligament is perforated, and the implant is brought through the conjoined tendon close to the midline on each side. The ends of the implant are tightened to allow approximately 2 cm between the urethra and the symphysis pubis, thus maintaining the space of Retzius. The ends of the implant are then fastened together beneath the aponeurosis of the external oblique at the level of the symphysis pubis. The implant is trimmed of excess at the ends.

The ESVS succeeds in establishing a competent urethra by fixation of the vesicourethral angle, prevention of urethral gaping, and by affording immediate and lasting support to the urethra. Physiologic pressure relationships between the urethra and bladder are restored (ie, the intraurethral pressure is greater than the intravesical pressure). ESVS, because it suspends the urethra from above, avoids the "too-loose-or-too-tight" application of the pin-up associated with sling procedures. Adverse foreign body reaction has also been less with the silicone implant (about 8%), and even these cases are salvageable when the implant is left in for 6 months. A fibroepithelial capsule forms about the implant as a normal physiologic response. In the event the implant must be removed, the capsule is often capable of maintaining the anatomical correction.[31] The long-term functional usefulness of the fibrous envelope has been extensively demonstrated in the orthopedic application of the Hunter tendon prostheses.[33] The same principle has been demonstrated with prosthetic repair of vaginal vault prolapse.

The cul-de-sac of Douglas is a particularly susceptible site for pelvic floor hernia, which may result from muscle and fascia weakness. The problem is aggravated in geriatric patients by further atrophy and loss of pelvic diaphragm tone. Increases in intra-abdominal pressure may be magnified after hysterectomy by changes in the axis of the vagina and its ligamentous supports. The end result may allow the pelvic viscera and cul-de-sac peritoneum to slide through the widened levator hiatus, resulting in complete vault prolapse.

Surgical procedures to treat this defect are numerous, and none has been fully accepted as satisfactory enough to exclude all others. In order to reestablish normal anatomy with normal anatomical direction of the vaginal canal, the upper vagina must be replaced over the levator plate. Both the vaginal sacrospinous ligament fixation and the abdominal sacropexy procedure reestablish this important anatomical relationship. But unless the pexy is combined with anatomical closure of the pelvic floor defect, recurrence is common. Closure of the levator defect and obliteration of the cul-de-sac frequently result in marked shortening and constriction of the vagina, which usually preclude satisfactory coitus for the patient. In addition, the hernial sac usually has a wide neck and the tissues with which to perform a cul-de-sac herniorrhaphy are inevitably disappointing.

The cul-de-sac implant under investigation is a molded silicone elastomer dome with a suture flange made of Dacron-reinforced silicone elastomer. The dome is 24.3 mm high and has an outer diameter of 54 mm at its widest area. The dome is 3 mm thick at the top and 5 mm thick at the bottom. The suture flange is a ring attached to the bottom of the dome and extending 5 mm beyond the dome's outer diameter about its entire circumference.

The device is implanted as an ambulatory procedure with the patient under general anesthesia. A vertical colpotomy incision is made over the protruding pelvic hernia to permit dissection of the pelvic viscera from the vaginal mucosa and reduction of the hernial sac so that the upper vagina is relocated above the levator plate. The dissection permits the implant to be placed manually over the levator plate, and #0 delayed absorbable sutures placed at the 12, 3, 6, and 9 o'clock positions for fixation of the implant at the upper third of the vagina. Excess vaginal tissue is excised, and the remaining flaps retract to the upper third of the vagina and location of the implant.

If the levator plate will not support the implant, a posterior colporrhaphy must be included in the operative procedure with particular emphasis on approximation of the levator ani muscles anterior to the rectum.

The implant is left in place for 6 months, sufficient time to stimulate an adequate fibrous envelope. For device removal, the patient is admitted as an ambulatory procedure and placed under local or general anesthesia. The implant is removed by making a small colpotomy incision over the cul-de-sac suture line. After device removal, the suture line is approximated with continuous delayed absorbable suture.

To date, 31 geriatric patients with vaginal vault prolapse have been managed by the cul-de-sac implant. The initial results are most encouraging, and more extensive investigation is pending.

Postoperative Bladder Drainage

All of the advantages of suprapubic bladder drainage take on increased significance in the context of geriatric patient care.

Many suprapubic catheters are available, and may be classified as either small caliber or large caliber catheters. The author prefers a #14/F Foley catheter inserted by open cystotomy during retropubic surgery and by closed cystotomy after vaginal plastic procedures. Regardless of the type of suprapubic catheter, if the patient is discharged before satisfactory voiding, dependent collection bags for attachment to leg and bed must be sent home to maintain a closed system and permit measurement of residual urine. Many geriatric patients are reluctant to be discharged before they are voiding comfortably, as the accessories make ambulation difficult. In addition, emptying the bag in such a way that the system remains closed may be difficult without professional help.

To simplify postoperative care and facilitate early ambulation and discharge from the hospital, the author developed a suprapubic cystotomy urine pump (SCUP). The SCUP—consisting of a proximal tubing segment, a duplex silicone and stainless steel antireflux valve/pump, and a distal tubing segment—is connected in-line between the catheter and conventional urinary drainage bag immediately postoperative. The proximal tubing segment includes a tapered, barbed nylon adapter that connects easily to both small- and large-caliber catheters. The antireflux valve permits rapid perfusion of urine and eliminates significant urinary retention during dependent drainage of the bladder. Independent drainage will begin 48 hours postoperative, at which time the distal tubing segment is detached from the collection bag and closed off with an integral plug. The patient is encouraged to void every two to four hours and check her own residual urine by opening the distal tubing segment and manually pumping residual urine into a measuring cup. Manual pumping is accomplished by repeatedly compressing the "pumping chamber," the soft rubber cylindrical area between the two valve components. The patient stops pumping when the chamber is sluggish in returning to its noncompressed state, indicating an empty bladder. The distal end is cleansed with alcohol or antiseptic solution and plugged after each residual measurement. The device is held in place on the patient with a universal, disposable waist belt made of Velcro. When the residual levels are acceptable to the attending doctor, the patient will return to the office for removal of the suprapubic catheter and the SCUP.

Results of bacteriology confirm a low incidence of both asymptomatic and symptomatic bacteriuria. No patients had prolonged hospital stay or readmission for the treatment of urinary tract infection. The average length of stay has been reduced 2.4 days since instituting the SCUP as a routine support system for postoperative suprapubic bladder drainage.

Results

Treatment modalities were applied to 151 patients in various combinations, according to the needs of the individual patient (Table 11-10). By careful clinical

Table 11-10 Treatment Modalities for the Types of Urinary Incontinence

Type	Treatment
Stress	Behavioral therapy Estrogen Alpha-adrenergic agonists Surgery to correct incompetent urethra
Urge	Behavioral therapy Bladder relaxants Estrogen Pessary or surgery for genital prolapse Antibiotics or surgery for intrinsic or extrinsic urethral or bladder disease
Overflow	Behavioral therapy Pessary or surgery for urethral obstruction owing to prolapse Intermittent catheterization
Reflex	Neurologic, depending on cause Bladder relaxants Intermittent catheterization

evaluation, the patients who would benefit from surgical treatment were separated from those who would benefit from other treatment modalities. These modalities were evaluated by a 2-year follow-up interview in which each patient rated the result of treatment as good, fair, or poor: a good result had relief of symptoms of urinary incontinence, a fair result was one that achieved a 50% relief of symptoms, and a poor result was one in which there was no significant relief of symptoms.

Surgery was clearly the most effective method of alleviating symptoms of stress incontinence. Thirty of 38 patients were treated surgically; 21 were primaries and 9 were secondaries. For patients with severe incontinence, the retropubic approach was favored over anterior colporrhaphy and afforded the best results.

Medical treatment of urge incontinence owing to the unstable bladder was of limited success: of 25 patients treated, just more than half reported a good result, and most of the remainder reported a poor result. In sharp contrast were the patients treated for urge incontinence owing to the irritable bladder: of these 47 patients, 41 reported a good result. Sixteen of these patients had surgery or pessary to alleviate symptoms caused by prolapse, and the other 25 responded well to medication.

All 16 patients with "mixed" incontinence were first treated with bladder relaxants. After this therapy 11 of the 16 were deemed suitable candidates for surgery. Of these 11, 5 reported a good result in follow-up, and the remaining 6, a fair result. Five patients with mixed incontinence had a dominant symptom of urge incontinence and were, therefore, not considered for surgery. All five experienced troublesome side effects from the medications and rated the results of treatment as poor.

Overflow incontinence was found in 12 patients, and generally the result of treatment was poor. This was in part due to associated lower motor neuron disease. Two patients were considered suitable candidates for surgery and were successfully operated: one had removal of a meningioma involving the posterior roots of the sacral cord and the other had chronic urethral obstruction owing to genital prolapse and was treated with the cul-de-sac implant. The remaining ten were treated with intermittent catheterization. Two patients with chronic outlet obstruction and one patient with peripheral neuropathy reported a fair result, and the remaining seven, with peripheral neuropathy, reported a poor result (Table 11-11).

CONCLUSION

Urinary incontinence takes its toll on nearly every area of life—social, psychological, and even financial. It discourages interaction, lowers self-esteem, and adds significantly to the cost of nursing care.[34] These are burdens that the elderly—many of whom are already struggling with these issues—do not need to bear.

Operative procedures for stress incontinence abound, and in many cases age is not a deterrent. Behavioral therapy, estrogens, and alpha-adrenergic agonists should be tried before surgery, as the combination may relieve symptoms of stress incontinence. If surgery is indicated, medical treatment will enhance the postoperative result.

There is still much room for improvement. Although urge incontinence caused by the irritable bladder has been amenable to medical treatment, this has not been the case with the unstable bladder.

Table 11-11 Results—151 Patients

Incontinence Type	Good	Fair	Poor
Stress (38 patients)	27	3	8
Urge (72 patients)			
Unstable bladder (25)	13	2	10
Irritable bladder (47)	41	2	4
Mixed (16 patients)	5	6	5
Overflow (12 patients)	2	3	7
Reflex (13 patients)	0	4	9
Total	88	20	43

The association of urge incontinence with stress incontinence (ie, "mixed") makes the results of surgery difficult to predict unless bladder relaxants are effective preoperatively. Therefore, patients with mixed incontinence should be treated medically to rule out a dominant symptom of urge incontinence, which generally prevents a successful surgical result.

Patients with overflow incontinence and reflex incontinence have benefited the least from current treatment modalities. Intermittent catheterization, always indicated in treatment of these disorders of evacuation, should be done in conjunction with other appropriate treatment modalities and with the assistance of a home health aide.

A better understanding of the pharmacology involved in treating incontinence is needed. New pharmacologic agents and drug combinations should be explored. As response to various drug therapies is better understood, specificity will be improved.

A great deal of development can also take place in the area of synthetic tissue supports. New medical-grade synthetics are continually being developed and new applications for them discovered. The field of gynecologic urology has only begun to explore the possibilities of these new technologies.

New behavioral therapies to modify incontinence through environmental changes also hold a great deal of promise.

In conclusion, several basic principles apply to treating the geriatric patient. First, patience on the part of the medical team is a prerequisite. Communicate deliberately and listen carefully during the history-taking interview. Be reassuring during the physical examination and any invasive urodynamic testing. Second, develop diagnostic skills to precisely identify the type of incontinence present. Urodynamic testing should be done as required to assure correct diagnosis. And finally, always consider combination therapies, and modify surgical materials and methods accordingly.

Clinicians and other health-care professionals are trying to dispel the long-held view that incontinence is to be tolerated as part of the aging process. Previously reluctant individuals are now discussing their problems and seeking medical help. Now the ultimate goal is to provide the kind of medical, technical, and psychologic help that will either resolve the condition or control it adequately so that the patient can lead a dignified and satisfying life.

REFERENCES

1. Bates P, Bradley WE, Glen E, et al: The standardization of terminology of lower urinary tract function. *J Urol* 1979;121:551.

2. Staskin DR, Zimmer PE, Hadley RH, et al: The pathophysiology of stress incontinence. *Urol Clin North Am* 1985;12:271–278.

3. Batra S: Estrogen and smooth muscle function. *Trends Pharmacol Sci* 1980;1:388.

4. Whitfield HN, Doyle PT, Mayo ME, et al: The effect of adrenergic blocking drugs on outflow resistance. *Br J Urol* 1976;47:823–827.

5. Kendall AR, Karofin L: Classification of neurogenic bladder disease. *Urol Clin North Am* 1974;1:37–44.

6. Bradley WE: The neurology of micturition, in Ostergard DR (ed): *Gynecologic Urology and Urodynamics: Theory and Practice*. Baltimore, Williams & Wilkins, 1980, pp 11–27.

7. Hodgkinson CP: Stress urinary incontinence. *Am J Obstet Gynecol* 1970;108:1149.

8. Hodgkinson CP, Cobert N: Direct urethrocystometry. *Am J Obstet Gynecol* 1960;79:648.

9. Drake WN: The uroflowmeter: An aid to the study of the lower urinary tract. *J Urol* 1948;59:650.

10. Siroky MB, Olsson CA, Krane RJ: The flowrate nomogram: II. Clinical correlation. *J Urol* 1980;123:208.

11. Robertson JR: Gynecologic urethroscopy. *Am J Obstet Gynecol* 1973;115:986.

12. Robertson JR: Gas cystometrogram with urethral pressure profile. *Obstet Gynecol* 1974;44:72.

13. Iosif CS, Batra S, Ek A, et al: Estrogen receptors in the human female lower urinary tract. *Am J Obstet Gynecol* 1981;141:817.

14. Rud T: The effects of estrogens and gestagens on the urethral pressure profile in urinary continent and stress incontinent women. *Acta Obstet Gynecol Scand* 1980;59:265.

15. Wein A: Drug therapy for detrusor hyperactivity: Where are we? *Neurourol Urodynam* 1985;4:337–351.

16. Benson GS, Sarshik SA, Raezer DM, et al: Bladder muscle contractility: Comparative effects and mechanisms of action of atropine, propantheline, flavoxate, and imipramine. *Urology* 1977;9:31–35.

17. Caine M, Raz S: Some clinical implications of adrenergic receptors in the urinary tract. *Arch Surg* 1975;110:247–250.

18. Frommer DA, Kulig KW, Marx JA, et al: Tricyclic antidepressant overdose. *JAMA* 1987;257:521–526.

19. Stewart BH, Banowsky LHW, Montague DK: Stress incontinence: Conservative therapy with sympathomimetic drugs. *J Urol* 1976;115:558–559.

20. Bhatia NN, Bergman A: Pessary test in women with urinary incontinence. *Obstet Gynecol* 1985;65:220.

21. Rahman MS, Way S: Polyglycolic acid surgical sutures in gynecological surgery. *J Obstet Gynecol Br Commonwealth* 1972;79:849–851.

22. Laufman H, Rubel T: Synthetic absorbable sutures. *Surg Gynecol Obstet* 1977;145:597–608.

23. Berhan RE, Butz GW, Ansell JS: Comparison of wound strength in normal, radiated and infected tissues with polyglycolic acid and chromic catgut sutures. *Surg Gynecol Obstet* 1978;146:901–907.

24. Trimbos JB, Van Rijssel EJC, Klopper PJ: Performance of sliding knots in monofilament and multifilament suture material. *Obstet Gynecol* 1986;68:425.

25. Frisch EE: Technology of silicones in biomedical applications, in Rubin LR (ed): *Biomaterials in Reconstructive Surgery*. St Louis, CV Mosby, 1983, pp 73–89.

26. Beck RP: Recurrent urinary stress incontinence treated by fascia lata sling procedure. *Am J Obstet Gynecol* 1974;120:613.

27. Prem KA: Personal communication. August 1976.

28. Williams TJ, Telinde RW: The sling operation for urinary incontinence using mersilene ribbon. *Am J Obstet Gynecol* 1962;19:241.

29. Braley S: The silicones as subdermal engineering materials. *Ann NY Acad Sci* 1968;146:148–157.

30. Gordon M, Bullough PG: Synovial and osseous inflammation in failed silicone-rubber prostheses. *J Bone Joint Surg* 1982;64-A:574–580.

31. Sexton GL: The epiurethral suprapubic vaginal suspension (ESVS) for urinary incontinence, in Slate WG (ed): *Disorders of the Female Urethra and Urinary Incontinence*. Baltimore, Williams & Wilkins, 1982, pp 200–209.

32. Sexton GL: Epiurethral suprapubic vaginal suspension operation (Sexton operation) for urinary incontinence, in Wheeless CR (ed): *Atlas of Pelvic Surgery*. Philadelphia, Lea & Febiger, 1981, pp 112–115.

33. Hunter JM, Jaeger SH, Matsui T, et al: The pseudo-synovial sheath—its characteristics in a primate model. *J Hand Surg* 1983;8:461–470.

34. Harris T: Aging in the eighties, prevalence and impact of urinary problems in individuals age 65 years and over. *Advance Data Vital Health Stat* 1986;121:1–6.

Chapter 12

Urology for the Elderly Female

Eugene A. Stulberger and Stanley Bloom

INTRODUCTION

Both gynecologists and urologists deal with dysfunction of the genitourinary tract in elderly females. A variety of these conditions include urinary tract infection, calculi, neoplasm, and urinary tract fistula, and these are discussed in this chapter. This clinically oriented review highlights common areas of urologic concern to both the gynecologist and the urologist.

Aging is a continuous process that occurs at various rates in different individuals and causes numerous changes in different organ systems, including the genitourinary system. The genitourinary system of the female often reflects the changes inflicted by the hormonal, anatomical, and systemic stresses of aging. A large number of urologic problems may affect the female geriatric patient. Approximately 10% of all hospitalized patients have a urologic problem, and most of these patients are in the older age groups. The urinary tract is greatly influenced by the effects of age-related changes and the accumulation of multifarious pathologic problems that tend to increase with age. It is extremely common for elderly women to manifest with symptoms of lower urinary tract dysfunction. These pathologic conditions should be accurately diagnosed and promptly and properly treated.

URINARY TRACT INFECTION

It is well documented that urinary tract infections are more common in the elderly female. In fact, the incidence of urinary tract infection in the elderly female is approximately 12% greater than at any other age. The increase in prevalence appears to be significantly related to the menopause. Factors that predispose to this increase in prevalence are only partially understood. However, of extreme importance are mechanical factors and manipulation of the lower urinary tract. One of the mechanical factors involved is pelvic relaxation, which may lead to increased residual urine after micturition. However, in order to more completely understand the cause of urinary tract infections in the elderly female, one must examine the genital flora. The normal bacteria flora of the female genital tract can both cause and inhibit infection. It has become apparent that a woman's genital flora changes with age and becomes less protective. Numerous classic studies have demonstrated that the vaginal lactobacilli are antagonistic to pathogenic organisms and are nourished by glycogen provided through the trophic effect of estrogen. The lactobacilli metabolize glycogen, producing copious amounts of acid that restricts the vaginal flora to only those organisms able to tolerate such extreme conditions. Both an acid pH and lactobacilli are known to be present in the vagina of premenopausal women. This is in contradistinction to that of the postmenopausal woman, who has far less lactobacilli present in the vagina. This decrease in lactobacilli tends to create a clinical situation more favorable to colonization of organisms responsible for urinary tract infection. Most researchers believe that lactobacilli and an acid pH play a significant role in inhibiting urinary tract infection. Therefore, one of the most important changes that affects the elderly female is the postmenopausal decline in estrogen. The bladder, urethra, and genital tract have a common embryologic origin, and the epithelium of all these tissues responds to hormonal changes. With a decrease in estrogen, the epithelium and supporting tissues of the pelvic area atrophy. This results in a friable mucosa that tends to prolapse. The lower glycogen content in the vaginal epithelium results in less lactic acid metabolism by Döderlein's bacilli and an increase in the pH of the vaginal secretions, and thereby an increase in susceptibility to infection. Parsons has noted that the elderly female first colonizes her vaginal introitus and urethra before the onset of cystitis and will be at risk for recurrent urinary tract infection until colonization reverses to a more normal situation. Normal is considered to be the Gram-positive bacteria, lactobacillus, and diphtheroids that grow poorly in urine. These observations play an important role in the postmenopausal female because, as already noted, they are more prone to develop a Gram-negative colonization. Both the vaginal vault and the urethra have antibacterial defense mechanisms that are important in preventing the microorganisms from progressing from the rectum to the bladder. There are several theories to explain the vaginal resistance to bacteria. The most common is the acidity of the vaginal secretions. The alkaline pH noted in the vaginal tract of most menopausal females seems to be associated with the growth of Gram-negative bacteria.

Parsons reported that bacterial adherence to mucosal cells is a widely accepted prerequisite to colonization and infection of mucosal surfaces of many systems, including the genitourinary tract. The bacterial and mucosal cells' interaction is probably dependent on both receptors on the mucosa and some form of attachment mechanism utilized by the bacteria. The bacteria have special types of surface structures called pili that are used as adhesions to allow the bacteria to affix themselves to the mucosal tissue in question. The bladder, however, is highly resistant to infection, and its main defense mechanism is the continuous washing effect of the urine plus a nonadherent surface. The bladder is lined by a glycosaminoglycan that most effectively reduces infection by decreasing the bacteria adherence to the bladder mucosa. It has been suggested that reduced quantities of glycosaminoglycan is also responsible for decreasing the bladder's resistance to bacterial colonization and urinary tract infection. The chronically catheterized patient is also at great risk of developing urinary tract infection because it has been well documented that one of the significant predisposing factors to urinary tract infection is the indwelling urinary catheter.

Galask stated that one must also take into account, when discussing urinary tract infection in elderly females, other age-related changes that also occur. These can include alterations in immune function, especially in the lower urinary tract, and may potentially play a role in disorders of this organ system. In addition, from the 50th decade on, there are numerous age-related problems of intercurrent illness, with maturity-onset diabetes, malignancies, and decreased pulmonary and cardiovascular function tending to adversely affect the course of infection. Inadequate nutrition in the elderly has also been thought to play a role in both the development and the resolution of infection.

Pathogenesis

There are three primary routes for urinary tract infection: hematogenous, lymphatic, and retrograde extension of organisms directly from the rectum.

The retrograde extension of organisms from the rectum to the vagina and then to the urethra and ultimately to the urinary bladder is the most frequent route for infection. Organisms ascend into the lower urinary tract by the direct extension from the rectum across the moist perineum (which allows for bacterial colonization) to the urethra and ultimately to the bladder. Elderly females with cystitis first colonize their vaginal introitus and urethra before the onset of cystitis. The postmenopausal female is frequently a difficult patient to treat because she may not only have frequent episodes of cystitis, but these episodes may recur with an ever-changing variety of bacterial species. The source of the infection is the perineal flora. Most postmenopausal women tend to grow their entire rectal flora in this area. The pH of their vaginal secretions is significantly elevated, usually in the range of 7.0, because of the lack of estrogen stimulation. This results in many different rectal organisms growing in the vaginal introitus.

Etiology—Clinical Course and Symptoms

Dysuria and urinary frequency are among the most common urinary complaints brought to the gynecologist's and urologist's office. When a woman had significant bacteriuria (more than 10^5 bacteria per milliliter of urine) and also complained of dysuria and urinary frequency, she usually was said to have cystitis. However, recent data have suggested a need to reevaluate such patients because vaginitis and urethritis have also been noted to cause these types of symptoms. Komaroff and associates have noted that vaginitis was probably the cause in more than 60% of women who complained of dysuria. The urethral syndrome can also manifest with dysuria. The urethral syndrome has been subdivided into the acute form, which is often associated with infectious agents, and the chronic form, which most often is not associated with infectious agents.

Noninfectious causes of urinary frequency and dysuria, such as allergic, chemical, psychologic, anatomical, and hormonal, have also been implicated. However, no proof that these factors cause these symptoms has ever been documented. It has become clear that the majority of elderly females with dysuria and urinary frequency have infections of the vagina, the urethra, or the bladder. Approximately two thirds of women with dysuria and frequency who do not have vaginitis have significant bacteriuria, and thus cystitis is the cause of their symptoms. The remaining one third have acute urethritis, which can be subdivided into three groups: urethral infection owing to coliforms or staphylococci; urethral infection with sterile pyuria often caused by chlamydial or gonococcal infection; and those with pyuria who usually have no demonstrable infection. Chronic urethral syndrome is found in females who present with chronic dysuria but in whom no infectious cause can be demonstrated.

The causative agents responsible for urinary frequency and dysuria noted in vaginitis are *Trichomonas vaginalis*, *Candida albicans*, and *Gardnerella vaginalis*. There is, however, a question as to whether these organisms cause dysuria because they also produce a urethritis or because they cause a significant vulvar and labial inflammation with resultant burning on urination. These three pathogens can readily be cultured from the urethra in addition to the vagina. Urethritis may also be caused by *Chlamydia trachomatis*, *Neisseria gonorrhoeae*, *Escherichia coli*, *Klebsiella*, and *Staphylococcus*. *E coli* and *Klebsiella* urethritis usually also involve the bladder, resulting in cystitis. However, *E coli* is the pathogen most commonly responsible for cystitis. The majority of the remaining bladder infections are caused by other Enterobacteriaceae, including *Proteus mirabilis*, *Citrobacter*, *Enterobacter*, *Klebsiella*, and *Pseudomonas aeruginosa*.

Gleckman believes that bacteriuria is an inevitable occurrence in the chronically catheterized patient. It has been commonly observed that indwelling catheterization is a cause of urosepsis, Gram-negative bacteremia, transmission of pathogens, and stone formation. The presence of bacteriuria approaches 100% in chronically catheterized patients. In addition, it is unfortunate that the flora is not only polymicrobial, but also continuously changing. This flora tends to select out organisms like *P aeruginosa*, *P mirabilis*, *Serratia marcescens*, and *Providencia stuartii*, which are noted to have multiple antibacterial-resistant profiles (including tetracycline, ampicillin, and cephalothin resistance). These drug-resistant organisms persist once they emerge. The most frequent uropathogens isolated on urine cultures from catheterized patients include the above-mentioned resistant species plus *E coli*.

It is necessary to understand the natural history of urinary tract infection in addition to its morbidity in order to provide satisfactory medical treatment and to avoid excessive medical therapy. Edward Kass has theorized that urinary tract infections were, in many instances, unnoted during one's lifetime but were histologically evident at autopsy. It was also noted that urinary tract infection was much more common than previously thought. He found a significant group of any female population had asymptomatic urinary tract infection. Anomalies or complications of the urinary tract (stones, fistulae, tumors) were also found to be predisposing factors. In addition, it was found that the primary route of infection was ascending; that *E coli* was the most common pathogen; and that manipulation, catheters, and systemic diseases such as diabetes mellitus increase susceptibility to urinary tract infection.

At this point some simple definitions of various terminology related to urinary tract infection may clarify this subject. Bacteriuria means the presence of bacteria in the urine. However, the mere presence of bacteria in the urine does not constitute a urinary tract infection. As Stamey and associates have stated, the mucosal surface of the anterior urethra is normally colonized by bacteria, as are the vaginal vestibule and perineum. Significant bacteriuria is generally thought to indicate a bacterial count of 100,000 colonies per milliliter of urine in a properly collected voided midstream specimen. Asymptomatic bacteriuria refers to the presence of urinary tract infection in a patient without clinical symptoms. By definition, two consecutive positive urine cultures are needed to make this diagnosis. Cystitis denotes infection localized to the urinary bladder. Persistence of bacteriuria indicates the continued presence of the same microorganisms that were isolated at the beginning of the infection and continue to be isolated while the patient is still on therapy. Superinfection refers to the appearance, during treatment, of an organism that is different from the original infecting organism for which treatment was initiated. Relapse means recurrence of significant bacteriuria with the same species and serologic strain of organism as was originally documented. Reinfection denotes an infection that occurs after therapy has been stopped and is a different strain of microorganism or different serologic type from the original infecting strain. Pyelonephritis is used to describe bacterial infection of the renal parenchymal and renal pelvicaliceal system. Acute pyelonephritis is a clinical syndrome characterized by fever, flank pain, and costovertebral angle tenderness, and it may be associated with lower urinary tract irritative symptoms such as urinary frequency and dysuria. Chronic pyelonephritis denotes the histologic changes of patchy interstitial nephritis, destruction of the tubules, cellular infiltration, and inflammatory changes in the renal pelvicaliceal system (Figure 12-1).

Urinary tract infection may be either acute or chronic. It may also be relapsing, that is, with the same organism, or be a reinfection with a different organism. Lower urinary tract infections are usually characterized by bladder irritation with urinary frequency, urgency, suprapubic discomfort, and pain in the bladder region. Hematuria may be present. All patients with hematuria and/or recurrent cystitis should have a thorough urologic evaluation, including intravenous pyelography (IVP) and cystoscopic evaluation. One must always recognize the possible coexistence of a bladder tumor in patients presenting with lower urinary tract irritative symptoms because these symptoms may be present in both inflam-

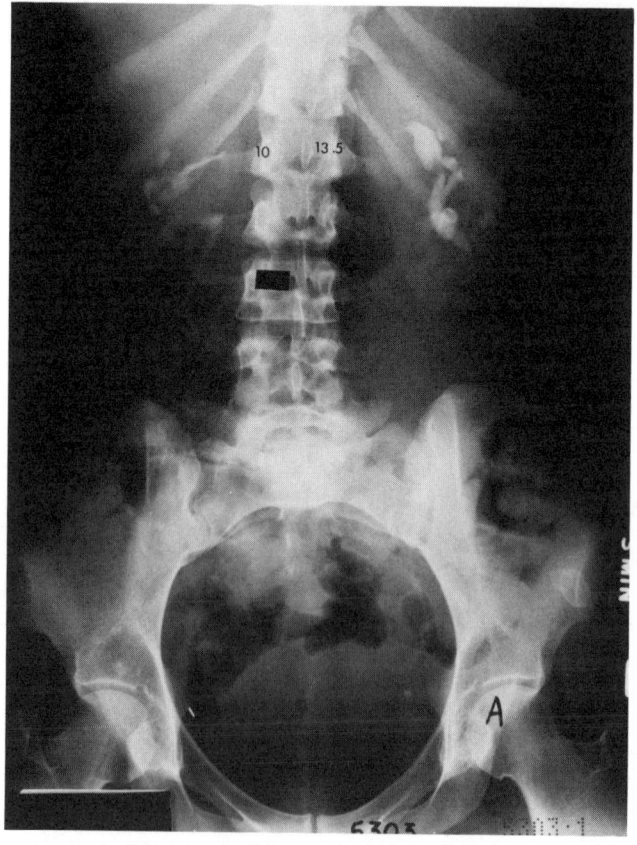

Figure 12-1 Pyelonephritis. Blunting of caliceal system with thinning of cortex of right kidney with calicectasis consistent with chronic pyelonephritis. *Source:* Courtesy of American College of Radiology Institute, Reston, VA.

matory and neoplastic diseases of the lower urinary tract. It is also important to remember that in the elderly female, urinary tract infections may only produce the nonspecific symptoms of weakness, unsteadiness, and confusion. However, when infection of the kidney (pyelonephritis) is also present, the patient may additionally present with fever, malaise, flank pain, and anorexia. Again, it is important to note that in the geriatric female, these symptoms may also be absent. It should also be noted that urinary incontinence is rarely caused by urinary tract infection.

Special problems arise with the elderly female patient who is either in a nursing home or hospitalized. Many of these patients are unable to care for themselves and are often thought to need an indwelling catheter on a long-term basis. As stated previously, approximately 100% of these patients will ultimately have infected urine. When it is necessary to use an indwelling catheter, one should use meticulous nursing care in addition to a closed urinary drainage system. The most significant factor concerning morbidity depends on the maintenance of free urine flow, intermittent catheter replacement to prevent the accumulation of amorphous material, and the development of aseptic techniques in caring for the indwelling catheter. The clinical manifestations of urosepsis in the chronically catheterized elderly female patient may at times simulate other disorders, such as intestinal obstruction. Shock has been reported in approximately one third of these female patients with catheter-associated urosepsis. Pyuria (10 or more leukocytes per high-power field) is commonly found in more than 90% of these patients. It is interesting, however, that the white blood cell count is normal in approximately 25% of these patients.

In most instances urinary tract infection is a benign condition. However, in some elderly females urosepsis produces disabling symptoms that necessitate hospitalization and, in some instances, can result in bacteremia, septic shock, adult respiratory distress syndrome (ARDS), and death. It has been demonstrated that the most commonly acquired infection that produces Gram-negative bacteremia in the elderly female is pyelonephritis. Classically, acute bacterial pyelonephritis manifests with flank pain, chills, fever, pyuria, and bacteriuria. These patients may manifest with mental confusion and with nonspecific abdominal complaints that may suggest a clinical diagnosis of intestinal obstruction or diverticulitis. It is also important to note that approximately 60% of elderly females with acute pyelonephritis will manifest with bacteremia. Of those females who develop bacteremia, approximately 25% will develop shock as a direct cause of the bacteremia.

Two other less commonly observed causes of urosepsis in the elderly female are papillary necrosis and emphysematous pyelonephritis. Papillary necrosis is a disease entity in which the renal papillae become necrotic, and slough off and obstruct the flow of urine. There are many causative factors that will enhance the development of papillary necrosis. One of the most common causes is the prolonged use of analgesic medication. Diabetes mellitus, arteriosclerotic disease, and sickle cell trait are also causative factors. One of the complications of acute bacterial pyelonephritis is also papillary necrosis. Diagnostically, this should be considered in all elderly females who present with one of the above-mentioned entities, especially if one also observes obstructive uropathy and/or progressive anemia. A patient with this disease will usually manifest with symptoms of flank pain, chills, and fever. She may also present with pyuria, hematuria, and leukocytosis. Pathognomonic, however, is the radiographic demonstration of a filling defect in the kidney (Figure 12-2).

Emphysematous pyelonephritis is an extremely rare and oftentimes life-threatening renal suppurative condition in which gas is demonstrated in one or both kidneys. This disorder may also be found as a complication of diabetes mellitus, especially in an elderly debilitated female patient. The patient is usually much

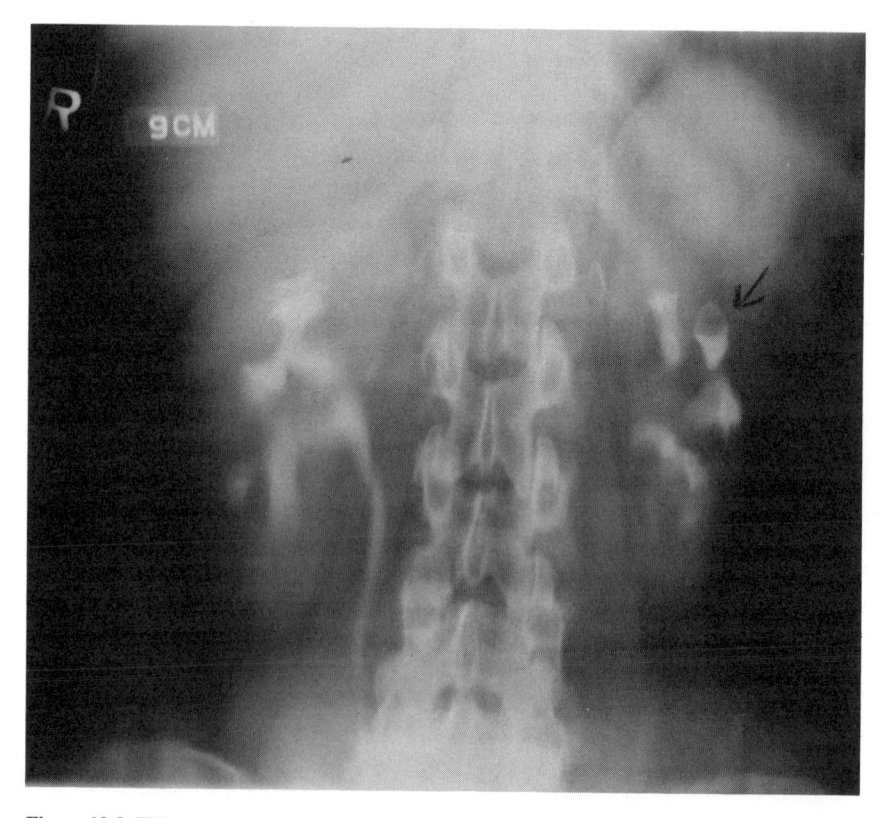

Figure 12-2 Filling defect of left upper renal caliceal group consistent with papillary necrosis. *Source:* Courtesy of Jan Levitan MD, St Barnabas Medical Center, Livingston, NJ.

sicker and presents with flank pain, vomiting, fever, and an extremely toxic appearance.

Other overwhelming infections of the upper urinary tract include renal abscess, perinephric abscess, and pyelonephrosis. These will usually present with chills, fever, leukocytosis, and a tender mass.

Vaginitis

A majority of genitourinary complaints in the elderly female are caused by vaginal infections. It is thought that the lack of estrogen causes the vaginal epithelium to become thin, dry, and friable and subject to various infectious processes. Symptoms and signs that favor this diagnosis include an associated history of a recent increase or change in vaginal discharge, vaginal odor, and vaginal and labial itching. These patients usually complain of pain as the urine passes over the labia. In most instances they do not complain of urinary frequency, urgency, hematuria, or suprapubic pain. The diagnosis of trichomoniasis or candidiasis can be proved by finding on microscopic examination the presence of trichomonads, or *C albicans* on wet-mount preparations of vaginal material. When clue cells are noted, this usually indicates nonspecific bacterial vaginitis.

Urethritis

After excluding vaginitis, the clinician should then consider the urethra and/or bladder as the sites for the patient's symptoms.

Acute urethritis is most often caused by *C trachomatis* or by *N gonorrhoeae*, which most commonly occurs in young, sexually active women as opposed to the geriatric patient. Examination may reveal a mucopurulent cervical discharge that contains many polymorphonuclear leukocytes. Urinalysis usually shows pyuria; however, coliforms are not usually found in Gram's stain. Special *Chlamydia* cultures are now also commonly available for office diagnosis.

One of the more perplexing individuals to diagnose is a patient with a nonbacterial form of urethritis, termed the urethral syndrome. Such individuals usually present with signs and symptoms of infection, but no bacteria or white blood cells are ever identified in the urine. This syndrome seems to include a spectrum of various nonspecific symptoms. The patient often complains of urinary urgency, frequency, and dysuria. Frequently these symptoms resolve spontaneously, but they may persist for months. On physical examination one may find a tender urethra; however, no white blood cells are noted on urinalysis and the urine culture is variably negative. No causative agent has ever been identified for this syndrome complex.

Cystitis

When symptomatic, this lower urinary tract infection is one of the most frequent problems of the ambulatory elderly female population. The symptoms of frequency and dysuria are not only bothersome, but also socially incapacitating and oftentimes lead to irritability and depression. Diagnosis of cystitis is most specifically made by urinalysis demonstrating pyuria (more than 10 leukocytes per high-power field) and a urine culture with at least 10^5 microorganisms of one species per milliliter of urine obtained by the clean-catch method. In approximately 50% of cases of coliform cystitis, pyuria is accompanied by hematuria. A presumptive diagnosis of significant bacteriuria can be made by examining a Gram's stain smear of uncentrifuged urine.

It is useful, when making a diagnosis, to classify cystitis as to its chronicity. Acute symptomatic cystitis in a female usually requires only a urinalysis and a urine culture for documentation. If a urine culture demonstrates infection to persist, the condition then falls into the category of chronic cystitis. Relapse (or reinfection) with a different organism of any frequency then requires further examination. On physical examination one must look for urethral outlet problems, such as urethral stenosis and cystoceles. An IVP should be done to detect any gross anatomical problem, such as bladder calculus, which may be a predisposing factor and is discussed later in this chapter. Finally, a cystoscopic examination should be performed. If abnormalities are found, successful treatment requires correction of these problems plus appropriate antibiotic coverage.

The classic concept that 10^5 organisms per milliliter are necessary to confirm the presence of urinary tract infection on a fresh aspirate from the bladder catheter lumen in patients who are chronically catheterized has recently been reappraised. Recent studies in catheterized patients reveal that, essentially, any quantity of bacteria from a catheterized patient can be consistent with early infection because progression to colony counts exceeding 10^5 per milliliter is a usual occurrence. Another observation is that urine obtained from the indwelling catheter can sometimes yield different microbial data from that information obtained by direct needle aspiration of the bladder. Therefore, for precise culturing, the urine should be obtained by either needle aspiration of the bladder or the introduction of a new urethral catheter. These two methods are much more accurate than obtaining a specimen directly from the indwelling Foley catheter.

A unique and oftentimes severe form of cystitis is interstitial cystitis. Its cause is poorly understood, but it may be a local autoimmune phenomenon. Recent theories have been advanced to suggest that in interstitial cystitis, there is a problem with the bladder surface. Diagnosis of interstitial cystitis is primarily made by cystoscopic examination under anesthesia. The findings are usually a reduced bladder capacity of less than 600 mL, diffuse petechial hemorrhages in the bladder mucosa, and pathopneumonically red erythematous patches of mucosa that split with bladder distention and are called Hunner's ulcers.

Pyelonephritis

Laboratory data usually include significant pyuria (more than 10 white blood cells per high-power field) and a positive urine culture of more than 10^5 bacteria per milliliter of urine. Blood studies frequently demonstrate a leukocytosis. Interestingly, however, in approximately one third of elderly patients, leukocytosis is absent. Blood cultures in approximately 60% of these women demonstrate a positive bacteremia. In pyelonephritis, however, even this tends to be inconsistent. Therefore, repeat blood cultures may be needed to demonstrate the presence of bacteremia in pyelonephritis because oftentimes the bacteria are inconsistently found in the blood. On the other hand, bacteriuria tends to be so common in the elderly female that its detection in the febrile geriatric patient is insufficient evidence to establish the diagnosis of acute symptomatic pyelonephritis. The findings, however, of a blood culture isolate identical to the urinary isolate provide strong confirmation that the urinary tract is the site of infection. Gleckman and Bergman have stated that the ACB (antibody-coated bacteria) immunofluorescence test is the preferred noninvasive test for determining the tissue source of a urinary tract infection. The test detects bacteria that are coated by human antibody directed against bacterial surface antigens. These antibodies are presumably kidney synthesized.

Treatment

Vaginitis

It would be inappropriate, and certainly unnecessary, for us, as urologists, to write anything about the proper treatment of vaginitis in a textbook geared to gynecologists. It is sufficient, however, to state in summary that trichomoniasis should be treated with metronidazole, candidiasis with nystatin (Mycostatin) vaginal suppositories, clotrimazole, or miconazole nitrate. In patients who are diagnosed as having nonspecific vaginitis, treatment is usually either ampicillin or metronidazole.

Urethritis

Women with chlamydial urethritis are usually treated with tetracycline, 500 mg, orally four times daily for seven days, or doxycycline, 100 mg, one to two times a day for seven to ten days.

In chronic nonbacterial urethritis (urethral syndrome), anticholinergic agents such as propantheline bromide (Pro-Banthine), 15 mg, four times a day, or phenazopyridine hydrochloride, 200 mg, orally three times a day are helpful. If these fail, urethral dilation may occasionally relieve symptoms; however, this is usually a temperizing method of treatment. Patients should be instructed to return to the office if their symptoms should not resolve. At that point another examination and evaluation for pyuria and a causative agent should be attempted. Cystoscopy and random biopsy of the bladder should also be considered if one suspects the possibility of in situ carcinoma of the bladder, which has, on occasion, been the causative factor for many of these ill-defined nonspecific symptoms.

Cystitis

Because cystitis is extremely common and there are numerous modalities of treatment, it is necessary to establish the following basic therapeutic goals before beginning therapy:

- The drugs should have as low a serum level as possible so that there is no disruption of the bacterial flora in other parts of the body.
- The principal place the drug should be found is in the urine.
- The antibiotic should, therefore, have a good urinary concentration.
- Of significant importance is the cost of the drug.

Asymptomatic bacteriuria is generally considered a benign condition in the elderly female who is free of a catheter. Most experts do not recommend treatment for asymptomatic bacteriuria in elderly females. In addition, they believe that treatment has no effect on morbidity or mortality and only hastens the development of resistant bacteria in the urinary tract. The benign nature of some of these infections should also lead to restraint in the use of antibiotics that have potentially dangerous side effects, particularly in the elderly. In addition, asymptomatic bacteriuria is not thought to cause progressive renal failure except in the presence of high-grade ureteral obstruction resulting in hydronephrosis. Patients with asymptomatic bacteriuria are, however, instructed to return for follow-up evaluation, especially if they become symptomatic. When the patient is symptomatic, the clinician may desire to begin initial therapy before the specific bacterial cause is known. In such circumstances the presence or absence of pyuria plays a critical role in determining appropriate therapy. Infection can nearly always be demonstrated in women with pyuria, making empiric therapy reasonable. Symptomatic infections in elderly women should be treated with an antibacterial agent that achieves high concentrations in the urine, such as ampicillin, tetracycline, sulfisoxazole, a cephalosporin, or nitrofurantoin. Courses of treatment over 1 to

3 days may cure some lower urinary tract infections in the younger female, but 7- to 14-day courses of antimicrobial therapy are probably more reasonable in the treatment of the elderly female.

Treatment of acute cystitis is directed against the specific pathogen in the urine culture, and sensitivity studies allow the choice of the specific antibacterial agent appropriate for treating the pathogen in question. The most commonly noted pathogen is *E coli*. In patients without renal dysfunction, sulfamethoxazole-trimethoprim, two 80- to 400-mg tablets twice a day, or nitrofurantoin macrocrystals, 50 to 100 mg four times a day, is a good choice. In patients with abnormal creatinine levels, ampicillin, 50 mg four times a day, or amoxicillin, 500 mg three times a day, may be used.

Follow-up cultures should be done in approximately 10 to 14 days to detect relapse of infection. Relapsing urinary tract infection in elderly females should be treated with a 2-week course of antibiotics. It is important to realize that chronic urinary tract infection usually does not result in renal failure. However, morbidity would be significant and may result in renal destruction if, in addition to chronic urinary tract infection, one finds an associated urinary tract obstruction or vesicoureteral reflux. If either of these is found, correction of the pathologic problem must accompany appropriate antibacterial therapy. Women with recurrent cystitis and no mechanical abnormalities are probably best managed with long-term, low-dose antibacterials. Two of the best drugs for this include nitrofurantoin macrocrystals and sulfamethoxazole-trimethoprim.

Patients with infrequent infections can probably be treated for a few days with each infection. However, those individuals who develop a severe and frequently relapsing series of lower urinary tract infections must be treated differently. If infections should occur more than five times a year or with an unusual organism, such as *P mirabilis*, in a patient in whom no structural abnormality is found, it is most likely that the source of the infection is the perineal area. This can be detected by performing a vaginal introital culture. In the management of these patients it is recommended that they have eradication of the bacteria with a full but short course of antibiotics and then the tendency for recurrence should be suppressed by giving a single dose of medication at bedtime for approximately 4 to 6 months. The most successful suppressive medication to date has been sulfamethoxazole-trimethoprim, one tablet at bedtime, or nitrofurantoin, 50 mg at bedtime. These have been demonstrated to significantly control recurrent episodes of cystitis. Most patients will become symptom-free and develop negative urine cultures. The theory for giving the bedtime dose of antibiotic is that the maximum benefit of the drug is obtained by having the bladder full of the antibiotic for the longest period. This usually occurs when the patient is asleep.

Parson has noted that another method of controlling chronic recurring infection is to change the alkaline pH of these elderly females to a more acid pH. This will partially control the problem by eliminating the abnormal flora from the vagina and the urethra. In most instances estrogen therapy will accomplish this within a short period of time. If the vaginal pH is over 5.0, a vaginal preparation using premarin, or dienestrol vaginal cream applied once a week will rapidly lower the pH of the vaginal secretion to 4.0. Once this occurs, the number of Gram-negative bacteria in the perineum will be reduced or disappear, thus allowing for easier control of recurrent bladder infections.

Interstitial Cystitis

There are a number of methods of treating interstitial cystitis, none of which have proved totally adequate. In a fairly large group of patients dimethyl sulfoxide (DMSO) therapy appears to be effective in controlling this disease. Therapy consists of 50 mL of DMSO instilled and left in the bladder for a 15- to 30-minute period. These bladder instillations are repeated on a weekly basis for approximately 3 months. If the patient does not respond to this therapy, other methods include hydrolic distention of the bladder and surgical procedures, such as cystolysis and bladder augmentation. If all of these modalities should fail, many of these patients ultimately will require some form of urinary diversion.

Urinary Tract Infections Secondary to Indwelling Foley Catheter

Adequate urinary output and free drainage are probably the most important factors in preventing symptomatic urinary tract infection in patients with chronic indwelling catheters. When urine specimens must be obtained from an indwelling Foley catheter, one must use aseptic techniques when handling, changing, or inserting the catheters, thus reducing the risk of infection.

Most authors do not recommend aggressive attempts at urinary sterilization in the asymptomatic chronically catheterized elderly female. This is because indiscriminant antibiotic administration can cause the emergence of drug-resistant strains. Antibacterial therapy, therefore, should be reserved for symptomatic infections. Treatment of a catheterized patient for urosepsis initially is the same as that of a noncatheterized patient. A 7- to 10-day course of treatment is usually adequate.

Pyelonephritis

Gleckman noted that urinary sterilization and defervescence in acute pyelonephritis can usually be expected within 72 hours of beginning appropriate drug therapy. An elderly female patient with normal renal function as established by creatinine clearance should be given intravenous gentamicin or tobramycin initially with a loading dose of 1.75 mg/kg of body weight followed by 1.5 mg/kg dosing every eight hours until serum drug assays are known. Drug assay monitoring is essential with these agents because of their potential for nephrotoxicity, ototoxicity, and vestibular dysfunction. However, Smith stated that tobramycin is less nephrotoxic than gentamicin. Gleckman has written that recommended peak serum concentrations for these agents are 6 to 8 µg/mL and trough values should be 2 µg/mL or less. The duration of therapy is usually 7 to 21 days. If fever fails to resolve in 92 hours, the following suspicions should be raised: presence of obstructed uropathy (calculus disease or papillary necrosis), inappropriate drug selection or dosing, adverse drug reaction, or intrarenal or perinephric abscess. Bacterial pyelonephritis may be complicated by shock, disseminated intravascular coagulation, or ARDS. Treatment of these complications includes vasoactive drugs, steroids, attention to intravascular volume requirements, respiratory support, and blood transfusions.

Papillary Necrosis

Papillary necrosis should be treated with appropriate antibiotics, supportive measures (food and electrolyte management), and, if needed, surgical removal of the obstruction. Nephrectomy is occasionally required for survival.

Emphysematous Pyelonephritis

Emphysematous pyelonephritis cannot usually be managed by antibiotics alone. Nephrectomy plus aggressive antibiotic therapy is usually required to treat this rather uncommon and oftentimes life-threatening renal suppurative condition.

RENAL CALCULI

Many advances have recently been made in the treatment of urinary calculi. As recently as 1978 it was suggested that as many as 50% of all stone patients may require some form of surgical intervention for treatment of their stone disease.

Advances in the medical management and the advent of extracorporeal shock wave lithotripsy (ESWL) and its adjunctive procedures (percutaneous ultrasonic lithotripsy and electrohydrolic lithotripsy) have reduced the necessity for open surgical intervention to less than 5% of all afflicted patients.

This is particularly significant when one considers that the peak incidence of urinary calculi in females occurs in the third to fifth decade. Indeed, the incidence of stone disease is less than three times as common in the male as in the female in the general population. Despite this ratio only 6% of males at age 50 compared with 25% of females are afflicted. This increased incidence of stone disease in females in this age group may be due in part to renal infections or metabolic diseases, especially hyperparathyroidism.

Despite these differences, Lonsdaler has noted that the incidence of upper urinary tract calculi is equally prevalent in males and females at autopsies, but the cause is different. In the male it is due to idiopathic calcifications or uric acid calculi, whereas in the female it is caused by urinary tract infections and metabolic defects.

Initial Presentation of Urinary Lithiasis

A urinary calculus will usually present with an acute episode of renal or ureteral colic, which may be associated with microscopic hematuria in the majority of cases and, less frequently, with gross hematuria.

A typical episode of colic begins suddenly with acute right or left flank pain with rising crescendo that courses laterally around the abdomen and generally radiates to the labia majora and round ligament in the female.

The pain is mediated by the autonomic nervous system and may cause other visceral symptoms, such as nausea, vomiting, and ileus. During the acute episode the patient is unable to lie still and frequently paces around the room or writhes in bed. Fever is rarely present. Pulse and blood pressure may be elevated, and there is evidence of respiratory distress.

Abdominal examination reveals some deep tenderness to palpation. In addition, the patient may show mild to moderate tenderness with fist percussion over the posterior flank. Urine analysis may show red blood cells, and a flat film of the abdomen may reveal the presence of a calcification in the area of kidneys, ureter, or bladder (Figure 12-3).

Management of Patients with Renal Colic

The first priority and therapy of a patient with severe renal colic is relief of pain. The diagnosis can quickly be established in most patients by doing a history and physical examination and checking the urine analysis for the presence of red blood cells.

Even in elderly patients as much as 100 mg of meperidine (Demerol) may be required for immediate relief. The amount of analgesic required varies from patient to patient, and recurrent episodes of colic may require additional analgesics in as short a period as two hours. Intravenous medications have been suggested by some physicians for immediate relief, although in most instances subcutaneous medication will suffice.

Confirming the diagnosis of the stone is relatively easy in a hospital setting. A urine analysis will have red blood cells at the time of colic, but the urine may clear within six hours. Kidney-ureter-bladder x-ray and an IVP will verify the diagnosis in most instances. Ultrasound is an alternative in the allergic patient (Figure 12-3).

Urology for the Elderly Female 263

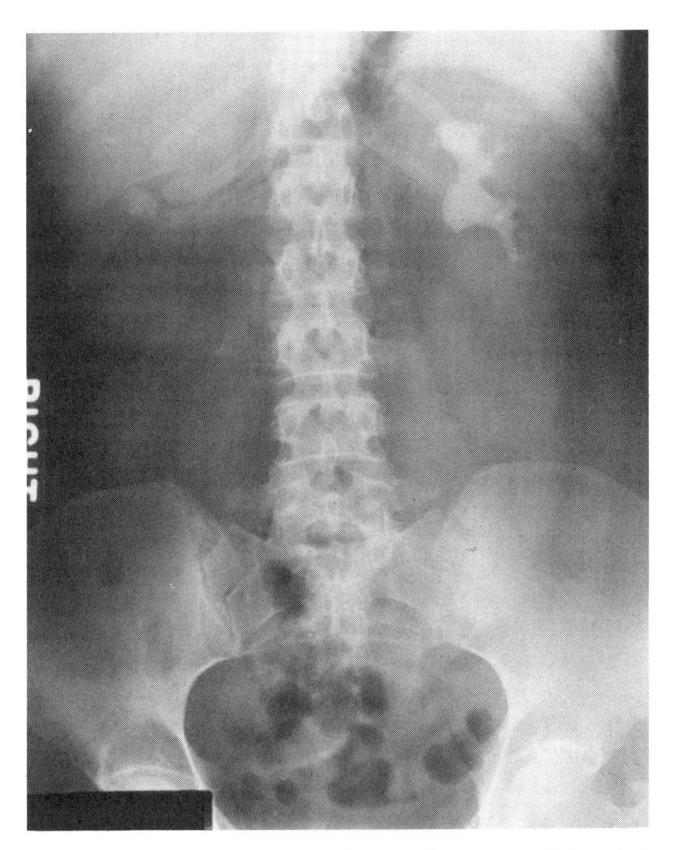

Figure 12-3 Intermediate phase of an arteriogram demonstrating an upper pole irregular hypervascular mass consistent with hypernephroma. *Source:* Courtesy of American College of Radiology Institute, Reston, VA.

Treatment of the patient with urinary stone in many cases may be expectant, since up to 60% of all stones will pass spontaneously. These patients are treated conservatively with hydration and appropriate analgesics, and their urines are strained to catch any stone fragments that may pass.

Current Kidney Stone Treatments

A number of methods are used to treat kidney stones, ranging from drug therapy to dissolve the stones to an open surgical procedure for stone removal. The type of treatment depends on the size and location of the stone and whether the stone is contributing to other urinary complications, such as blockage and infection.

Drug Therapy

If a stone remains small, usually less than 3 or 4 mm, it usually passes spontaneously in the urine, and the patient can be treated with drugs to reduce discomfort. Sometimes larger stones can be shrunk by appropriate drugs and will pass spontaneously or dissolve in the urinary tract. This is particularly true of pure uric acid calculi, which respond quite readily to treatment with alkalinization and reduction of uric acid levels.

The principles of conservative drug therapy are as follows:

- Identify the type of stone that is present.
- Test the patient for risk factors that exist in predisposed patients to new stone formation.
- Treat with appropriate medication to reduce these risk factors, and thereby reduce the possibility of stone recurrence.

Several new drugs hold promise in the treatment of kidney stone disease. Among them are cellulosodium phosphate (CSP), approved by the Food and Drug Administration (FDA) in 1982. This drug prevents calcium oxalate stone formation and is marketed under the name of Calcibine. It is an ion exchange resin that has a high affinity for calcium. CSP prevents the excessive absorption of dietary calcium, thought to encourage the formation of calcium stones.

Acetohydroxamic acid (AHA) was approved by the FDA in 1983 for the prevention of struvite stones. AHA, marketed under the name of Lithostat, is a bacterial enzyme blocker that prevents the formation of struvite stones that occur in patients with chronic urinary tract infections.

A third drug being looked at is potassium citrate, which inhibits the formation of stones associated with abnormally low levels of urinary citrate. Urine citrate normally prevents stone formation by inhibiting the crystalization of calcium salt. These drugs are now on the market and are expected to aid in the control of recurrent stones. As more experience is gained they may prove to be beneficial when used in combination with other, more familiar drugs for kidney stone treatment.

Surgical Treatment

As mentioned earlier, most stones that are small will pass spontaneously and require no intervention. In fact, about 60% of all urinary stones pass spontaneously within 1 to 2 weeks. The other 40% require some form of medical or surgical treatment. Treatment depends on the size and location of the stone as well as its mobility. Intervention can take the form of open surgical procedures, endoscopic procedures, percutaneous lithotripsy, or ESWL.

The traditional form of surgery for kidney stones is an open surgical procedure performed through the flank, which often required a 12-inch incision and sometimes required the removal of a portion of the 12th or 11th rib. A surgical procedure is reserved for stones in the kidney, renal pelvis, or upper ureter that could not be removed in any other fashion. The average convalescent time after this type of procedure is 6 weeks, and the procedure is often followed by a kidney stone recurrence rate as high as 40% to 50%. Up to one third of all patients required a secondary procedure to have additional or new stones removed at a later time.

Open surgery was also used for lower ureteral and bladder stones that could not be removed any other way. Patients similarly often required 4 to 6 weeks to convalesce after such surgical intervention.

Endoscopic Procedures

A number of methods were always available to urologists to extract stones from the lower urinary tract and bladder. One of the simplest was a standard cystoscopy combined with catheterization to bypass the ureteral stone. Very often leaving a ureteral catheter in place for 48 hours would dilate the ureter sufficiently to allow the stone to pass spontaneously after removal of the catheter. Other methods that have been used with moderate success have been extraction of ureteral stones with a stone basket and crushing of bladder stones mechanically with a special stone instrument. This could be carried out through the cystoscope.

New developments in endoscopy have provided alternative surgical methods for removal of stones in the lower and upper urinary tract.

Ureteroscopy. The passage of the ureteroscope into the ureter allows the urologist to directly visualize the stones that are present in any portion in the ureter. These stones may be grasped with special forceps or fragmented with an ultrasonic or electrohydraulic probe. These probes, called lithotrites—literally stone breakers—can be inserted into the ureteroscope and will disintegrate the stone under direct vision. In some instances this endoscopic procedure, which is called transurethral lithotripsy, can be successfully carried out for upper ureteral or even renal pelvic stones. However, stones lodged within the kidney cannot normally be recovered or removed by this method.

Percutaneous Lithotripsy. Another new endoscopic technique for kidney stone removal is percutaneous lithotripsy. This method allows the urologist to remove stones from the kidney, renal pelvis, and upper urinary tract through a percutaneous channel. An initial tract is formed by doing a percutaneous nephrostomy, usually under fluoroscopic control in the radiology suite or operating room. A fine needle is inserted into the kidney, and a tract is established that is gradually dilated. A nephroscope is introduced into this tract under general anesthesia and provides direct vision and direct access to the kidney and the renal pelvis. Stones that are visualized through this nephroscope can be removed by various types of loops, baskets, or forceps. Larger stones can be fragmented with an ultrasonic lithotrite probe, and then the fragments are irrigated free through the established tract. This procedure is essentially a closed procedure and shortens the hospitalization as compared with open surgery, which may require 2 weeks. Patients may leave the hospital within 72 hours after percutaneous stone removal. Postoperative recuperation is also much faster, and patients may return to work within 1 week after discharge from the hospital, compared with the standard 4 to 6 weeks after open surgery. One disadvantage of the percutaneous approach is bleeding. This can often be controlled by introduction of a catheter through the percutaneous tract after removal.

Extracorporeal Shock Wave Lithotripsy. ESWL, introduced in the United States in 1984, is the most significant advance in urology in the past several decades. It uses acoustic shock waves to disintegrate kidney stones noninvasively. The patient is immersed into a special tank of water, and the shock waves are generated by high-voltage underwater sparks that are focused on the kidney area. Under fluoroscopy control, the patient is positioned over the focus and, with general or local anesthesia, anywhere from 500 to 2,500 shocks are passed through the water. These shocks pass through the tissue and impact on the stones, fragmenting them into many small pieces. These pieces then may pass spontaneously over a period of several days to several weeks, usually without significant pain or morbidity. The shock waves are generated and regulated by a special electrocardiograph monitor that prevents the generation of the shock wave during the sensitive period of the cardiac cycle. It takes about 60 minutes to completely disintegrate a stone.

Many of these procedures are performed in an outpatient setting, and in some centers as many as 85% of the patients will be discharged on the day of the procedure and may return to work within 3 to 4 days.

A second-generation shock wave lithotripsy is currently being introduced. This machine no longer requires immersion in a water bath, but has the patient lying on a bubble of fluid on a regular operating room–type table. In the second-generation unit the shock waves are generated in sequence with the patient's respirations, and high-power fluoroscopy and imaging have improved the visualization and localization of the stones.

Initially ESWL was reserved for removing kidney and renal pelvic stones. It can now be used for upper ureteral and even lower ureteral stones, thereby obviating the need for surgery in most stone patients. As of the end of 1987, more than 250,000 patients had been successfully treated with ESWL worldwide, with well over 85% of patients being stone-free after one or, in some instances, two treatments. Only 5% of patients require open surgery.

One of the most significant benefits of shock wave lithotripsy is that patients can be discharged a day or two after treatment and resume normal activity, as compared with percutaneous lithotripsy, which requires approximately five days to a week of convalescence, and open surgical procedures, which may require up to 6 weeks of convalescence. In addition, complications are far less than that of an open surgical procedure or percutaneous procedures, and the risk to elderly patients is far less. These recent medical and surgical advances will be refined in the next several years and will lead to a continued success for resolution of treatment of kidney stones and reduce the complications and dangers of this disease.

URINARY VAGINAL FISTULA

The causes of urinary vaginal fistula have changed over the years. Birth trauma was the most common cause. Today, particularly in the older age group, the most common occurrence is after abdominal hysterectomy in patients who have had large fibroid tumors or who have had preoperative radiation for carcinoma of the cervix. In Kettle's series 77% occurred after some type of abdominal hysterectomy, whereas 19.8% occurred after some type of vaginal operative procedure.

Vesicovaginal fistula is the most common type of radiation injury to the bladder, accounting for up to 2% of the patients treated for cervical cancer. The factors that predispose to the occurrence of fistula after gynecologic surgery are as follows:

- Problems with circulation
- Use of preoperative radiotherapy, particularly radium with a variable dose to the bladder
- Bladder destruction by large tumors or previous surgery
- Lack of experience by the surgeon

Symptoms and Diagnosis

Patients who develop symptoms after surgery usually do so within the first 14 days, and the patient complains of painless leakage of urine through the vagina. The amount depends on the size of the fistula. With a small fistula the urinary leakage may be slight. With a large fistula all the patient's urine may exit through the vagina.

Patients may experience frequent vaginal leaks that require constant changing of pads. The odor of urine may be offensive to the patient and may be a cause for considerable consternation.

A Foley catheter may be inserted into the bladder, and if the fistula is not too large and is in a favorable position, the amount of urinary leakage may be limited.

Localization

At the time of the examination, demonstration of the lesion may be obtained by instilling a color dye such as methylene blue, which will appear in the vagina. Retrograde urethrography and IVP should also be performed to rule out the presence of a concomitant ureterovaginal fistula.

Once a diagnosis of urinary fistula has been made, a large Foley catheter should be inserted to reduce the occurrence of vaginal drainage. If the fistula is small, an attempt to endoscopically coagulate the lesion should be considered. This can be carried out by using a Bugby electrode, which is placed into the fistula through the cystoscope. The Bugby should be introduced into the entire channel of the fistula so that coagulation fibrosis may occur. After this procedure a Foley catheter is left indwelling for 3 to 4 weeks. When the fistula does not respond to this conservative measure, an open surgical procedure is indicated.

Here the timing of the surgery is all important. Most surgeons recommend a waiting period of 6 to 12 months to allow for the edema and inflammatory changes to subside. During this period the patient is advised to use estrogen cream in the vagina and oral corticosteroids.

In previously radiated patients or in radiation-induced fistulas, a waiting period greater than 1 year may be necessary for sloughing to cease and inflammation to resolve.

Treatment

In a patient suspected of having a vesicovaginal fistula, cystoscopy should be carried out as soon as possible to allow definite diagnosis. Small fistulas may be managed by tampons, pads, or adult diapers. A contraceptive diaphragm often provides additional protection when pads are not effective, but it must completely cover the fistula and should be properly fitted.

The standard management is to delay surgery for at least 3 months. Some believe that the uncomplicated fistula that is pliable on both bladder and vaginal sides without inflamed epithelial tissue may be suitable for earlier wound repair.

Some surgeons perform surgery within 4 weeks of injury when the repair was preceded by four to six days of phenylbutazone, 400 to 600 mg/day. Collins and Jones recommend use of oral hydrocortisone to decrease inflammation followed by early repair.

Postmenopausal or elderly patients are placed on estrogen replacement to aid in healing the vaginal side of the fistula. In the patient that still has a uterus, progestational agents should be given in addition to estrogen to prevent endometrial hypoplasia.

Each case must be individualized by the surgeon, bearing in mind that the best chance of success is the first attempt at surgical repair.

The surgical management of the fistula should be determined by its type and location and the experience of the surgeon.

The vaginal approach may be used for those fistulas that are low-lying and occur on the anterior aspect of the vaginal cuff near the midline.

Cure Rates

Vaginal repairs of simple posthysterectomy vesicovaginal fistulas are greater than 90% successful.

An abdominal repair is performed when multiple fistulas are present, or when organs other than the bladder and vagina are involved, or when the experience of the surgeon dictates an abdominal route.

Overall, cure rates are slightly lower than for vaginal repairs.

O'Connor believes that the following six factors generally are responsible for failure of vesicovaginal surgery:

1. Premature closure
2. Poor exposure
3. Inadequate dissection
4. Inadequate mobilization
5. Infection
6. Tension on the suture lines

He further believes that when these are avoided, vaginal closures should be at least 90% successful. He generally removes the urethral Foley catheter after 2 weeks.

TUMORS

Kidney Tumors

Renal cell carcinoma is increasing in incidence in the United States, and the death rate has risen to 2.76 per 100,000 annually. There is a distinct difference in incidence in this tumor between the sexes, with males outnumbering females by a ratio of 2 to 1. Soloway supports the concept that hormonal influence may be involved in the histogenesis of renal cell carcinoma. This is predominantly a tumor of adults with a peak incidence occurring in the sixth decade of life. The etiology is unclear, and there may be genetic, viral, hormonal, or chemical carinogenic factors as a cause. The tumors are usually unilateral and have no predilection for one side or the other, but in some instances they may present as bilateral tumors.

Clinical Presentation

The classic signs and symptoms of nephrocarcinoma include abdominal mass, flank pain, gross or microscopic hematuria, and a palpable tumor mass. However, it is not uncommon for the tumor to grow quite large without any symptoms appearing. In fact, many renal tumors are discovered incidentally in the course of various diagnostic studies or other conditions. When pain is present, it can be dull and confined to the flank area. Hematuria is usually microscopic, and this does not occur unless the tumor has invaded the renal pelvis. On occasion significant gross hematuria may be noted with a clot formation. It should be noted, however, that 50% of all patients will not exhibit hematuria in any form at any time.

Other presenting symptoms include elevated temperature owing to hemorrhage and tumor necrosis, and hypertension in the older age group, which can be due to vascular compression or arteriovenous shunting within the tumor mass itself. Other nonspecific signs include weight loss, anorexia, nausea, vomiting, constipation, and weakness.

Laboratory Findings

Anemia may be present in about one third of the patients owing to chronic blood loss. Polycythemia is not uncommon as well as eosinophilia, thrombocytosis, and hypercalcemia. If the tumor has invaded the collecting system, urinary cytology may be abnormal as well.

Uroradiologic diagnosis can be made with IVP, retrograde pyelography, ultrasonography, computed tomography, or renal arteriography (Figures 12-4, 12-5, 12-6). If a renal cyst is identified on ultrasound and this lesion is thought to be benign, cyst puncture may be carried out. One should recognize the risk of violating an unsuspected carcinoma in these instances and before this is done, further definitive arteriography and computed tomography should be carried out in an attempt to make the diagnosis of malignancy without violating the lesion.

Of particular importance in aspirating an apparent benign cyst is the cytologic evidence of malignancy from the fluid obtained or the presence of a bloody aspirate, which may be suggestive of a malignancy.

Metastatic Spread

Renal cell carcinoma is spread by direct extension beyond the renal capsule into the perinephric fat. It invades nearby structures, including the renal vasculature

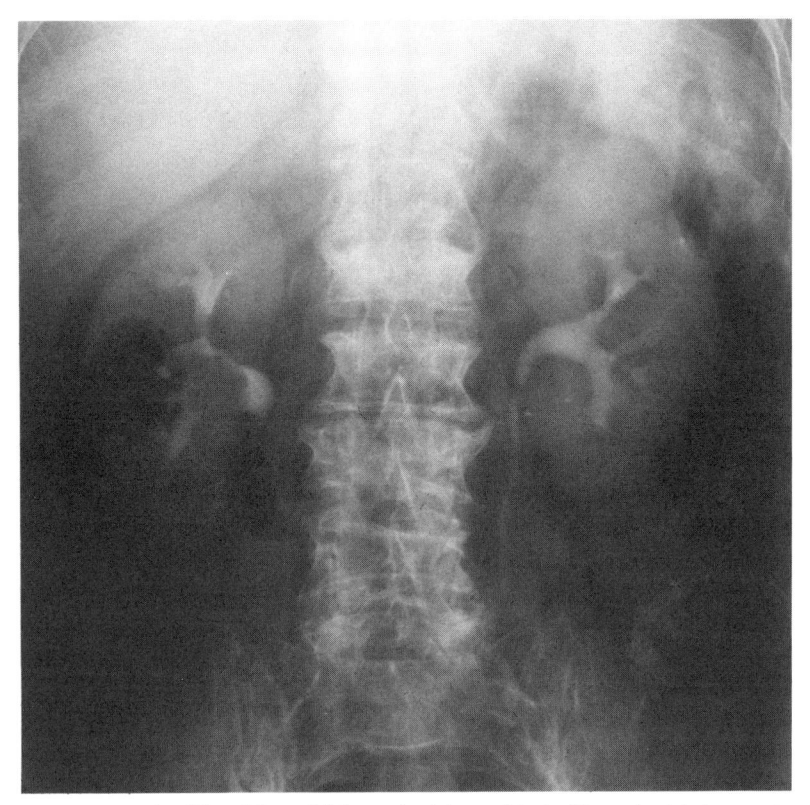

Figure 12-4 Irregular filling defect of right renal pelvis consistent with renal pelvic tumor—transitional cell type. *Source:* Courtesy of American College of Radiology Institute, Reston, VA.

and lymphatics. Up to one third of patients will have this type of local spreading at the time the diagnosis is made. The most common sites of distance spread are lymph nodes, lung, liver, and bone. It is not unusual to encounter patients with multiple metastatic involvement.

Staging System

The tumor is classified according to the degree of spread. Stage I tumor is limited to the kidneys. In stage II tumor the renal pedicle or renal fat or both are invaded. In stage III tumor there is regional lymph node involvement. In stage IV tumor there is distant metastatic disease.

Treatment

The optimal treatment for renal carcinoma, regardless of the stage, is radical nephrectomy with regional lymph node dissection. This offers the only certain

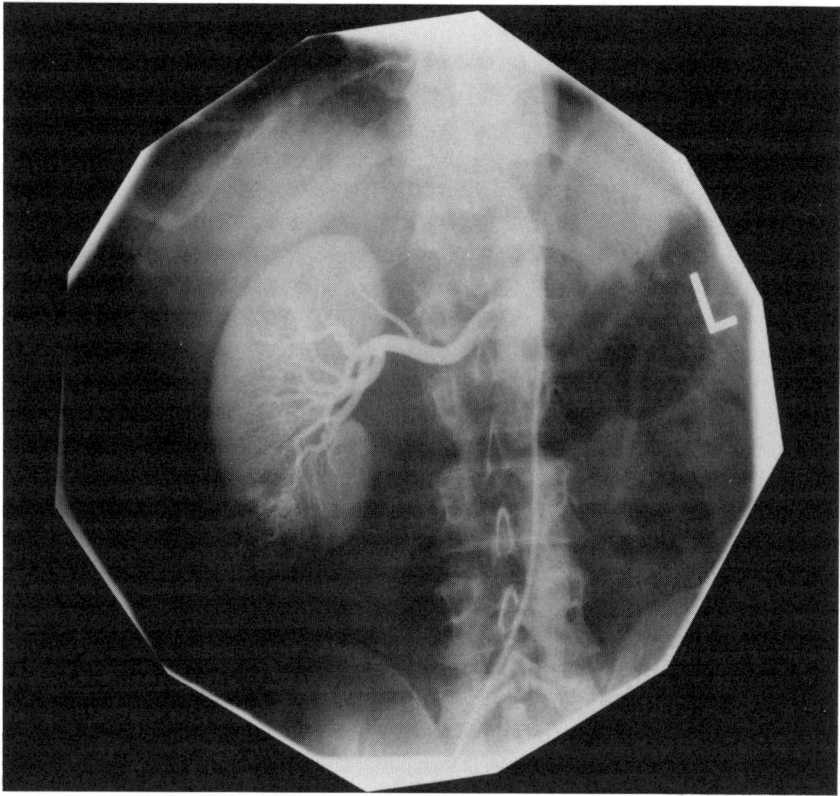

Figure 12-5 Arteriogram demonstrating a hypervascular mass of the inferior pole of the right kidney consistent with hypernephroma. *Source:* Courtesy of American College of Radiology Institute, Reston, VA.

cure for this type of tumor. Metastatic renal cell carcinoma has remained a disease that is resistant to all modes of therapy, and treatment of patients with this disease has been the subject of considerable debate for a decade.

Prompted by the occasional disappearance of metastases after removal of the primary tumor, urologists have long advocated so-called palliative nephrectomy to induce regression of metastatic lesions. In the literature there have been anecdotal reports citing such cases, although this treatment has been challenged by many urologists. Nevertheless, palliative nephrectomy for this group of patients can be carried out. Nephrectomy for those patients with significant pain caused by their tumor is an indication for palliative nephrectomy, and up to 50% of all cases require nephrectomy for local pain. There does not seem to be any increase in longevity of metastatic tumor patients whether the tumor is surgically removed or left in place.

Urology for the Elderly Female 273

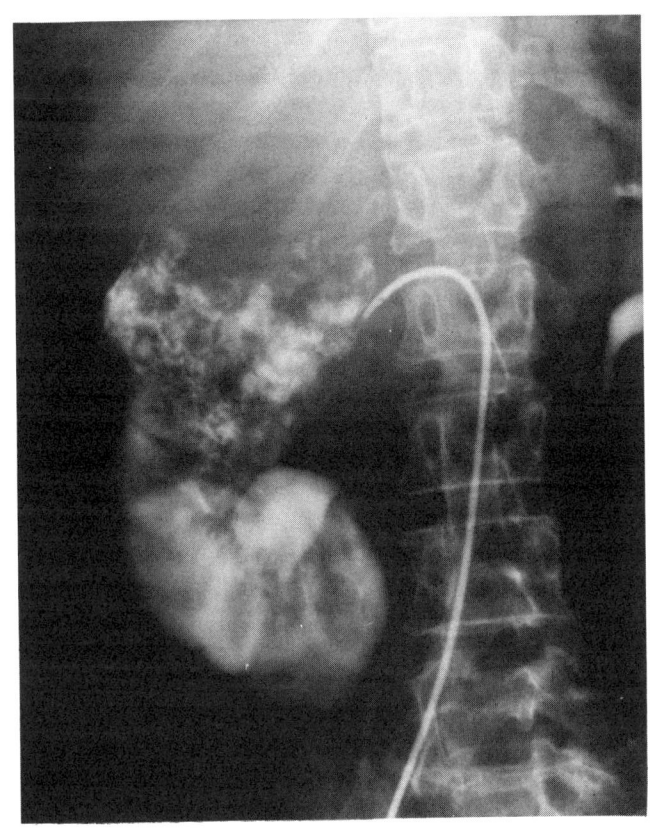

Figure 12-6 Kidney-ureter-bladder film demonstrating a large staghorn calculus of the left kidney. *Source:* Courtesy of American College of Radiology Institute, Reston, VA.

A third category of patients who may undergo surgery are those with only one or two concomitant metastases that are surgically resectable. The 5-year survival rate of this group of patients is in the range of 30%.

As pointed out earlier, the surgical treatment as well as radiation therapy, hormonal therapy, chemotherapy, and immunotherapy have all been tried for treatment of metastatic renal disease with not very satisfying results. Recent attention has been drawn to the possibility of immunotherapeutic strategies for the control of this tumor. Rosenberger and colleagues have used intravenous interleukin-2 (IL-2) therapy, and suppressor cell–depleted T cells have been tried. Belldegrun and co-workers have reported on tumor-infiltrating lymphocytes (TILs) in a number of human renal tumors. They were able to mix renal tumor with IL-2 and expand the TIL population while the tumor cells died. In several metastatic murine tumor models, treatment with expanded TILs provided complete resolution of pulmonary metastases, and a clinical trial of TIL therapy in patients with metastatic renal cell disease will begin shortly.

Bladder Cancer

Bladder cancer has a predilection for older people more than any other urologic cancer. In individuals aged 35 to 39 the incidence is 3 per 100,000, whereas in individuals aged 75 to 79, the incidence increases to 155 cases per 100,000. The average age diagnosed is 68 years, with men being affected by bladder cancer three times more often than women.

Cancer Risk Factors

Numerous carcinogens have been implicated as causative factors in bladder cancer. Among them are aromatic aramines used in leather and dye industries, the amino acid tryptophan, and artificial sweeteners such as saccharin and cyclomates.

Cigarette smoke is imputed to have a twofold increased risk of bladder cancer. There has been no direct evidence implicating artificial sweeteners as a carcinogen related to bladder tumors; however, there may be a long latency period between exposure and occurrence. Therefore, it may take years before we are really sure whether sweeteners are implicated.

Signs and Symptoms

The most common symptom present in bladder cancer is hematuria. Seventy percent of all patients who present with this complaint usually have gross, painless hematuria. This should never be ignored when seen in an elderly patient. Because hematuria often coexists with urinary tract infections, it must be investigated, especially in older patients. They must be carefully evaluated in order not to overlook a cancer. The initial presentation is usually due to a localized lesion on the bladder mucosa or superficial muscle layers, and therefore physical examination is usually unrevealing. Only with advanced disease may a suprapubic mass be felt. Rectal examination is usually of little value, and IVP (Figure 12-7) routinely done on many of these patients may not demonstrate the lesion. Therefore, cystoscopy is obligatory, often with biopsy and urine cytology. It is important to remember that the entire bladder mucosa is at risk for the occurrence of neoplasm, and therefore it is important to obtain a biopsy specimen of irritated or inflamed bladder mucosal areas that may not seem to be typical of the tumorous lesions. Often a random biopsy in an elderly patient with urinary irritative symptoms will uncover a bladder tumor.

Bladder washings and urinary cytology are central parts of patient evaluation. Another useful technique is flow cystometry. In this cytologic method the bladder is vigorously irrigated after it is emptied five times with 50 mL of saline through a

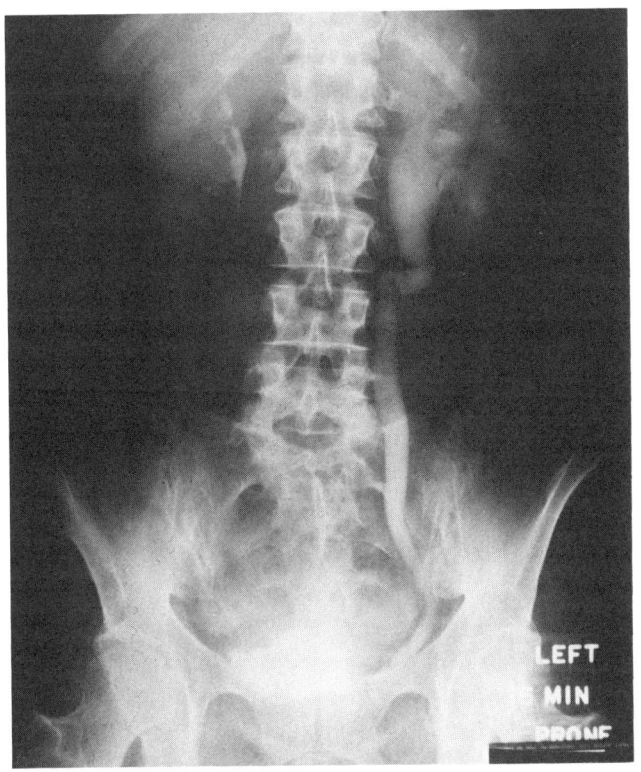

Figure 12-7 Obstruction in the distal left ureter with irregular filling defect of bladder consistent with bladder tumor. *Source:* Courtesy of American College of Radiology Institute, Reston, VA.

Foley catheter or cystoscope. The irrigant is then immediately placed in 50 mL of 50% alcohol and sent to the laboratory for evaluation.

Pathology and Natural History

Most bladder tumors are transitional cell carcinomas, constituting 95% of all lesions. The other 5% are made up of epidermoid and squamous cell carcinomas and adenocarcinomas. Transitional cell carcinoma of bladder typically may appear anywhere within the bladder, and the entire urothelial lining of the urinary tract is at risk to develop tumors, including renal pelvis, ureters, or urothelial lining of the urethra. Recurrences of bladder tumors are common, and often they occur in locations within the bladder other than the initial site. At least 30% of patients who have one bladder cancer will develop a new or recurrent tumor within 5 years of the original diagnosis.

The risk of recurrence of bladder tumors is directly related to their cytologic dedifferentiation, and the greater the dedifferentiation of the tumor, the more likely the recurrence. Patients who develop one bladder tumor must have mandatory follow-up and vigorous follow-up throughout their lives at regular intervals in order to detect and treat recurrences at the earliest possible time.

Staging

Stage or extent of disease is also important, as the bladder tumors are staged according to the depth of penetration within the walls of the bladder. The deeper the penetration, the higher the stage and the more invasive the tumor. Superficial tumors can be managed quite well by cystoscopy or local chemotherapy. Deeply invasive tumors have a higher risk of local and disseminated recurrence and often make transurethral techniques inadequate.

Management

Superficial tumors are generally well-differentiated papillary. They are confined to the urothelium and do not enter the deep muscle layer. These may be adequately controlled with transurethral resection alone. These patients should be cystoscoped at regular intervals, initially every 3 months and thereafter less frequently, depending on the rate of recurrence. Eighty percent of such patients will be free of disease and alive in 5 years.

Patients with multifocal superficial tumors in the bladder are more likely to develop recurrent disease. One third of the recurrences are at a more advanced stage than those seen when initially diagnosed. Consequently transurethral resection alone may be insufficient for those tumors. In these patients intravesical chemotherapy may be of distinct benefit. Among the agents used with success are thiotepa, which is triethylenethiophosphoramide and an alkylating agent, as well as doxorubicin (Adriamycin) and mithramycin. Work is currently being done with bacille Calmette-Guérin instillations. This has been shown to have considerable promise, although it was not yet approved by the FDA at the time of this writing. The side effects of agents such as these include bladder irritation and myelosupression, and therefore these patients should have their blood counts monitored before treatment.

In single isolated lesions it is possible to perform a simple resection of the lesion and follow the patient cystoscopically. Patients who undergo segmental cystectomy have a 50% to 80% 5-year survival rate. Encouraging results have been reported with the use of external beam radiation therapy for superficial transitional cell carcinoma.

For tumors that are more invasive a transurethral resection of the bladder and topical chemotherapy are inadequate. The 5-year survival rate of such treatment is only in the range of 10% to 20%. In these patients radical cystectomy or high-dose external beam radiation therapy yields higher 5-year survival rates. The morbidity and mortality of radical cystectomy and radiation therapy are a concern in older patients with bladder cancer. Operative morbidity and mortality with combined therapy is 3% to 5% and postoperative complications are as high as 25%. Although appreciable, these risks are often justifiable, given the overall dismal prognosis of stage B-2 and C bladder cancers treated with more conservative measures. Adjunctive radiotherapy is often used in combination with cystectomy and bladder diversion. One modality of treatment is to give 4,500 rad followed by cystectomy and then completing radiotherapy to 6,000 rad after surgery.

Another method is to give a quick course of 6,000 rad over a five-day period and then operate immediately after this therapy. More recently chemotherapy has been used in conjunction with radical surgery, and results have been promising.

Metastatic Disease

Most common sites of metastases from the bladder cancer are the lungs, bone, and liver. Patients should have a complete evaluation for disease in those organs before undergoing a cystectomy and ileal conduit diversion for cure. There is also an appreciable incidence of infiltration of the rectal, vaginal, and pelvic soft tissues and involvement of the retroperitoneal nodes.

Many regimens have been designed to exploit the efficacy of a number of chemotherapeutic agents. The most used drugs are cis-platinum, Adriamycin, vinblastine, methotrexate, and cyclophosphamide. Used in various combinations they are known by acronyms such as M-Vax, Cisca, and CMV, and are found to have effectiveness ranging as high as 70% in partial response for variable periods of time. In some instances complete responses have been documented after such treatment. Now some institutions suggest the use of one of these regimens preoperatively with follow-up evaluation of the bladder by computed tomography and cystoscopy with biopsies, and then to proceed with radical cystectomy.

There is so much to be learned about the efficacy of these various drug combinations, and in view of the substantial toxicity that exists for many of them, selection of patients appropriate for such treatment is of major importance. Patients who may not have metastases at the time of surgery may be spared the potential side effects of these vigorous regimens by eliminating them before surgery.

REFERENCES AND SUGGESTED READINGS

Urinary Tract Infection

Akhtar AJ, Andrews GR, Cairo FI, et al: Urinary tract infection in the elderly. A population study. *Age Ageing* 1972;1:48.

Asscher AW: Urinary tract infection. *Lancet* 1974;2:1365.

Asscher AW, Chick S, Radford N, et al: Natural history of asymptomatic bacteriuria (ASB) in non-pregnant women, in Brumfitt W, Asscher AW (eds): *Urinary Tract Infection*. London, Oxford University Press, 1973, p 51.

Asscher AW, Susman M, Waters WE, et al: Asymptomatic significant bacteriuria in the non-pregnant woman: 2. Response to treatment and follow up. *Br Med J* 1969;1:804.

Bergqvist D, Brönnestam R, Hedelin H, et al: The relevance of urinary sampling methods in patients with indwelling Foley catheters. *Br J Urol* 1980;52:92.

Cox CE, Lact SS, Hinman F Jr: The urethra and its relationship to urinary tract infection: 2. The urethral flora of the female with recurrent urinary infection. *J Urol* 1968;99:632.

Cruickshank R, Sharman A: The biology of the vagina in the human subject: 1. Glycogen in the vaginal epithelium and its relation to ovarian activity. *J Obstet Gynaec Br Com* 1934;41:190.

Cruickshank R, Sharman A: The biology of the human vagina: 2. The bacterial flora and secretion of the vagina in relation to glycogen in the vaginal epithelium. *J Obstet Gynaec Br Commonw* 1934;41:208.

Dickerson J, Bressler R, Christian CO, et al: Efficacy of estradiol vaginal cream in postmenopausal women. *Clin Pharmacol Ther* 1979;25:502.

Engel G, Schaeffer AJ, Grayhack JT, et al: The role of excretory urography and cystoscopy in the evaluation and management of women with recurrent urinary tract infection. *J Urol* 1980;123:190.

Forland M, Thomas V, Shelokov A: Urinary tract infections in patients with diabetes mellitus. *JAMA* 1977;238:1924.

Fowler JE: Urinary tract infections in women. *Urol Clin North Am* 1986;13:673.

Fowler JE, Stamey TA: Studies of introital colonization in women with recurrent urinary infection: 7. The role of bacterial adherence. *J Urol* 1977;117:472.

Galeck RP, Larsen B: Identifying and treating genital tract infection in postmenopausal women. *Geriatrics* 1981;3G:69.

Garibaldi RA, Burke JP, Dickman ML, et al: Factors predisposing to bacteriuria during indwelling urethral catheterization. *N Engl J Med* 1974;291:215.

Gladstone JL, Friedman SA: Bacteriuria in the aged: A study of its prevalence and predisposing lesions in a chronically ill population. *J Urol* 1971;106:745.

Gladstone JL, Recco R: Host factors and infectious diseases in the elderly. *Med Clin North Am* 1976;60:1226.

Gleckman RA, Bergman MM: Community acquired bacterial urosepsis in elderly women. *Geriatr Med Today* 1986;5:73.

Gleckman R, Blagg N, Hibert D, et al: Catheter-related urosepsis in the elderly: A prospective study of community-derived infections. *J Am Geriatr Soc* 1982;4:255.

Gleckman R, Bradley P, et al: Therapy of symptomatic pyelonephritis in women. *J Urol* 1985;133:176.

Gutti RA, Good RA: Aging, immunity, and malignancy. *Geriatrics* 1970;25(September):158.

Harding GKM, Ronald AR: A controlled study of antimicrobial prophylaxis of recurrent urinary infection in women. *N Engl J Med* 1974;291:597.

Harding GKM, Ronald AR, Nicolle LE, et al: Long-term antimicrobial prophylaxis for recurrent urinary tract infection in women. *Rev Infect Dis* 1982;4:438.

Kass EH: Asymptomatic infection of the urinary tract. *Trans Assoc Am Physicians* 1956;69:56.

Kass EH: The role of asymptomatic bacteriuria in the pathogenesis of pyelonephritis, in Quinn EL, Kass EH (eds): *Biology of Pyelonephritis*. Boston, Little, Brown, 1960, p 399.

Kass EH, Savage W, Santamarina BA: The significance of bacteriuria preventive medicine, in Kass EH (ed): *Progress in Pyelonephritis*. Philadelphia, FA Davis, 1965, p 3.

Komaroff AL, Pass TM, McCue JD, et al: Management strategies for urinary and vaginal infections. *Arch Intern Med* 1978;138:1069.

Kraft JK, Stamey TA: The natural history of symptomatic recurrent bacteriuria in women. *Medicine* 1977;56:55.

Kunin CM: *Detection, Prevention, and Management of Urinary Tract Infections.* Philadelphia, Lea & Febiger, 1979.

Kurtz SB: UTI in the elderly; seeking solutions for special problems. *Geriatrics* 1980;8:97.

Nagami P: Management of common infections in the elderly outpatient. *Geriatrics* 1986;41:67.

Notelovitz M: When and how to use estrogen therapy in women over 60. *Geriatrics* 1980;35:113.

Ouslander JG: Lower urinary tract disorders in the elderly female, in Raz S, *Female Urology.* Philadelphia, WB Saunders, 1983, p 308.

Parsons CL: Prevention of urinary tract infection by the exogenous glycosaminoglycan sodium pentosanpolysulfate. *J Urol* 1982;127:167.

Parsons CL: Urinary tract infection in the female patient. *Urol Clin North Am* 1985;12:355.

Parsons CL, Greenspan C, Moore SW, et al: Role of surface mucin in primary antibacterial defense of bladder. *Urology* 1977;9:48.

Parsons CL, Schmidt JD: In vitro bacterial adherence to vaginal cells of normal and cystitis-prone women. *J Urol* 1980;123:184.

Riehle RA, Vaughan ED: Genitourinary disease in the elderly. *Symp Clin Geriatr Med* 1983;67:445.

Smith CR, Lipsky JJ, Laskin OL, et al: Double-blind comparison of the nephrotoxicity and auditory toxicity of gentamicin and tobramycin. *N Engl J Med* 1980;302:1106.

Stamey TA: *Pathogenesis and Treatment of Urinary Tract Infections.* Baltimore, Williams & Wilkins, 1980.

Stamey TA, Condy M, Minara G: Prophylactic efficacy of nitrofurantoin macrocrystals and trimethoprim-sulfamethoxazole in urinary infection. *N Engl J Med* 1977;296:780.

Stamey TA, Sexton CC: The role of vaginal colonization with Enterobacteriaceae in recurrent urinary infections. *J Urol* 1975;113:214.

Stamey TA, Timothy MM: Studies of introital colonizations in women with recurrent urinary infections: 1. The role of vaginal pH. *J Urol* 1975;114:261.

Stamm WE: Guidelines for prevention of catheter-associated urinary tract infections. *Ann Intern Med* 1975;82:386.

Stamm WE: Management of the acute urethral syndrome. *Drug Therapy* 1982;12:155.

Stamm WE, Counts GW, Running KF, et al: Diagnosis of coliforms infection in acutely dysuric women. *N Engl J Med* 1982;307:463.

Stamm WE, Running K, McKevitt M, et al: Treatment of the acute urethral syndrome. *N Engl J Med* 1981;304:956.

Stark RP, Maki DG, Bacteriuria in the catheterized patient. What quantitative level of bacteriuria is relevant? *N Engl J Med* 1984;311:560.

Svensson R, Larson P, Lincoln K: Low-dose trimethoprim prophylaxis in long-term control of chronic recurrent urinary infection. *Scand J Infect Dis* 1982;14:139.

Warren JW, Muncie HL Jr, Bergquist EJ, et al: Sequelae and management of urinary infection in the patient requiring chronic catheterization. *J Urol* 1981;125:1.

Weigel JW: Diagnosis and management of urologic problems. *Geriatr Consult* 1984;2:14.

Yoshikawa TT, Guze LB: UTI: Special problems in the elderly. *Geriatrics* 1982;37:109.

Renal Calculi

Brannen GE, Bush WH: Ultrasonic destruction of kidney stones. *West J Med* 1984;140:227.

Brannen GE, Bush WH, Correa RJ, et al: Kidney stone removal: Percutaneous versus surgical lithotomy. *J Urol* 1985;133:1.

Bush WH, Gibbons RP, Lewis GP, et al: Impact of extracorporeal shock wave lithotripsy on percutaneous stone procedures. *Am Roentgen Ray Soc* 1986;147:89.

Chaussey C, Schmiedt D, Jocham V, et al: Extracorporeal shock wave lithotripsy: New aspects in the treatment of kidney stone disease. Basel, NY, Karger, 1982.

Coe FL, Parks JH: Recurrent renal calculi causes and prevention. *Hosp Pract* 1986;21:49.

Coe FL, et al: *Nephrolithiasis: Pathogenesis and Treatment.* Chicago, Year Book Medical, 1978.

Coe FL, et al: Effects of low-calcium diet on urine calcium excretion, parathyroid function and serum 1,25 $(OH)_2D_3$ levels in patients with idiopathic hypercalciuria and in normal subjects. *Am J Med* 1982;72:25.

Feit RM, Fair WR: The treatment of infection stones with penicillin. *J Urol* 1979;122:592.

Griffith DP: Struvite stones. *Kidney Int* 1978;13:372.

Griffith DP, Gibson JR, Clinton CW, et al: Acetohydroxamic acid: Clinical studies of a urese inhibitor in patients with staghorn renal calculi. *J Urol* 1978;119:9.

Hutschenreiter G, Alken P, Gunther R, et al: Percutaneous stone manipulation. *J Urol* 1981;125:463.

Lingeman JE, Newman D, Mertz JHO, et al: Extracorporeal shock wave lithotripsy: The Methodist Hospital of Indiana experience. *J Urol* 1986;135:1134.

Mitchell MD, Ker WS Jr: Experience with the electrohydraulic disintegrator. *J Urol* 1977;117:159.

Moores WK: The surgical significance of the proteus stone. *Br J Urol* 1976;48(suppl 6):399.

Nemoy NJ, Stamey TA: Surgical, bacteriological, and biochemical management of "infection stones." *JAMA* 1971;215:1470.

Pak CYC: A critical evaluation of treatment of calcium stones, in Massry SG, Ritz E, Jahn H (eds): *Phosphate and Minerals in Health and Disease.* New York, Plenum Press, 1980, p 451.

Pak CYC, Delea CS, Bartter FC: Successful treatment of recurrent nephrolithiasis (calcium stones) with cellulose phosphate. *N Engl J Med* 1974;290:175.

Pak CYC, Fetner C, Townsend J, et al: Evaluation of calcium urolithiasis in ambulatory patients: Comparison of results with those of inpatient evaluation. *Am J Med* 1978;64:979.

Pak CYC, Kaplan R, Bone H, et al: A simple test for the diagnosis of absorptive, resorptive and renal hypercalciurias. *N Engl J Med* 1975;292:497.

Parfitt AM, Higgins BA, Nassim JR, et al: Metabolic studies in patients with hypercalciuria. *Clin Sci* 1964;27:463.

Schulze H, Hertle L, Graff J, et al: Combined treatment of branched calculi by percutaneous nephrolithotomy and extracorporeal shock wave lithotripsy. *J Urol* 1986;135:1138.

Smith LH: Medical evaluation and urolithiasis: Etiologic aspects and diagnosis evaluation. *Urol Clin North Am* 1974;1:241:260.

Smith LH: Urolithiasis, in Earley LE, Gottshalk GW (eds): *Strauss and Welt's Disease of the Kidney,* vol 2, ed 3. Boston, Little, Brown, 1979, p 911.

Strauss AL, Coe FL, Deutsch L, et al: Factors that predict relapse of calcium nephrolithiasis during treatment: A prospective study. *Am J Med* 1982;72:17–24.

Wickham JEA, Ford TF: Transurethral ureteroscopic stone extraction. *Br J Surg* 1984;71:777.

Urinary Vaginal Fistula

Alfert HJ, Gillenwater JY: The consequences of ureteral irradiation with special reference to subsequent ureteral injury. *J Urol* 1972;107:369.

Collins GG, Jones FB: Preoperative cortisone for vaginal fistulas. *Obstet Gynecol* 1957;9:533.

Counseller VS, Haigler FH: Management of urinary vaginal fistula in 253 cases. *Am J Obstet Gynecol* 1956;72:367.

Graham JB: Vaginal fistulas following radiotherapy. *Surg Gynecol Obstet* 1965;120:1019.

Graham JB, Abad RS: Ureteral obstruction due to radiation. *Am J Obstet Gynecol* 1967;99:409.

Hebert DB, Vaughn ED: Vesicovaginal fistula: A therapeutic challenge. *Infect Surg* 1985;4:130.

Kaplan AL: Postradiation ureteral obstruction. *Obstet Gynecol Surv* 1977;32:1.

Keetal WC, Laube DW: Vaginal repair of vesicovaginal fistula, in Buchsbaum HJ, Schmidt JD (eds): *Gynecology and Obstetric Urology*. Philadelphia, WB Saunders, 1982, p 318.

Kline JC, Buchler DA, Boone ML, et al: The relationship of reactions to complications in the radiation therapy of cancer of the cervix. *Radiology* 1972;105:413.

O'Conor VJ: Review of experience with vesicovaginal fistula repair. *J Urol* 1980;123:367–369.

Patil U, Waterhouse K, Laungan G: Management of 18 difficult vesicovaginal and urethrovaginal fistulas with modified Ingleman-Sundberg and Martius operations. *J Urol* 1980;123:653.

Stockbine MF, Hancock JE, Fletcher GH: Complications in 831 patients with squamous cell carcinoma of the intact uterine cervix treated with 3000 rads or more whole pelvis irradiation. *Am J Roentgenol Radium Ther Nucl Med* 1970;108:293.

Tancer ML: The post-total hysterectomy (vault) vesicovaginal fistula. *J Urol* 1980;123:839.

Teham TJ, Nardi JA, Baker R: Complications associated with surgical repair of urethrovaginal fistula. *Urology* 1980;15:31.

Watson EM, Herger CC, Sauer HR: Irradiation reactions in the bladder: Their occurrence and clinical course following the use of X-ray and radium in the treatment of female pelvic disease. *J Urol* 1947;57:1038.

White AJ, Buchsbaum HJ: Cecovesicovaginal fistula. *Urology* 1973;2:559.

Wolff HD, Gililland NA: Vaginal diaphragm catheters. *J Urol* 1957;78:681.

Yenen E, Babuna C: Genital fistulas. *Obstet Gynecol* 1965;26:219.

Renal Cell Carcinoma

Bailey MJ, Williams JE, Riddle PR: Metastatic deposits from a previously treated carcinoma of the lung presenting as a renal cell carcinoma. *Br J Radiol* 1986;59:333.

Belldegrun A, Linehan WM, Robertson CN, et al: Tumor-infiltrating lymphocytes (TILs). *Surg Forum* 1986;37:671.

Campbell MF, Harrison JH, et al: *Urology*. Philadelphia, Saunders, 1970, vol. 3 p 1957.

DeKernion JB: Renal cell carcinoma (editorial). *J Urol* 1986;136:805.

Fein AB, Lee JK, Balfe DM, et al: Diagnosis and staging of renal cell carcinoma: A comparison of MR imaging and CT. *Am J Radiology* 1987;148:480.

Fowler JE Jr: Failure of immunotherapy for metastatic renal cell carcinoma. *J Urol* 1986;135:22.

Golimbu M, Al-Askari S, et al: Aggressive treatment of metastatic renal cancer. *J Urol* 1986;136:805.

Golimbu M, Joshi P, Sperper A, et al: Renal cell carcinoma: Survival and prognostic factors. *Urology* 1986;27:291.

Rosenberg, et al: Observation on the systematic administration of autologous lymphokine-activated killer cells and recombinant interleukin-2 to patients with metastatic cancer. *N Engl J Med* 1985; 313:1485.

Rotolo JE, O'Brien WM, Lynch JH: Renal cell carcinoma. *Hosp Pract* 1987;22:59.

Sarna G, Figlin R, et al: Interferon in renal cell carcinoma. The UCLA experience. *Cancer* 1987; 59:610.

Tosi P, Luzi P, et al: Nuclear morphometry as an important prognostic factor in stage I renal cell carcinoma. *Cancer* 1986;58:2512.

Bladder Cancer

Bloom HJG, Hendry WF, Wallace DM, et al: Treatment of T_3 bladder cancer: Controlled trial of preoperative radiotherapy and radical cystectomy vs radical radiotherapy. Second report and review (for the Clinical Trials Group, Institute of Urology). *Br J Urol* 1982;54:136.

Droller MJ: Therapies and potential therapies in bladder cancer. *Mediguide to Urology* 1986;2(1).

Fisher B, Slack N, Katrych D, et al: Ten-year follow-up results of patients with carcinoma of the breast in cooperative clinical trial evaluating surgical adjuvant chemotherapy. *Surg Gynecol Obstet* 1975; 140:528.

Harris MF, Schwinn CP, Morrow JW, et al: Exfoliative cytology of the urinary bladder irrigation specimen. *Acta Cytol* 1971;15:385.

Mostofi FK, Sorbin LH, Torloni H: Histological typing of urinary bladder tumors, in *International Classification of Tumors*. Geneva, WHO, 1973.

Murphy WM, Soloway MS: Developing carcinoma (dysplasia) of the urinary bladder. *Pathol Annu* 1982;17:197.

Murphy WM, Webb JN: Pathology of bladder cancer, in Skrabanek P, Geneva AW (eds): *Bladder Cancer: UICC Technical Report Series,* vol 60, ch 1.

Perez CA: Preoperative irradiation in the treatment of cancer. Experimental observation and clinical implications. *Front Radiat Ther Oncol* 1970;5:1.

Richie JP, Weichselbaum RR, Dahlberg W, et al: Effects of ionizing radiation on human bladder cell lines: An in vitro radiobiologic study. *Surg Forum* 1983;34:674–675.

Soloway MS: The role of intravesical therapy in the management of urothelial cancer. *J Urol* 1985; 26(4).

Soloway MS, Ikard M, Scheinberg M, et al: Concurrent radiation and cisplatin in the treatment of advanced bladder cancer: Preliminary report. *J Urology* 1982;128:1031.

Steinberg CN, Yogada A, Scher HI, et al: Preliminary results of M-Vac (methotrexate, vinblastine, doxorubicin and cisplatin) for transitional cell carcinoma of the urothelium. *J Urol* 1985;133:1.

Tannock IF, Gospodarowicz M, Evans WK: Chemotherapy for metastatic transitional carcinoma of the urinary tract. *Cancer* 1983;51:216.

Whitmore WF Jr: Management of bladder cancer. *Curr Prob Cancer* 1979;4:1.

Whitmore WF: Integrated irradiation and cystectomy for bladder cancer. *Br J Urol* 1980;52:1.

Yagoda A: Future implications of phase 2 chemotherapy trials in ninety-five patients with measurable advanced bladder cancer. *Cancer Res* 1977;37:2775.

Yagoda A: Progress in the chemotherapeutic treatment of advanced bladder cancer, in Dennis L, Smith PH, Pavone-Macaluse M (eds): *Clinical Bladder Cancer*. New York, Plenum Press, 1982, p 113.

Chapter 13

Vulvar Changes with Aging

James. A. Wilson II

INTRODUCTION

The aging vulva can be described in both physiological and pathological terms. The physiology of vulvar aging requires an understanding of the morphological changes that occur in skin over time. The molecular events that underlie these changes are currently obscure, although productive research in molecular biology is being made.[1,2] Despite our inability to define a biochemical mechanism for aging, distinct changes are observable, both histologically and grossly. These are discussed below. Dermatoheliosis, a term used to describe sun-induced aging, is not discussed, since the vulva is not usually exposed in the same manner as skin elsewhere on the body. However, it should be recognized that no explanation of the aging process of skin would be complete without reference to the changes that occur with solar exposure.

Pathological conditions that affect the vulva may be viewed from the standpoint of those conditions that are the direct result of the aging process, and those that are merely associated with it. Some lesions primarily seen in postmenopausal women are also encountered in younger women and are also addressed here. This does not imply that they occur solely in older women, but that they contribute to the pathology that is seen in older women.

THE NORMAL AGING PROCESS

Embryologically, the vulva is formed in response to the factors that regulate normal sexual development. In 46,XX individuals the Y chromosome is not present, and development will occur along female lines.

Before 10 weeks' gestation a bipotential state of development of the external genitalia exists. Without the masculinizing effects of the Y chromosome the urogenital sinus remains open and forms the vagina and urethra. In addition, the genital tubercle becomes the clitoris, the genital swellings become the labia majora, and the genital folds evolve into the labia minora. This process occurs from the 10th through the 14th week of gestation.

At puberty an increase in adrenal androgens results in the appearance of pubic hair on the vulva. This commences at a median age of 10.5 years. Once begun, pubic hair growth continues even under modest conditions of androgen stimulation. In addition to vulvar hair growth, enlargement of the labia majora and mons pubis, owing to proliferation of the subcutaneous fat layer, is seen, along with increased labial pigmentation.

Before discussing the age-related changes in the vulva, a review of the components of normal skin is offered.

The skin consists of three separate layers: (1) the epidermis, (2) the dermis, and (3) the subcutaneous fat layer. The epidermis is chiefly composed of stratified squamous cells, which make up approximately 85% of the cells of this 0.2-mm layer. Epidermal appendages such as hair follicles, and sebaceous, eccrine, and aprocrine glands are derived from these squamous cells during embryological development. The second major cell type is the melanocyte, of neural crest derivation. This cell is responsible for the production of melanin pigment and makes up 3% of epidermal cells. The third major cell type are the Langerhans' cells, approximately 2% of the epidermis, which are of bone marrow origin. Langerhans' cells are believed to function in the role of antigen recognition.

The dermis is a complex layer consisting of fibroblasts, mast cells, histiocytes, and macrophages. The fibroblast produces collagen and elastin, which contribute both tensile strength and elasticity to the layer. Also seen in the dermis are blood vessels, lymphatic channels, nerves, glands, and hair follicles, which are all surrounded by a mucopolysaccharide gel.

The subcutaneous fat is mainly composed of adipose cells and serves as a mechanical and thermal barrier. This layer varies in thickness form 3 to 25 mm.

The aging process causes several morphological changes in vulvar skin. Generally the skin becomes dry and rough, more susceptible to trauma, and becomes wrinkled. Skin turgor is appreciably decreased, and areas of uneven pigmentation are noted.

One of the most striking age-related changes is a flattening of the epidermal-dermal junction. An effacement of both the epidermal rete pegs and the dermal papillae results in more than a 50% reduction in the number of these interdigitations per unit of skin.[3] The smaller surface area undoubtedly contributes to the general reduced adhesion between the two layers and the tendency for older skin to tear and form bullae.[4-6] Other epidermal changes associated with aging include a decrease in the number of melanocytes[7] and Langerhans' cells[8] and a decrease in the epidermal turnover rate.[9,10]

The dermis is also subject to many age-related changes. Dermal thickness is reduced by 20%,[11,12] with noted reductions in both vasculature and cellularity.[13,14] This gives the skin an almost transparent appearance.[15] Dermal appendages, such as hair follicles, decrease in number,[16] and the hair itself is thinner. Grayness results from the progressive loss of melanocytes from the hair bulb.[17-19] Eccrine sweat glands decrease by 15%.[20,21] A significant reduction in the number of neurocutaneous end-organs is noted. Pacinian corpuscles, responsible for pressure perception and vibration, and Meissner's corpuscles, responsible for light touch, are both reduced to less than 50% of their original number.[22] Free nerve endings do not appear to change with aging. The decrease in the neural complement to the skin is undoubtedly responsible, at least in part, for the increase in cutaneous pain threshold that is seen later in life.[23-26]

Collagen, elastin, and dermal ground substance show age-related changes. Several studies demonstrate cross-linking changes in both collagen[27-29] and elastin,[30] but how this relates to the properties of aging skin is yet to be determined. Mucopolysaccharide ground substance has not been well studied, but it is thought to be decreased with age.[31,32] One study implies that this may account, in part, for a decrease in skin turgor with age.[33]

AGE-ASSOCIATED VULVAR PATHOLOGY

Contact Dermatitis

Contact dermatitis, also called reactive vulvitis, is caused by irritants or allergens that come into contact with sensitive vulvar skin. Some of the more common physical irritants would include mechanical trauma, such as bike or horseback riding, walking with tight, irritating clothing, and exposure to irritating synthetic fabrics. Chemical irritants are also commonly seen. These include soaps and detergents, perfumes and oils, fabric dyes, feminine hygiene sprays and powders, spermicidal jellies and foam, condom lubrication, precoital lubricants, and a variety of douches.[34(p112)] Certain medicines have the potential to cause irritation, and these are both fluorinated and unfluorinated corticosteroid creams, estrogen creams, gentian violet, podophyllin, and antifungal imidazole creams. Some women have claimed irritation to such innocuous substances as petroleum jelly and vitamins A and D ointment. The relationship between oral-genital contact, saliva, and vulvitis has also been described.[35]

The gross appearance is that of a diffuse, erythematous, often symmetrical lesion with slightly raised, irregular borders. Depending on where and how extensive the initial insult is, the lesion may be seen localized to the vaginal introitus, or it may involve the entire vulva. Saddle-shaped lesions suggest contact in the sitting position. Gradation of color intensity is seen with severer lesions, and in these cases bullae formation can occur.[36]

Microscopically, contact dermatitis may be seen in acute, subacute, and chronic forms. The histologic picture of acute dermatitis is that of variable intercellular and intracellular epidermal edema. Epidermal lymphocytes, neutrophils, and eosinophils are seen. As acute dermatitis goes to subacute and chronic dermatitis, less epidermal vesicles and edema will be seen with a graduate increase in the amount of acanthosis and hyperkeratosis. As the chronic condition persists, the number of lymphocytes decreases, and neutrophils will no longer be seen.

Usually the first symptom is pruritus. Scratching will exacerbate the lesions and may lead to secondary bacterial infection. An accurate history is absolutely essential, since it is the only means to gain insight into the sometimes strange and various insulting agents. In the geriatric population an accurate history is often difficult to obtain, and questions should be directed to changes in daily routines and new products.

The therapy for contact dermatitis is to first remove the primary reactant. If an insulting agent or mechanism cannot be found, it is best to advise a "blanket"-type approach. This would include warm soaks four times daily with a 1:40 Burow's solution followed by cool drying; no medications, sprays, powders, creams, ointments, or home remedies; and the use of only 100% cotton undergarments. The wearing of dresses and skirts should be encouraged. For patients who will only wear pants, it should be advised that they be worn loosely. For severer cases, soaks should be used as above. In addition, the use of corticosteroid lotion or cream applied three times daily, coupled with oral analgesics, may be necessary. For severe cases with bullae formation, the use of systemic corticosteroids is necessary. Prednisone, 20 mg twice daily tapered to nothing over a 2-week period, has been suggested.[36] Nearly complete resolution should occur over a 3-week period with proper treatment and elimination of the primary irritant.

Seborrheic Dermatitis

Seborrheic dermatitis is a relatively common inflammatory condition seen most often as a chronic, erythematous, diffuse lesion with irregular borders. The lesion may appear scaly and oily. In addition to the vulva, common areas of involvement are the nasolabial folds, eyebrows, scalp, sternum, and the region of the scapula. Although this condition is seen in areas where sebaceous glands are numerous, the lesion is not necessarily the result of the sebaceous cells themselves.[34(p114)] Interestingly, when lesions are noted on the vulva, the labia minora are not usually involved, perhaps because of the decreased number of dermal appendages in this area.[37]

Seborrheic dermatitis is a chronic condition of unknown cause. Recurrences seem to be associated with emotional stress, mechanical trauma, fatigue, or chemical and infective insult.

Treatment has been best achieved with the use of hydrocortisone cream topically applied three times daily. Severer cases require wet soaks three times daily with 1:40 Burow's solution, along with an oral antihistamine, such as hydroxyzine. If pruritus is present, Friedrich[34(p114)] has found that a mixture of seven parts betamethasone valerate (Valisone) cream and three parts crotamiton (Eurax) applied twice daily not only gives significant symptomatic relief from itching, but also improves the rash.

Vulvovaginal Candidiasis

Vulvovaginal candidiasis is extremely common. It is seen in women of all ages and in various areas of the body. In an overwhelming majority of these infections the causative agent is the fungus *Candida albicans*. *Candida glabrata*, formerly known as *Torulopsis glabrata*,[38] is found in only 5% of cases. Infections are found with increased frequency in association with periodic coitus, anemia, diabetes mellitus, a recent history of antibiotic usage, the use of corticosteroids, and a subadequate immune response.[39] If found on the vulva, it is virtually always present in the vagina.

Candidiasis is characteristically seen with large areas of irregularly bordered vulvar erythema. The redness, in some cases, can be intense. The dominant symptom is pruritus, which may be most acute on the medial surfaces of the labia minora. Patients complain of dysuria and dyspareunia. The associated vaginal discharge ranges from being thick and white-yellow to being thin, watery, and gray-white. Malodor is not a prominent feature.

A diagnosis of vulvovaginal candidiasis is usually straightforward. In uncomplicated cases the pH of the vagina as measured from secretions of the lateral vaginal wall will be less than 5.0. A fresh saline or KOH microscopic preparation often reveals the presence of branched and budding mycelial filaments and spores. KOH accentuates the microscopic presentation of the fungus by lysing epithelial and inflammatory cells, thereby blanching the background. An abundance of Döderlein's bacilli can be seen. Saline preparations reveal numerous polymorphonuclear leukocytes and cellular debris. *C albicans* can also be detected through Gram's staining and the use of a Papanicolaou smear, or through a fungal culture using Sabouraud's medium. The fungal culture does not need to be incubated.

Proper therapy consists of recognizing and treating underlying systemic illness such as diabetes mellitus and anemia, or realizing that systemic antibiotics or corticosteroids can precipitate candidiasis. The imidazole (miconazole, clotrimazole) creams and suppositories have been effective as topical agents. These are usually used nightly for three to seven nights. A longer period is sometimes needed for refractory cases. For particularly tenacious infections the detection of an occult anemia with adequate treatment has been rewarded with a quick and efficacious cure of the infection. Oral preparations, such as ketoconazole and nystatin, can be used in particularly difficult cases, although the use of ketoconazole has been associated with hepatotoxicity and anaphylaxis. The benefits versus potential risk with the use of this medication must be carefully weighed. An excellent drug for the treatment of all candidal species is topical gentian violet 1%. A one-time application to the involved vulvar or vaginal area will usually suffice. After treatment with gentian violet 1%, the patient should be advised that staining will occur unless proper precautions are taken.

Psoriasis

Psoriasis is a chronic, recurrent disorder characterized by focal areas of epidermal proliferation. Inheritance is almost certainly a factor in the transmission of this disease, and patients with psoriasis have a much greater incidence of rheumatoid arthritis than the general population. Interestingly, serologic tests for rheumatoid factor are usually negative. Vulvar psoriasis is usually seen in the area between the labia majora and the inguinal folds. When found on the vulva, it should also be searched for on the extensor surfaces of extremities, the scalp, back, buttocks, and nails.

The characteristic appearance of psoriasis is that of an erythematous, well-circumscribed plaque or papule with a white or silvery scalelike appearance. Vulvar psoriasis may appear less scaly than psoriasis in other areas of the body. Microscopic features include acanthosis and parakeratosis, elongation of the rete pegs and dermal papillae, intraepidermal microabscesses (Munroe microabscesses), a nonspecific inflammation with edema of the upper dermis, and dilated venules.

Treatment involves the suppression of the altered epidermal growth rate and can best be controlled with the intermittent use of fluorinated corticosteroids. These may be topically applied twice to three times daily on a short-term basis to avoid the development of atrophy. Coal tar preparations should be avoided, since they are not well tolerated in the vulvar region.

Pemphigus Vulgaris

Pemphigus vulgaris is a bullous disease of the skin and mucous membranes. Through the use of sophisticated indirect immunofluorescent studies, we now know that pemphigus vulgaris is a disease of autoimmune etiology. IgG-type autoantibodies react with antigens located in the intercellular spaces between individual epidermal cells. The nature of the antigens remains controversial, and their true nature needs further clarification. The antigen does, however, appear to be produced by the stratified squamous epithelial cells.

Characteristically, pemphigus vulgaris is especially evident on vulvar and oral regions of the body. The lesions grossly appear as flaccid and weeping bullae that leave large, denuded areas of skin. Because the bullae rupture easily, the initial presentation may be that of an erythematous, suppurative ulcer. The widespread nature of the disease can be a frightening observation for the clinician, especially if secondary bacterial infection has begun.

Histopathologically, the bullae are suprabasally, intraepidermally located with a loss of cohesion between epidermal cells, a process known as acantholysis. This process is pathopneumonic for pemphigus vulgaris. The entire pemphigus vulgaris bullae is composed of epidermal cells.

The diagnosis for pemphigus vulgaris is made from a biopsy of a fresh specimen and the appropriate IgG histochemical studies.

The treatment of pemphigus vulgaris requires an early aggressive approach with a physician skilled in the long-term use of systemic corticosteroids and immunosuppressive agents. The therapy is difficult and potentially hazardous to the patient, but it must be kept in mind that before the advent of systemic corticosteroids, pemphigus vulgaris was nearly always fatal. Other regimens, such as intramuscular gold sodium thiomalate, have been advocated by some, and proper consultation should be obtained to arrive at the best possible treatment plan for the patient.[40]

Bullous Pemphigoid

Bullous pemphigoid is a bullous disease of the skin of antoimmune etiology. It differs from pemphigus vulgaris in that no acantholytic process is demonstrated. The lesions of bullous pemphigoid, while having the ability to attain considerable size, show a good tendency toward healing. Diagnosis may be made through biopsy of a fresh specimen with a demonstration of IgG antibody using indirect immunofluorescent studies.

The treatment for bullous pemphigoid is similar to that for pemphigus vulgaris and involves the use of systemic corticosteroids and immunosuppressive agents. The therapeutic dosages in the treatment of bullous pemphigoid are usually lower than those used for pemphigus vulgaris. Sulfapyridine and sulfones may also be of value in the treatment of this disease. Warm compresses of 1:40 Burow's solution three times daily and silver sulfadiazine cream will reduce the risk of infection. Topical steroids may be beneficial with bullous pemphigoid, whereas with pemphigus vulgaris they are not.

Intertrigo

Intertrigo is a nonspecific inflammatory eruption of intertriginous areas. This is most often seen between the labia majora and labia minora, at the crease between the upper extremity and the abdomen, and at the opposing skin surfaces beneath an abdominal panniculus. Often seen with intertrigo are candidiasis, tinea, psoriasis, and seborrheic dermatitis. These conditions should be considered before making a diagnosis of intertrigo.

Characteristically, intertrigo appears as a mildly glistening, white-on-red widespread lesion on opposing surfaces where skin comes together. Its borders are often indistinct, and edema is usually present. Patients will primarily complain of pruritus and soreness.

Treatment consists of either hydrocortisone 1% cream or iodochlorhydroxyquin applied topically as necessary. Proper hygiene is important to minimize aggravating factors. Weight loss programs should be strongly suggested, along with "breathable" cotton undergarments and talcum. Acute excoriation of the skin is best treated with warm soaks followed by proper air exposure until the acute insult has subsided.

Urethral Caruncle

Urethral caruncles are inflammatory, nonneoplastic lesions of the distal urethra and urethral meatus. They generally present as a single, small red tissue mass located on the posterior margin of the external urethral meatus. They are rarely found in an anterior position or as multiple lesions. Urethral caruncles appear to arise from a localized ectropion of the urethral mucosa, and are bright red with a smooth or papillary surface. They are considered to be friable, highly vascular lesions and bleed easily when touched. Pain may be associated with micturition, coitus, and pressure on the lesion from either walking or sitting.

Microscopically, edematous granulation tissue is seen with a rich infiltration of lymphocytes and plasma cells. Abundant vascularity is noted. The differential diagnosis must include urethral carcinoma.

The most efficacious treatment for a large urethral caruncle is surgical excision. Once a biopsy has established the diagnosis, surgery can be undertaken with either electrocautery or cold-knife excision. The type of anesthesia is a surgical decision, but many procedures can be accomplished with a local infiltration of lidocaine 1%. If the caruncle is small, topical estrogen cream applied in small amounts twice daily may effect resolution. Before beginning hormonal therapy, a biopsy must be taken to rule out urethral carcinoma.

Nevi

Nevi, more commonly referred to as moles, are clusters of neural crest cells that are present from birth at the basal layer of the epithelium. This particular abnormality is on a time continuum, and when encountered at the basal layer is referred to as a junctional nevus. These may grossly appear as round, flat macules. As time progresses the cells of the nevi occupy areas above and below the basement membrane, and if biopsy specimens are examined at this time, they are referred to as compound nevi. Eventually the cells will occupy a completely intradermal position. As the cells become more intradermal, there is less likelihood for them to be transformed into a melanoma. In actuality few nevi become melanomas. It is interesting to note, however, that approximately one third of all melanomas arise from preexisting nevi.

Nevi are light to dark brown and may be fleshy and crustlike with a scaly texture. Diagnosis by biopsy is mandatory, since many entities resemble the nevi, including melanoma, lentigo, extramammary breast tissue, granular cell myoblastoma, acrochordon, and hydradenoma.

The treatment for nevi is excisional bioposy, which provides both the diagnosis and the cure. A generous biopsy should be used, to include the dermal layers.

Seborrheic Keratoses

Seborrheic keratoses are pigmented lesions that may be found on the vulva of postmenopausal women, although they are more prominent on other areas of the skin. These lesions are papulary and well circumscribed and comprise proliferating basal cells, intermixed with varying numbers of melanocytes. A histologic diagnosis is needed to distinguish this lesion from malignant melanoma and carcinoma. Sometimes seborrheic keratoses are seen in conjunction with malignancy elsewhere in the body but are, of themselves, not thought to have malignant potential.

The treatment for seborrheic keratoses is excisional biopsy, which is both diagnostic and curative. This may be carried out in the usual manner with local anesthesia.

Lentigo

Lentigo, a common, dark lesion of the vulva, can be found as single or multiple (lentigines) lesions. They are usually seen as flat, well-circumscribed discrete areas of approximately 1 cm in diameter. They are caused by an abnormal production of melanin from the melanocytes in the basal layer. Care must be taken to distinguish this lesion from nevi, melanomas, pigmented basal cell carcinomas, and squamous cell carcinomas.

There is no specific treatment with regard to lentigo. A biopsy is mandatory to establish the diagnosis, and if a solitary lesion is encountered, an excisional biopsy is curative. If several lesions are encountered and biopsies establish the diagnosis, no further treatment is necessary. A diagnosis of carcinoma should always be entertained when dark lesions of the vulva are encountered.

VULVAR DYSTROPHY

The vulvar dystrophies as a group are extremely common. They present as white lesions on the vulva and for years were referred to as leukoplakia, which, to many clinicians, implied cancer or a premalignant condition. It is now clear that vulvar dystrophy is not a premalignant condition, and although carcinoma can exist with vulvar dystrophy, it most probably does so as a separate entity not arising from the dystrophy.

The present nomenclature for vulvar dystrophy defines two basic forms: lichen sclerosus and hyperplastic dystrophy.[41] A third classification known as mixed dystrophy occurs when both lichen sclerosus and hyperplastic dystrophy occur together. Atypia may occasionally be seen with hyperplastic dystrophy in its pure form or in mixed dystrophy. When this occurs it is graded as mild, moderate, or severe. When severe atypia is present it is best approached as carcinoma in situ.

Lichen Sclerosus

Through the years lichen sclerosus, one of the vulvar dystrophies, has been noted by several names, which include lichen sclerosus et atrophicus, kraurosis vulvae, and atrophic leukoplakia. Some of the dermatologic literature still refers to lichen sclerosus as lichen sclerosus et atrophicus, but lichen sclerosus does not relate to a true atrophic condition, and gynecologists have rightfully dropped the "et atrophicus" from the formal name of this disease.

The cause of lichen sclerosus is unknown. Inheritance may play a role under certain circumstances, and certain studies may indicate an association between lichen sclerosus, pernicious anemia, and autoimmune diseases.[42] Some recent reports indicate that there is a partial deficiency in plasma testosterone and an elevation in androstenedione that may be correlated with patients afflicted with lichen sclerosus.[43] Other studies indicate a reduction in elastic fibers in the tissues of patients with lichen sclerosus.[44] Despite this ongoing research, the cause for lichen sclerosus is yet to be elucidated.

Lichen sclerosus may be seen in women of all ages and anywhere on the skin surface. However, it is seen most frequently in postmenopausal women, and the vulva is the most common site. In a large study by Wallace,[45] 190 of 200 women with lichen sclerosus had genital disease. Lichen sclerosus is more common in whites and is only infrequently reported in blacks and orientals. The same lesion in males, termed balanitis xerotica obliterans, is much less common.

The most common presenting complaint is pruritus. In cases of longer duration, patients may complain of vaginal soreness and dyspareunia. As the process advances further, complaints referable to the urinary tract, such as incontinence and dysuria, may be heard.

The gross appearance of lichen sclerosus is one of a white, confluent "atrophic-appearing" skin lesion. It is usually wrinkled, and described in terms of parchment or cigarette paper. Cracks and fissures owing to both the disease and scratching can lead to bleeding and ecchymosis. The changes are usually symmetrical and involve the entire vulva in a figure-eight or butterfly fashion. Advanced cases show a dissolution of the labia minora and clitoris.

Histologically, the changes seen with lichen sclerosus are a thinning of the epithelium with loss of the rete pegs. Below the basal layer of the epidermis is a homogenous band of dermis of variable thickness. Inflammatory cells, mostly lymphocytes, are frequently seen in this layer and may be due to secondary infection from the cracks and fissures. Surface covering will reveal hyperkeratosis, which is slightly acanthotic. Special stains reveal that elastic fibers are less apparent with varying degrees of dermal edema.

The treatment of lichen sclerosus involves the topical application of steroids. Friedrich[34(pp51-52,136)] has noted consistent relief and improvement with the twice-weekly application of 2% testosterone propionate in petroleum jelly. Initially the medication is applied two to three times daily and should be continued for 6 weeks, after which time the dosage may be tapered according to the patient's symptoms. A maintenance dosage of one application one to two times weekly for life is recommended. If the patient cannot tolerate testosterone well, topical progesterone creams have been helpful. This therapy is well tolerated and free of masculinizing effects associated with testosterone.

Surgery is not a viable alternative. Friedrich[34(p136)] has studied the surgical response with regard to lichen sclerosus and has determined that more than 50% of patients treated with a total vulvectomy had a recurrence. So, too, a majority of patients with deep vulvar laser vaporization were seen to have recurrences. From this information, and with biopsy-proven lichen sclerosus, the surgical option should be reconsidered.

Hyperplastic Dystrophy

Hyperplastic dystrophy, or lichen simplex chronicus, as it is known in the dermatologic literature, is the second of the vulvar dystrophies. Repeated local insult, together with longstanding chronic dermatitis, appears to be the mechanism in this disease. Patients universally complain of pruritus, and the itch-scratch cycle contributes to the local insult with inflammation and possibly secondary infection. Patients range from reproductive age to postmenopausal.

The gross appearance is that of a vulvar white lesion. Unlike lichen sclerosus, this lesion appears more localized with a thicker-appearing epithelium. The architecture of the labia minora and clitoris is usually retained in hyperplastic dystrophy, and ecchymotic ulcerative-appearing areas are usually not seen. The overall white appearance of the lesion is primarily due to an increased layer of keratin on top of the epithelium and the thickened epithelium itself with the basal melanocytes quite removed from the skin surface, thereby negating their color contributions.

Histologically, the cardinal feature of hyperplastic dystrophy is acanthosis, a thickening and widening of the rete pegs, and a generalized thickening of the epithelium. The broad and deep rete pegs of squamous cells usually show normal maturation from the basal cell layer to the keratinized zone. When atypia is present it is categorized as mild, moderate, or severe, in the usual manner, depending on how high the depolarization reaches. Atypia within hyperplastic dystrophy should be regarded in the same manner as atypia anywhere else on the vulva. As previously stated, hyperkeratosis is present. Inflammatory cells are almost invariably found in the dermal layer.

The treatment of hyperplastic dystrophy is aimed at obtaining resolution of the lesion and reducing the patient's symptoms. Toward this end, topical, fluorinated corticosteroids have produced a rapid response. To obtain the best response, a combination of three parts crotamiton (Eurax) is mixed with seven parts of a fluorinated corticosteroid, such as betamethasone valerate (Valisone). Crotamiton offers immediate relief from the itch, and when this combination is used twice daily for approximately 3 months, remarkable resolution usually occurs. Unlike lichen sclerosus, when resolution has occurred, it is not likely to return unless the previous insulting factors are reestablished. Efforts should be made to remove irritants from the area, which have included at times tight clothing, laundry detergent or body soap, feminine hygiene sprays, and certain douches. Some patients have complained that the lesions are aggravated with the ingestion of acidic fruits and vegetables. If this is the case, these foods should be avoided. Surgery is, again, inappropriate, and is frequently followed by a recurrence, since surgery per se does not remove the causative factors.

Mixed Dystrophy

Mixed dystrophy is the condition when both lichen sclerosus and hyperplastic dystrophy occur on the same vulva. Of all dystrophies, mixed vulvar dystrophy occurs from 10% to 15% of the time. The components of mixed dystrophy, both lichen sclerosus and hyperplastic dystrophy, will appear from a histologic standpoint as they do singly. The gross appearance of mixed dystrophy is difficult to tell from both hyperplastic dystrophy and lichen sclerosus in that all three appear as a vulvar white lesion. On occasion, however, biopsy of slight areas of parchmentlike tissue will reveal lichen sclerosus. Atypia is seen at a slightly higher rate when mixed dystrophy is present, and will be seen in conjunction with the hyperplastic portion of the dystrophy. Atypia for the mixed dystrophy is categorized as mild, moderate, or severe. As in the case of hyperplastic dystrophy, severe atypia is best managed as carcinoma in situ. Mild and moderate atypia usually resolve with treatment of the underlying dystrophy. Diagnosis is usually made through numerous punch biopsies, and it is advised that prior staining with toluidine blue be done in order to facilitate the directed biopsy.

Treatment of mixed dystrophy must accomplish the twofold purpose of eradicating the hyperplastic dystrophy and reducing and controlling lichen sclerosus. This may be accomplished in the first place with a 6-week course of corticosteroid cream applied topically twice daily. This may be followed by testosterone therapy. The testosterone therapy should proceed as if lichen sclerosus were present alone. The same concerns that apply to testosterone therapy with lichen sclerosus should be kept in mind with mixed dystrophy. Friedrich[34(p140)] has suggested an alternative method of using corticosteroid cream and testosterone preparations on alternative days. Using this method will delay resolution, but it has the advantage of fewer testosterone side effects.

REFERENCES

1. Finch CE, Hayflick L: *Handbook of the Biology of Aging*. New York, Van Nostrand Rheinhold, 1977.

2. Gilchrest BA: *The Skin and Aging Process*. Boca Raton, FL, CRC Press, 1984.

3. Andrews W et al: Changes with advancing age in the cell population of human dermis. *Gerontologia* 1965;10:1.

4. Katzberg AK: The area of the dermo-epidermal junction of human skin. *Anat Rec* 1958;131:717.

5. Kiistala U: Dermal-epidermal separation: 1. The influence of age, sex, and body region on suction blister formation in human skin. *Ann Clin Res* 1972;4:10.

6. Grove GL et al: Use of non-intrusive tests to monitor age-associated changes in human skin. *J Soc Cosmet Chem* 1981;32:15.

7. Fitzpatrick TB et al: Age changes in the human melanocyte system, in *Advances in the Biology of Skin. Aging*, vol 6; Montagna W (ed). Oxford, Pergamon Press, 1965, p 35.

8. Gilchrest BA et al: Effects of chronologic aging and ultraviolet irradiation on Langerhans cells in human skin. *J Invest Dermatol* 1982;79:85.

9. Grove GL, Kligman AM: Age-associated changes in human epidermal cell renewal. *J Gerontol* 1983;38:137.

10. Leyden JJ et al: Age-related differences in the rate of desquamation of skin surface cells, in Adelman RD et al (eds): *Pharmacological Intervention of the Aging Process*. New York, Plenum Press, 1978, p 297.

11. Black MM: A modified radiographic method for measuring skin thickness. *Br J Dermatol* 1969;81:661.

12. Tan CY et al: Skin thickness measurement by pulsed ultrasound: Its reproducibility, validation and variability. *Br J Dermatol* 1982;106:657.

13. Montagna W, Carlisle K: Structural changes in aging human skin. *J Invest Dermatol* 1979;73:47.

14. Andrews W et al: Changes with advancing age in the cell population of human dermis. *Gerontologia* 1965;10:1.

15. Fitzpatrick TB et al: *Dermatology in General Medicine*, ed 3. New York, McGraw-Hill, 1987, pp 146–150.

16. Giacometti L: The anatomy of the human scalp, in *Advances in the Biology of Skin. Aging*, vol 6; Montagna W (ed). Oxford, Pergamon Press, 1965, p 97.

17. Fitzpatrick TB et al: HA changes in human melanocyte system, in *Advances in the Biology of Skin. Aging*, vol 6; Montagna W (ed). Oxford, Pergamon Press, 1965, p 35.

18. Keogh EV, Walsh RJ: Rate of greying of human hair. *Nature* 1965;207:877.

19. Birch PRJ et al: The age-prevalence of arcus senilis, greying of hair, and baldness. Etiological considerations. *J Gerontol* 1971;29:364.

20. Silver AF et al: The effect of age on human eccrine sweating, in *Advances in the Biology of Skin. Aging*, vol 6; Montagna W (ed). Oxford, Pergamon Press, 1965, p 129.

21. Montagna W: Morphology of the aging skin: The cutaneous appendages, in *Advances in the Biology of Skin. Aging*, vol 6; Montagna W (ed). Oxford, Pergamon Press, 1965, p 1.

22. Winkelmann RK: Nerve changes in aging skin, in *Advances in the Biology of Skin. Aging*, vol 6; Montagna W (ed). Oxford, Pergamon Press, 1965, p 51.

23. Cauna N: The effects of aging on the receptor organs of human dermis, in *Advances in the Biology of Skin*. Aging, vol 6; Montagna W (ed). Oxford, Pergamon Press, 1965, p 63.

24. Sherman ED, Robillard E: Sensitivity to pain in relationship to age. *J Am Geriatr Soc* 1964;12:1037.

25. Procacci P et al: The cutaneous pricking pain threshold in old age. *Gerontol Clin* 1970;12:213.

26. Procacci P et al: Pain threshold measurement in man, in Bonica JJ et al (eds): *Recent Advances on Pain: Pathophysiology and Clinical Aspects*. Springfield, IL, Charles C Thomas, 1974, p 105.

27. Bentley JB: Aging of collagen. *J Invest Dermatol* 1982;78:444.

28. Bakerman S: Quantitative extraction of acid-soluble human skin collagen with age. *Nature* 1962;196:375.

29. Miyahara T et al: Age-related differences in human skin collagen: Solubility in solvent, susceptibility of pepsin digestion, and the spectrum of the solubilized polymeric collagen molecules. *J Gerontol* 1982;37:651.

30. Patridge SM: Biological role of cutaneous elastin, in *Advances in the Biology of Skin. The Dermis*, vol 10; Montagna W et al (eds). New York, Merideth, 1965, p 69.

31. Breen M et al: Acidic glucosaminoglycans in human skin during fetal development and adult life. *Biochim Biophys Acta* 1970;201:54.

32. Fleischmajer R et al: Human dermal glycosaminoglycans and aging. *Biochim Biophys Acta* 1972;279:265.

33. Silbert JE: Mucopolysaccharides and ground substances, in Fitzpatrick TB et al (eds): *Dermatology in General Medicine*, ed 2. New York, McGraw-Hill, 1979, p 189.

34. Friedrich EG: *Vulvar Disease*, ed 2. Philadelphia, WB Saunders, 1983.

35. Davis BA: Salivary vulvitis. *Obstet Gynecol* 1971;37:238.

36. Rossman I: *Clinical Geriatrics*, ed 3. Philadelphia, JB Lippincott, 1986, p 379.

37. Derbes VJ: Seborrheic dermatitis. *Cutis* 1968;4:553.

38. Boquet-Jimenez E, San Cristobal AA: Cytologic and microbiologic aspects of vaginal torulopsis. *Acta Cytol* 1978;22:331.

39. Syverson RE, Buckley H, Gibian J, et al: Cellular and humoral immune status in women with chronic *Candida* vaginitis. *Am J Obstet Gynecol* 1979;134:624.

40. Ahmed AR, Graham J, Jordan RE, et al: Pemphigus: Current concepts. *Ann Intern Med* 1980;92:396.

41. International Society for the Study of Vulvar Disease: New nomenclature for vulvar disease. *Obstet Gynecol* 1976;47:122.

42. Harrington CI, Dunsmore IR: An investigation into the incidence of autoimmune disorders in patients with lichen sclerosus et atrophicus. *Br J Dermatol* 1981;104:563.

43. Friedrich EG, Kalra PS: Serum levels of sex hormones in vulvar lichen sclerosus and the effect of topical testosterone. *N Engl J Med* 1984;310:488.

44. Godeau G et al: Isolation and partial characterization of an elastase-type protease in human vulva fibroblasts: Its possible involvement in vulvar elastic tissue destruction of patients with lichen sclerosus et atrophicus. *J Invest Dermatol* 1982;78:270.

45. Wallace HJ: Lichen sclerosus et atrophicus. *Trans St Johns Hosp Dermatol Soc* 1971;57:9.

Chapter 14

Vaginal Changes with Aging

Paul A. Bergh

INTRODUCTION

This chapter describes the normal anatomy, physiology, and ecology of the vagina and the changes that occur with aging. It presents the pathophysiology of vaginitis as it relates to the estrogen deprivation of menopause. Also, it reviews the prevalent types of vaginitis common to all ages of women.

Vaginitis, an inflammatory condition of the vagina, may manifest itself by a variety of signs and symptoms, including copious discharge, malodor, pruritus, burning, dysuria, and dyspareunia. These symptoms may range in severity from mild irritation to marked discomfort leading to sexual dysfunction and an impaired quality of life. In the postmenopausal woman vaginitis accounts for the majority of gynecologic complaints and is therefore one of the most common reasons for outpatient therapy. Correct diagnosis and treatment of this common and potentially debilitating condition require an understanding of its pathophysiology.

ATROPHIC VAGINITIS

With the advent of recent physiologic and microbiological studies the vagina has become recognized as an organ exquisitely sensitive to estrogen, undergoing marked hormonal-dependent changes and containing a dynamic ecosystem comprising numerous organisms. The onset of menopause, and its resultant estrogen deprivation, leads to physical, physiologic, and microbiological changes in the vagina. These changes are often the cause of many of the symptoms and sexual problems experienced by postmenopausal patients.

ANATOMY

The vaginal wall is composed of three coats: the tunica externa, the muscularis, and the mucosa. The tunica externa or adventitia is made up of dense connective tissue with many coarse elastic fibers. It contains numerous vessels and nerves, and offers support by itself and its connections with the rectovaginal fascia and vesicovaginal fascia. The muscularis makes up the bulk of the vaginal wall and mainly consists of a mixture of smooth muscle and dense connective tissue. The muscle bundles are primarily arranged longitudinally with a smaller inner portion of circular fibers.[1] The mucosa is composed of the epithelium with a basement membrane and lamina propria. The lamina propria is a dense, thin layer of connective tissue with an interlacing network of elastic fibers. There are numerous interspersed blood vessels but no glands except for occasional epidermal inclusion cysts, displaced endocervical glands, or mesonephric duct remnants.[2] Above the basement membrane lies the epithelium, consisting of six to ten layers of stratified squamous epithelium subdivided into four parts: the basal, parabasal, intermediate, and superficial layers.[3] The hormonal milieu determines the relative proportion of each of the three outer layers.

The vagina begins as a potential cavity, with the walls of the nulliparous patient in a normal state of apposition. A cross section of the midportion of the vagina is H-shaped with a moderate medial convexity of the lateral walls. With the tearing and stretching of childbirth or the senescent loss of vaginal support, the potential space of the vagina becomes a persistent cavity in the multiparous or postmenopausal patient.

In the nulliparous woman the vaginal epithelium contains numerous rugae. These are secondary to elevation of surface epithelium over the dermis. These rugae are lost with multiparity and senescence, resulting in the smooth and shiny appearance of the postmenopausal vagina.

PHYSIOLOGY

The vagina remains remarkably sensitive to estrogen throughout its lifetime. Cytosol receptors have been demonstrated within the vaginal tissue, with the highest concentration found in the basal and parabasal cells. These receptors are characterized by a low capacity but high affinity for estradiol. The concentration of these receptors is independent of the patient's age or menopausal status.[4] Thus the vaginal changes seen in the postmenopausal patient can be attributed, for the most part, to the vagina's lack of hormonal support.

Vaginal lubrication is important in maintaining a baseline level of protective moisture and in providing adequate lubrication for sexual arousal and intercourse. The vaginal dryness experienced by postmenopausal women leads to symptoms of vaginitis, vaginismus, and dyspareunia, with possible loss of sexual interest. In the reproductive age group the normal vaginal discharge is produced at a rate of 3 to 4 g/4 h.[5,6] These secretions originate predominantly from the vagina, and consist of transudate and exfoliated cells from the vaginal epithelium.[7]

The transudate of the vagina is dependent on an adequate blood flow, and appears to be related to both the hemodynamics of blood flow in subepithelial tissues as well as the vascular-dependent active transport mechanism of the vaginal epithelium. Semmens and colleagues evaluated the vaginal physiology in postmenopausal women before and after estrogen replacement therapy. They found that the maintenance of vaginal blood flow at levels necessary for adequate production of baseline protective moisture and coital lubrication is estrogen dependent.[5,6] In the estrogen-deprived postmenopausal woman the mean quantity of vaginal fluid produced was 1.7 g/4 h. Cyclic estrogen therapy (oral or topical) was found to be effective in restoring the vaginal fluid production to premenopausal levels. Although cytologic and hormone levels reach a maximum response within 30 days, the physiologic response to exogenous estrogen therapy occurs more slowly. The maximum effects on vaginal perfusion and production of transudate with postmenopausal estrogen replacement was not seen until 18 to 24 months of regular therapy. Intermittent or inadequate duration of hormone replacement may explain why estrogen therapy does not always appear to resolve menopause-related complaints, especially those of sexual dysfunction.

Exfoliating epithelial cells constitute a significant portion of the vaginal secretions.[7] Four cell types may be recognized and the proportion of each is dependent on the degree of estrogen stimulation.

Those cells originating from the germinal layer of the vaginal epithelium are called basal cells. They are small and cylindrical with scant cytoplasm and are not seen in the vaginal smear under normal circumstances. Basal cells are found only after extensive trauma or radiation exposure. Parabasal cells are round with large vesicular nuclei. They originate from the deep portion of the spinal cell layer of the vaginal epithelium and are the predominant cell in the hypoestrogenic patient. Intermediate cells are polygonal and are larger than the parabasal cells. Their nuclei are vesicular but smaller than those of basal cells. They originate from the outer portion of the spinal cell layer. Superficial cells are polyhedral and flat with an eosinophilic cytoplasm. They have the largest surface of all the vaginal epithelial cells. Their nuclei are small, dark, and pyknotic. Folding and clumping of the superficial cells in association with intermediate cells is seen with a progestational effect. The intermediate cells contain increased glycogen and often appear boat-shaped (navicular cells) with eccentric nuclei.

The first sign of estrogen stimulation is an increase in the mitotic activity of the basal layer.[3] This results in the proliferation and maturation of the squamous cells and an increased thickness in the vaginal mucosa. The vaginal smear, therefore, can be used for hormonal evaluation. The three most commonly used methods of describing hormonal effect are as follows:[3,8]

1. *Karyopyknotic index* is the percentage of mature superficial cells having pyknotic nuclei.

ie, Atrophic smear = karyopyknotic index <10%
Mature smear = karyopyknotic index >40%
2. *Maturation index* is based on the evaluation of at least 200 cells. The superficial, intermediate, and parabasal cell types are expressed as a percentage of the total cell count.
ie, Atrophic smear = maturation index with parabasal cells >20%
Mature smear = maturation index with superficial cells >40%
3. *Maturation value* expresses the maturation index as one number by multiplying the cell types by a constant and adding the total: Maturation value = sum of (% cell type × unit value), where unit value is a function of cell type.

Cell Type	Unit Value
Superficial	1.0
Large intermediate	0.6
Small intermediate	0.5
Parabasal	0.0

ie, Atrophic smear = maturation value <50
Moderate smear = maturation index >50 and <65
Mature smear = maturation index >65

Vaginal smears for hormonal evaluation should always be gathered from the lateral wall of the upper portion of the vagina. If the samples are contaminated with cervical material or inflammatory infiltrates, a hormonal interpretation should not be attempted.[9] Although hormonal vaginal cytology has lost some of its importance with the advent of radioimmunochemical assays, it remains an easy and inexpensive preliminary method of evaluation in daily practice. This is especially true for the extreme patterns of maximum proliferation and atrophy. The intermediate patterns are less reliable and may be subject to multiple interpretations. Although numerical values are used to report the maturation indexes, they do not directly reflect serum hormone levels.[3,8,10] This discrepancy can be partially explained by individual variability of target organ response to hormone stimulation and the effect of local factors such as inflammation and medication. One should always interpret these vaginal smears in light of all the clinical data.

In the postmenopausal patient the lack of estrogen produces a progressive atrophy of the vaginal epithelium. This is reflected by the vaginal smear that consists of predominantly parabasal cells in addition to frequent evidence of secondary inflammatory lesions. Cellular necrosis and degenerative changes may cause problems in differentiating dysplasias and carcinomas. A brief period of estrogen therapy should clear up these worrisome changes if they are truly of atrophic origin.[9]

As mentioned earlier, there is a lag time of up to 2 years between cytologic findings and physiologic response with postmenopausal replacement therapy.[5,6] This also appears to be the case in patients who are initially experiencing postmenopausal estrogen withdrawal symptoms. Recent data indicate that postmenopausal dyspareunia may precede any cytologic evidence of vaginal atrophy.[11] These findings suggest that impairment of vaginal transudation of fluids may precede cytologic changes and emphasize the importance of considering relevant clinical data when evaluating vaginal smears.

ECOLOGY

The ecosystem of the vagina is made up of a dynamic microbial flora that is under the influence of multiple factors, including the glycogen content of the epithelial cells, pH, hormonal support, trauma, and coitus. In 1892 Döderlein first described the abundance of facultative Gram-positive rods in the normal vaginal flora.[12] Although these Döderlein bacilli are referred to as *Lactobacillus* species, they constitute a heterogeneous group of acidophilic Gram-positive bacilli. In addition to the more abundant lactobacilli, the vaginal flora is made up of high concentrations of many other facultative and obligate anaerobic organisms.[7]

The superficial cells produced under the influence of estrogen have a high glycogen content. The metabolism of this rich supply of glycogen by the Döderlein bacteria produces organic acids and results in the acidic environment of the vagina. The normal vaginal pH in menstruating women ranges from 3.5 to 5.0, and favors the growth of the lactobacillus and other acidophiles while inhibiting the overgrowth of pathogens. The primary acids produced are acetic, lactic, and propionic.[13] The sensitivity of this ecosystem to the hormonal milieu is reflected by the variation in vaginal pH with each menstrual cycle. The production of organic acids normally increases during midcycle and falls during the luteal phase.[7]

The hypoestrogenic state of menopause brings about a great reduction in the epithelial thickness, with a dramatic drop in cellular glycogen content. This lack of substrate for the vaginal flora leads to a decrease in acid production (pH of 7.0 is common) and depletion of lactobacilli with an increase in colonization of anaerobic organisms. The vagina is, therefore, vulnerable to infection and trauma. Exogenous estrogen therapy (oral or topical) has been shown to restore the vaginal epithelium and pH to premenopausal levels. Although short-term therapy has resulted in dramatic improvement in vaginal ecology, the maximum effect in pH normalization is seen only after 1 year of regular treatment.[5,6]

In postmenopausal women who are undergoing estrogen replacement, a lower vaginal pH was found in those who were regularly sexually active.[5,6,14] This finding suggests an enhancement of the therapeutic effects of postmenopausal estrogen replacement by continued sexual activity, and is somewhat paradoxical in that semen is a known buffer. After ejaculation there is a rapid, temporary rise in the vaginal pH to a neutral level. This permits the replication of pathogenic organisms with an increased potential for infection.[13,15] The benefit of regular sexual activity is thought to be related to promotion of local vascularity and appears to outweigh any semen-related alterations in vaginal pH.

The mixture of low-molecular-weight fatty acids that are produced by the vaginal flora is also responsible for vaginal odor. This odor is dependent on the vapor pressures of these acids at body temperature and their pKa at the vaginal pH. Because these acids are largely bacterial by-products, the vaginal odor reflects the predominant microbial flora.[12]

VAGINAL INFECTIONS

Vaginitis in the postmenopausal patient should not always be assumed to be secondary to the lack of estrogen. Vaginal infections and vaginitis owing to certain organisms may occur with or without atrophic changes. Therefore, every patient, regardless of her menopausal status, deserves a thorough evaluation and specific diagnosis with directed treatment.

Bacterial Vaginosis

Bacterial vaginosis is the current and preferred term for what has formerly been called *Gardnerella vaginalis*, *Hemophilus vaginalis*, and *Corynebacterium vaginale*, or nonspecific vaginitis. This is the most common type of infectious vaginite, accounting for 45% of symptomatic cases and estimated to be present in 15% of asymptomatic sexually active women.[15,16] *G vaginalis*, a small, nonmotile, Gram-variable coccobacillus, was thought to be the causative organism of this condition, since it can be found in almost all women with bacterial vaginosis. However, 40% of asymptomatic women and 40% of women successfully treated for bacterial vaginosis have positive cultures for *G vaginalis*. Also, in symptomatic women, *G vaginalis* is accompanied in the vaginal flora by 100- to 1,000-fold higher concentrations of anaerobes, predominantly of the *Bacteroides* and *Peptococcus* species.[16] No single causative agent is responsible for bacterial vaginosis, and although not well understood, the overgrowth of the normal vaginal flora appears to be related to some unique interactions of these organisms.

The most frequent complaint associated with bacterial vaginosis is a fishy amine odor and a homogenous, creamy, gray or light yellow leukorrhea that often causes a nonpruritic irritation of the vulva. The characteristic odor reflects the altered vaginal flora and vaginal pH (pH>5.0). This alkaline environment allows the release of the bacterial by-products putrescine and cadaverine.[13]

The clinical diagnosis can be established by the following criteria:[13,17]

- A pH greater than 5.0 with a homogenous leukorrhea.
- A fishy amine odor that can be easily elicited by adding 10% potassium hydroxide to the discharge (sniff test).
- The presence of clue cells and a paucity of white blood cells on wet-mount examination. Clue cells are epithelial cells that have large numbers of coccobacilli (*Gardnerella* organisms) attached to their surface, obscuring their normally distinct borders.

The treatment of bacterial vaginosis is recommended only for symptomatic women. Of the various modalities that have been tried, metronidazole has consistently been the most effective. One double-blind study unequivocally found metronidazole (500 mg bid × seven days) the most effective in treatment of bacterial vaginosis when compared with triple sulfa cream, ampicillin, and doxycycline.[18] Similar results were found in another study comparing metronidazole (500 mg bid × seven days) with tetracycline.[19] Tetracycline, ampicillin, and ampicillin with triple sulfa cream were effective in only 50% of the cases of bacterial vaginosis.[18,19] Evaluation of a single 2-g dose of metronidazole found it to be significantly less effective than the usual seven-day course.[20,21] Good results have been reported using douches with either benzydamine or povidone-iodine.[22,23]

There is no place for the use of sulfa (sulfanilamide and sulfisoxazole) vaginal creams in vaginitis. A recent Food and Drug Administration bulletin reports that there is no evidence that sulfa creams are more effective than bland vaginal creams in the treatment of vaginitis.[24] This finding has been confirmed by several unblinded and double-blinded studies.[18,25,26] Any effect that these sulfa preparations have is probably due to the low pH of the cream. Sulfonamides are weakly active against anaerobes[27] and have no activity against *G vaginalis*.[26,28] In fact, the use of these sulfa creams has been associated with the development of serious dermatologic disorders, including erythema multiforme and photosensitivity dermatitis.[29] It is therefore difficult to justify the use of these sulfa preparations for vaginitis in light of their questionable efficacy and potential toxicity.

G vaginalis has been isolated from the bulk of the male partners of females with bacterial vaginosis. Although a specific causative organism is unknown, the data lead to the conclusion that bacterial vaginosis is sexually transmitted. Current recommendations are that the sexual partners of infected patients be treated concurrently with metronidazole therapy.[13,15]

Monilial Vulvovaginitis

Monilial vulvovaginitis, a frequent and often recurrent vaginal infection, accounts for approximately 27% of symptomatic vaginitis.[13,16] The most common causative organism is *Candida albicans*, followed by *Candida glabrata*.[13,30] The former organism forms both hyphae and spores, whereas the later forms only spores.

Patients most commonly complain of vulvar and vaginal burning and pruritus associated with varying amounts of an odorless, thick, yellow-white, cream cheese–like discharge. Often the vulvovaginal irritation is severe, despite minimal leukorrhea. These symptoms may be so debilitating as to interfere with daily activities, sleep, and intercourse.

The yeast organisms grow optimally in a slightly acid environment with a pH range of 4.5 to 6.5. Their growth is thought to be antagonized by the presence of other organisms of the normal vaginal flora, particularly Gram-negative bacteria.[13,15,30] Thus monilial vulvovaginitis is a common occurrence after the depletion of the normal vaginal flora by the use of broad-spectrum antibiotics, particularly tetracycline. Immunosuppressive disorders or conditions, particularly lymphoma, and corticosteroid use predispose to this vaginitis. The increased vaginal glycogen seen in estrogen replacement therapy as well as pregnancy and oral contraceptive use has also been correlated with an increased incidence of vaginal fungus. There is a well-known association between diabetes mellitus and monilial vaginitis, although the exact relationship is not understood. *Candida* is found in the gastrointestinal tract, and may act as a reservoir. Also, clothing that results in poor ventilation with increased temperature and moisture encourages the proliferation of yeast. Thus improper perineal hygiene is also a causal factor involved in the development of candidal vaginitis. *Candida* can be sexually communicated. Because the organism may be harbored by the male genitourinary system or the saliva, it may be transmitted by way of coitus or cunnilingus.

The diagnosis is suggested by the history and physical findings. One usually finds a hyperemic vulva with evidence of scratching. Vaginal examination often reveals the typical thick, cheesy discharge with an underlying inflamed and tender mucosa. The pH is acid, and the vaginal smear generally shows mature epithelial cells. A wet mount with the addition of a drop of potassium hydroxide frequently confirms the diagnosis with the identification of the mycelia, that is, entangled masses of branching fiberlike hyphae and clusters of attached, budding cells known as conidia or spores. Further confirmation is made within 48 hours by a culture for *Candida* with Nickerson's medium. These cultures are available for office use and do not require incubation.

Therapy for *Candida* vaginitis includes one of many efficacious regimens. Vaginal suppositories containing nystatin (Mycostatin) are administered twice daily for ten days. Imidazole derivatives, including miconazole (Monistat) and clotrimazole (Mycelex-G, Gyne-Lotrimin), have a more rapid action and require a shorter duration of treatment. Therapeutic regimens vary with the dosage and mode of administration of the drug. Excellent results have been obtained with both the one-time administration of 500 mg of clotrimazole suppositories and the multiple-day regimen of miconazole or clotrimazole (200-mg suppository each day for three days or 100-mg suppository or cream each day for seven days).[13,15,30,31] When vulvar irritation is also present, the concurrent topical use of one of these agents in cream form is indicated. Older and seldom used therapy includes the application to the vaginal mucosa of 0.5% to 1% gentian violet solution or 0.5% acriflavine in glycerin by douche or vaginal paint.[2,13,15]

Recurrent *Candida* vulvovaginitis necessitates evaluation for any underlying causative factors. Although rarely positive, a fasting or postprandial serum glucose should be checked. The patient should be instructed in proper perineal hygiene, including the wiping from front to back and the use of loose-fitting clothing and cotton-lined underwear. The role of sexual transmission should be brought to the patient's attention. The use of oral nystatin, two tablets (500,000 units per tablet) tid to qid for seven days, for the patient and her sexual partner is often effective in recurrent infections. When other underlying causes have been ruled out, those women who experience recurrent infection with estrogen replacement therapy may require the use of local prophylactic therapy 1 week each month with one of the drugs mentioned earlier. Similarly, those patients with a history of infection after receiving broad-spectrum antibiotic therapy will benefit from the prophylactic concurrent use of vaginal antifungal therapy.

Over-the-counter douches, used once or twice a week, may be beneficial in recurrent infection. These products either contain the antifungal agent potassium sorbate (Summer's Eve) or inhibit the growth of *Candida* by helping to restore the normal vaginal flora. The latter type of douches utilize such ingredients as yogurt, acidophilus culture (carried by most health food stores), and vinegar. A commonly used douche can be prepared by mixing 2 tbsp of white vinegar and 2 tbsp of acidophilus culture into 1 qt of warm water.[32]

Trichomonas Vaginitis

Vaginitis caused by *Trichomonas vaginalis* is common, with a frequency similar to that of monilial vaginitis. It is caused by a flagellated protozoa with optimal growth at an alkaline pH (5.0 to 7.0), similar to that seen with bacterial vaginosis. Although infection with this organism usually results in a fulminant vaginitis, it is estimated that 20% of women who harbor *T vaginalis* are asymptomatic.[2] Symptomatic patients complain of a profuse, frothy, yellow discharge that frequently causes an irritating pruritic vulvitis. Symptoms may be so severe as to cause marked discomfort and dyspareunia.

Physical examination usually reveals a distinctive leukorrhea and alkaline pH with reddening of the labia minora and a tender and inflamed vaginal mucosa and cervix. Occasionally (25% to 35% of patients) this results in multiple petechia involving the vagina and cervix, giving the classic "strawberry sign."[17] Diagnosis is confirmed in 75% of cases by identification of the motile, almond-shaped, flagellated organisms on a wet mount of normal saline.[33] Although rarely necessary and not routine, the diagnosis can also be confirmed by culture. The trichomonads are about one half the size of mature epithelial cells but larger than leukocytes. To ensure motility is observed, care should be taken to examine the slide immediately after preparation. Excessive cold should be avoided, and normal saline, not water, should be used in the wet mount. In addition to the motile protozoa, numerous white blood cells will be seen because of the associated inflammation of the vaginal mucosa. The vaginal flora present in the background of a *T vaginalis* infection includes a wide range of organisms with the predominant bacteria being obligate anaerobes.[13,15,17]

Unlike most other sexually transmitted organisms, *T vaginalis* can survive outside the vagina for one to three hours. Protozoa have been recovered from contaminated douche equipment, splashed toilet water, and chlorinated swimming pools.[2,13,15] Thus, although sexual communication is common, there is an endless number of potential sources of transmission.

The standard treatment of trichomonas vaginitis is with metronidazole. The obligate anaerobes associated with this vaginitis are also sensitive to this drug. The routine dosage schedule has been 250 mg tid or 500 mg bid for seven days. The cure rate and incidence of side effects, however, have been similar with a 2-g single-dose regimen.[34-37] The latter dosage schedule has the advantage of less cost, less total drug, and improved patient compliance. The incidence of infection in male partners of affected females is high, although usually asymptomatic. Therefore, both partners must be treated concurrently. The major cause of treatment failure is the omission of therapy for the sexual partner.[38,39]

NONINFECTIOUS VAGINITIS

Mechanical and Chemical Vaginitis

Acute and chronic inflammation of the vaginal mucosa can be caused by mechanical irritation and an assortment of chemical substances. Examples include pessaries, contraceptive devices, foreign bodies, irradiation, and various antiseptics. Surgery, specifically hysterectomy, has been followed by a local granulation reaction of the vaginal vault. In addition, the use of superabsorbent tampons has been associated with vaginal mucosal drying, leading to mucosal ulcers, bleeding, and discharge.[9]

On physical examination the vaginal mucosa is erythematous, inflamed, and edematous, and the surface is often granular.[9] A diagnosis is made by the history and physical examination and after other causes of vaginitis have been ruled out.

Emphysematous Vaginitis

Emphysematous vaginitis, a rare disorder, is also called cystic vaginitis, gaseous cysts of the vagina, and emphysematous copitis. It is most often reported in association with pregnancy or cardiopulmonary disease, particularly congestive heart failure.[9,40] Emphysematous vaginitis involves the ectocervix and the upper portion of the vagina. On physical examination one characteristically sees small liquid- or gas-containing cysts within the mucosa. These cysts may rupture and give rise to the appearance of a red, superficially ulcerated mucosa. The cause of this vaginitis is not clear, but it has been theorized that the cysts are secondary to gaseous by-products of anaerobic bacteria.[9] This theory is suggested by the presence of foreign-body giant cells within the walls of these mucosal cavities and by the frequent association with other vaginal infections, particularly trichomonas vaginitis.[40]

REFERENCES

1. Hollinshead WH: *Textbook of Anatomy*. New York, Harper & Row, 1974, pp 702–704.

2. Kistner RW: *Gynecology: Principles and Practice*. Chicago, Year Book Medical Pub, 1986, pp 71–82.

3. Sedlis A, Chen P: Cytology, in Sciarra JJ (ed): *Gynecology and Obstetrics*. New York, Harper & Row, 1986, vol 1, chap 29, pp 1-25.

4. Weigerinck MAHM, Poortman J, Agema AR, Thijssen JHH: Estrogen receptors in human vaginal tissue. *Maturitas* 1980;2:59

5. Semmens JP, Wagner G: Estrogen deprivation and vaginal function in postmenopausal women. *JAMA* 1982;248:445.

6. Semmens JP, Tsai CC, Semmens EC, Loadholt CB: Effects of estrogen therapy on vaginal physiology during menopause. *Obstet Gynecol* 1985;66:15.

7. Paavonen J: Physiology and ecology of the vagina. *Scand J Infect Dis* 1983;40(Suppl):31.

8. Benjamin F, Deutsch S: Immunoreactive plasma estrogens and vaginal hormone cytology in postmenopausal women. *Int J Gynaecol Obstet* 1980;17:546.

9. Gompel C, Silverberg S: *Pathology in Gynecology and Obstetrics*. Philadelphia, JB Lippincott, 1985, pp 46–52.

10. Weid GL: Terminology of cytologic reporting of endocrinologic conditions. *Acta Cytol* 1964;9:383.

11. Semmens JP: Vaginal function in postmenopausal women, reply to letter. *JAMA* 1983;249:195.

12. Döderlein A: Die Scheidensekretuntersuchungen. *Zentralbl Gynakol* 1894;18:10.

13. Kempers RD: Vaginitis. *Postgrad Obstet Gynecol* 1985;5:1–5.

14. Leiblum S, Bachmann G, Kemmann E, et al: Vaginal atrophy in the postmenopausal woman; the importance of sexual activity and hormones. *JAMA* 1983;249:2195.

15. Weinstein L: Vaginitis: An overview of a common condition, in Sciarra JJ (ed): *Gynecology and Obstetrics*. New York, Harper & Row, 1986, vol 1, chap 40, pp 1–7.

16. Eschenbach DA: Diagnosis of bacterial vaginosis (nonspecific vaginitis): Role of the laboratory. *Clinical Microbiology Newsletter*, June 18, 1984, p 134.

17. Sweet RL: Importance of differential diagnosis in acute vaginitis. *Am J Obstet Gynecol* 1985;152:921.

18. Malouf M, Fortier M, Morin G, Dube JL: Treatment of *Hemophilus vaginalis* vaginitis. *Obstet Gynecol* 1981;57:711.

19. Balsdon MJ, Taylor GE, Pead L, Maskell R: *Corynebacterium vaginale* and vaginitis: A controlled trial of treatment. *Lancet* 1980;1:501.

20. Blackwell AL, Fox AR, Phillips I, Barlow D: Anaerobic vaginosis (non-specific vaginitis): Clinical, microbiological, and therapeutic findings. *Lancet* 1983;2:1379.

21. Bardi M, Manenti G, Mattioni D, Lassala L: Metronidazole for non-specific vaginitis. [Letter] *Lancet* 1980;1:1029.

22. Singha HS: The use of a vaginal cleansing kit in non-specific vaginitis. *Practitioner* 1979;223:403.

23. Mega M, Marcolin D, Magginot T, DeGregorio M: Therapeutic effects of topical benzydamine in gynecology. *Clin Exp Obstet Gynecol* 1980;7:25.

24. Sulfa vaginal creams. *FDA Drug Bulletin* 1980;10:6.

25. Piot P, Van Dyck E, et al: A placebo-controlled, double-blind comparison of tinidazole and triple sulfonamide cream for the treatment of nonspecific vaginitis. *Obstet Gynecol* 1983;147:85.

26. Pheifer TA, Forsyth PS, et al: Nonspecific vaginitis. Role of *Haemophilus vaginalis* and treatment with metronidazole. *N Engl J Med* 1978;298:1429.

27. Rosenblatt JE, Stewart PR: Lack of activity of sulfamethoxazole and trimethoprim against anaerobic bacteria. *Antimicrob Agents Chemother* 1974;6:93.

28. McCarthy LR, Mickelsen PR, Smith EG: Antibiotic susceptibility of *Haemophilus vaginalis* (*Corynebacterium vaginale*) to 21 antibiotics. *Antimicrob Agents Chemother* 1979;16:1986.

29. Goette DK, Odom RB: Vaginal medications as a cause for varied widespread dermatitides. *Cutis* 1980;26:406.

30. Sobel JD: Epidemiology and pathogenesis of recurrent vulvovaginal candidiasis. *Am J Obstet Gynecol* 1985;152:924.

31. Ritter W: Pharmacokinetic fundamentals of vaginal treatment with clotrimazole. *Am J Obstet Gynecol* 1985;152:945.

32. Vaginitis. Planned Parenthood Federation of America, 1985 (810 Seventh Ave., NY, NY).

33. Brockmann J, Hohne C: Bacteriological aspects of trichomonal vaginitis. *Zentralbl Gynakol* 1979;101:722.

34. Thin RN, Symonds MA, et al: Double-blind comparison of a single dose and a five-day course of metronidazole in the treatment of trichomoniasis. *Br J Vener Dis* 1979;55:354.

35. Hager WD, Brown ST, et al: Metronidazole for vaginal trichomoniasis: Seven-day vs single-dose regimens. *JAMA* 1980;244:1219.

36. Lossick JG: Single-dose metronidazole treatment for vaginal trichomoniasis. *Obstet Gynecol* 1980;56:508.

37. Aubert JM, Sesta HJ: Treatment of vaginal trichomoniasis; Single 2gm dose of metronidazole as compared with a seven-day course. *J Reprod Med* 1982;27:743.

38. Norgaard M, Lyng J: Treatment of trichomoniasis in women with a single dose of tinidazole. *Ugeskr Laeger* 1975;137:672.

39. Lyng J, Christensen J: A double-blind study of the value of treatment with a single dose tinidazole of partners to females with trichomoniasis. *Acta Obstet Gynecol Scand* 1981;60:199.

40. Jones HW, Jones GS: *Novak's Textbook of Gynecology*. Baltimore, Williams & Wilkins, 1981, pp 270–271.

Chapter 15

Anesthesia for the Aging Gynecologic Patient*

Norman J. Zeig

INTRODUCTION

Changing patterns of practice have been and are altering the traditional procedures for caring for the surgical patient. The cost containment measures instituted by the federal government continue to force patients out of hospital beds and into ambulatory care facilities and home care situations. The physician is pummeled by requirements imposed by health maintenance organizations, preferred provider organizations, and other third party payers, demanding that he or she modify procedures for testing, preparing patients, and performing surgical procedures. On the other hand the genuine desire to deliver optimum care to the patient and the threat of malpractice suits generate confusion for many physicians.

This chapter puts in perspective for the gynecologic surgeon the considerations and responsibilities that have fallen to him or her in order to maintain a high standard of care for patients and the limitations imposed by the changes in practice patterns, particularly as it relates to the aging patient.

AGING AND ANESTHETIC RISK

The gynecologist in today's health care environment is in the position of having to plan care and schedule surgery without the benefit of the once-traditional in-hospital preoperative evaluation. Consequently, in order to deliver optimal care to the patient and at the same time avoid last-minute cancellation of surgical procedures resulting from inadequate preanesthetic preparation, the surgeon is required to devote additional effort to ensure that the patient is properly prepared for the impact of anesthesia and surgery. Consultations, when necessary, must be obtained well in advance of the contemplated surgery, and remedial measures must be dealt with, usually on an outpatient basis.

---

*Throughout this chapter, use of the term *we* refers to the Department of Anesthesiology at St. Barnabas Medical Center, Livingston, NJ.

The anesthesiologist is available for consultation or discussion of preoperative problems, when necessary, so that they do not present any surprises on the day of surgery, forcing delays and cancellation of the scheduled procedure. Relying on an internist for "clearance of surgery" does not always result in an adequate opinion relative to anesthetic risks and/or management.

The normal decline in physiologic function with age is portrayed in Figure 15-1. In the healthy aged patient the natural decline in physiologic function of the major organ systems leads to decreased organ reserves, making this group more susceptible to the stress of anesthesia and surgery, with the margin for error decreased as well.

Diminished reserves accompanied by a greater incidence of superimposed disease in the geriatric age group constitute a rationale for maintaining preoperative screening tests that are being modified for younger healthy patients in the cost containment atmosphere we find ourselves in the midst of.

Women are less prone than men to cardiovascular disease, particularly coronary heart disease. This relative immunity decreases with aging. Menopause in particular, whether spontaneous or induced, increases the risk of coronary heart disease.

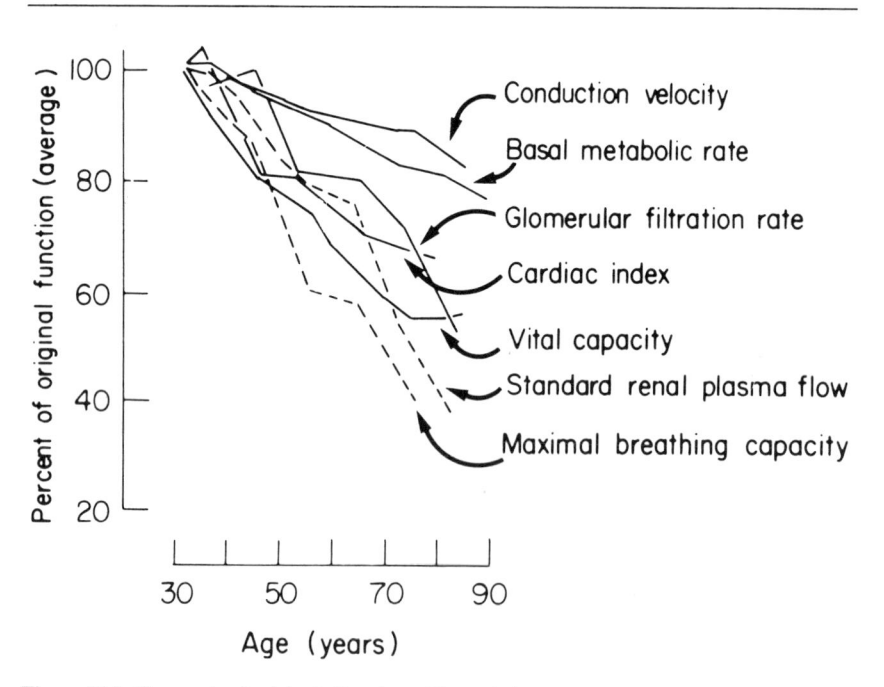

Figure 15-1 Changes in physiologic function with age in humans expressed as percentage of mean value at age 30 years. *Source:* Reprinted from *Anesthesia*, ed 2, vol 3 (p 1802) by RD Miller (Ed) with permission of Churchill Livingstone Inc, © 1986.

Hysterectomy, with or without oophorectomy, predisposes to coronary heart disease, which is not reduced by the administration of estrogens.[1(pp34–38),2]

Hypertension, which occurs in 35% of women between ages 65 and 84, is an ominous risk factor regarding mortality per se.[1(p48)] Hypertensive patients should be treated and well controlled before surgery. Medications should not be discontinued before surgery, but should be given even on the morning of the scheduled procedure.

ANESTHETIC RISK

Guidelines for assessing physical status established by the American Society of Anesthesiologists (ASA)[3] are listed in Table 15-1. The descriptions in Table 15-1 do not classify anesthetic risk, but they are useful guidelines for assessing the type of facility, extent of preoperative testing that might be in order, or for determining in what type of facility the procedure may be safely scheduled (eg, in-hospital ambulatory facility versus freestanding ambulatory care facility).

In assessing anesthetic risk, age must certainly be considered as a contributory factor. Although many senior citizens appear to be in excellent physical condition, the normal physiologic decline in organ function or reserve looms as an increased risk factor in the face of surgical and anesthetic stress.

Wilson and associates[4] studied 200 geriatric patients admitted to the hospital. They found that 78% suffered from at least four major diseases, 38% suffered from six or more diseases, and 13% were noted to have eight or more disease processes.

For this reason we arbitrarily select age 65 as a point where we consider all patients to represent at least a physical status 2, and require more extensive preoperative screening for our ambulatory care patients, including assessment by their internist relative to his or her opinion of their health and ability to withstand surgical stress.

Table 15-1 ASA Guidelines for Assessing Physical Status

1	Normal healthy patient
2	Patient with mild systemic disease
3	Patient with severe systemic disease that limits activity but is not incapacitating
4	Patient with incapacitating systemic disease that is a constant threat to life
5	Moribund patient not expected to survive 24 hours with or without surgery
E	Added to the above if emergency

Source: *Surgical Clinics of North America* (1983;63:1113), Copyright © 1983, WB Saunders Company.

The internist should limit himself or herself to providing information and suggestions relative to the existence or management of coexisting diseases, rather than suggest the anesthetic technique or offer such suggestions as "avoid hypoxia, hypotension, and hypercapnia."

Some of the factors that tend to increase anesthetic risk are diseases of the cardiovascular, renal, hepatic, respiratory, and immune systems, as well as the type and duration of the surgical procedure, the skill of the surgical team, and the skill and experience of the anesthesiologist. The ambitious nature of the surgical procedure relative to the facility's resources and monitoring abilities must be considered as well.

Many patients, particularly the elderly, are taking medications for concurrent conditions. A number of these pharmacologic agents interact with anesthetic agents or adjuncts, and surgeons as well as anesthesiologists should be aware of this.

Of particular importance is a group of psychoactive drugs. Monoamine oxidase (MAO) inhibitors interact with meperidine (Demerol) and indirect-acting sympathomimetics, and can produce marked hypertension and/or hyperpyrexic coma. Some of these MAO inhibitors are listed in Table 15-2.

It is generally recommended that for elective surgery, it is wise to discontinue these drugs for at least 2 to 3 weeks before surgery. Emergency surgery, of course, cannot be postponed, and the patient must be carefully managed with narcotics being avoided. Postoperative pain after major surgery may be dealt with by using carefully administered continuous epidural regional block.

Other mood-altering drugs that may commonly be encountered in the aging female—since depression is commonly seen in this group—are the tricyclic antidepressants. (See Table 15-3.)

Care must be taken if one attempts to switch patients from an MAO inhibitor to a tricyclic antidepressant. It is recommended to wait at least 14 days after discontinuing the MAO inhibitor. This time lapse is necessary because concurrent administration of a tricyclic antidepressant and an MAO inhibitor have produced hyperpyretic crises, severe convulsions, and death.

Side effects of tricyclic antidepressants include atropinelike reactions (eg, dry mouth, delirium, tachycardia, urinary retention, and constipation). Electrocardiographic (ECG) changes that may occur include prolongation of the QRS

Table 15-2 MAO Inhibitors

Isocarboxazid (Marplan)
Phenelzine sulfate (Nardil)
Tranylcypromine sulfate (Parnate)
Pargyline (Eutonyl)

Table 15-3 Tricyclic Antidepressants

Imipramine (Tofranil, Presamine, Imavate)
Amitriptyline (Elavil, Endep)
Desipramine (Norpramin, Pertofrane)
Doxepin (Adapin, Sinequan)
Nortriptyline (Aventyl, Pamelor)
Amoxapine (Asendin)
Trimipramine (Surmontil)
Protriptyline (Vivactil)

---

complex, bundle branch block or other conduction abnormalities, and premature ventricular contractions.

Tricyclic antidepressants interfere with the action of guanethidine, and fatal dysrhythmias have been reported after the use of halothane and pancuronium.[5,6] Glisson and co-workers[7] reported an increased incidence of cardiac dysrhythmias in patients taking tricyclic antidepressants during reversal of neuromuscular blockade.

Ketamine and pressor drugs may cause hypertension and tachycardia. It is generally considered safe to continue these drugs for the benefit of the patient and to work around them during anesthesia.

Lithium carbonate, which has traditionally been used to treat manic-depressive illness, is being used more frequently now as an antidepressant or as an adjuvant to other antidepressants. Patients who receive lithium may experience prolonged neuromuscular blockade and may exhibit reduced anesthetic requirements.[8,9]

A number of other classes of drugs are encountered in the older age group and should be continued, for example, steroids, beta blockers, anticonvulsants, antihypertensives, insulin, and central alpha agonists (clonidine and α-methyldopa).

Patients who take diuretics should have careful screening of their electrolytes, since they frequently have decreased serum potassium and sodium levels. Low potassium levels are generally better treated by the oral administration of potassium chloride elixir several days before surgery. Attempts to correct low serum potassium levels intravenously are limited by the maximum rate of 10 mEq/h while monitoring the ECG. Intravenous potassium is very irritating to veins, and patients frequently complain of pain during infusions.

Although, ideally, the patient for elective surgery should have normal serum potassium levels, I do not delay surgery if the serum potassium is over 3.2 or under 5.3 mEq/L, or the cause for the discrepancy is known.

Because this situation is somewhat arbitrary, one must defer to the limits with which the anesthesiologist responsible for the case feels comfortable.

AMBULATORY CARE OF THE AGED SURGICAL GYNECOLOGICAL PATIENT

As Medicare administrators ratchet down on the ability to hospitalize patients for procedures they deem suitable for ambulatory surgery, physicians must modify their traditional procedures for caring for these patients.

We have attempted to produce guidelines for the management of these cases. Physical status 1 and 2 patients may be treated at our satellite ambulatory care unit, which is in proximity to, but not part of, the hospital. Physical status 3 patients and AM admission patients (admitted on day of surgery) are treated in the hospital's ambulatory care unit.

The geriatric patient is required to have a preoperative evaluation consisting of a letter from her internist relative to her ability to tolerate surgery, and preoperative testing including CBC, SMA-12, an ECG, and a chest x-ray if clinically indicated.

Aside from written instructions distributed by the surgeon, the patient receives an extensive interview regarding her medical history from a perioperative nurse. Any important facts relevant to the patient are communicated to the anesthesiologist medical director, who decides if further testing is required, if medications should be taken, or if the surgeon should be contacted for a particular problem. Instructions are given relative to the importance of arriving in a timely manner, being assured of someone available to accompany the patient home, and reinforcing that the patient is to take nothing by mouth the day of surgery. If the patient seems confused or has difficulty with the language, the responsible family member or friend who will accompany the patient is given the information.

The patient arrives one hour before surgery, is interviewed extensively by the perioperative nurse, and then is seen, interviewed, and examined by the anesthesiologist. Preoperative medication is avoided and has presented no problems to date. Undoubtedly the concentrated attention given by caring nurses and physicians is responsible for the calming effect noted.

Carefully administered short-acting drugs and agents are used for anesthesia, and the patient proceeds to the acute recovery room postoperatively, where she remains for approximately an hour. Analgesics are seldom necessary in the recovery room. If needed, however, they are prescribed by the anesthesiologist.

The patient is then transferred to the advanced recovery room, placed in a comfortable reclining lounge chair, and given some clear liquids to drink and some crackers. An accompanying family member or friend is invited to stay with her. When the patient is alert, has voided, has retained oral fluids, and can ambulate, she is accompanied to her transportation by a nurse.

The next day the perioperative nurse from the advanced recovery room calls the patient and notes any complications and her condition.

Each patient is given two questionnaires to answer and return to the center. One questionnaire deals with the treatment by the facility and the other deals with the anesthesia care. The medical director and the administrative director review the returned questionnaires as part of the quality assurance program.

After 3½ years' experience dealing with some 15,000 patients, we have found our procedures to be exceedingly gratifying for all concerned—patients, physicians, and nurses.

MONITORING

In August of 1986 the Department of Anesthesiology at the Harvard Medical School in Boston published its standards for normal patient monitoring in the *Journal of the American Medical Association*.[10] These standards were the result of a major risk management/patient safety effort.

In October of 1986 the ASA adopted these basic monitoring standards (Table 15-4). The standards were recommended as minimal, since the realization of the increased use of the pulse oximeter, mass spectrometry, and end-tidal carbon dioxide measurements would result in one or more of these modalities being included in a future revision of the standards.

Although the authors were careful to state that these standards may not be applicable verbatim to all departments of anesthesia, they stated that the process by which they were promulgated was. I feel that these standards will be widely accepted.

At a meeting of the New York State Society of Anesthesiologists Post Graduate Assembly held in December 1986, Dr. Ronald Katz, speaking in a panel entitled "Lessons Learned from Malpractice Lawsuits," stated that his statement regarding the use of pulse oximetry as a monitor has made it a standard of care.

Tight budgets in many hospitals, brought about by cost containment legislation and reimbursement patterns, will have to yield in order to meet these standards.

It behooves the surgeon to support, encourage, and insist that the necessary funds be made available to ensure that monitoring capabilities and quality of anesthesia care be commensurate with at least the minimal standards mentioned, although at this time encouraging the routine use of pulse oximetry and end-tidal carbon dioxide measurements alone, or as part of mass spectrometry monitoring, is recommended.

The pulse oximeter, which measures arterial oxygen saturation, reflects the adequacy of oxygen delivery to the tissues, which is a more sensitive measurement of the true oxygen availability to the patient rather than the usual measurement of the amount of oxygen delivered to the lungs.

Table 15-4 American Society of Anesthesiologists Standards for Basic Intra-Operative Monitoring (Approved by House of Delegates on October 21, 1986)

These standards apply to all anesthesia care although, in emergency circumstances, appropriate life support measures take precedence. These standards may be exceeded at any time based on the judgment of the responsible anesthesiologist. They are intended to encourage high quality patient care, but observing them cannot guarantee any specific patient outcome. They are subject to revision from time to time, as warranted by the evolution of technology and practice. This set of standards addresses only the issue of basic intra-operative monitoring, which is one component of anesthesia care. In certain rare or unusual circumstances, (1) some of these methods of monitoring may be clinically impractical, and (2) appropriate use of the described monitoring methods may fail to detect untoward clinical developments. Brief interruptions of continual† monitoring may be unavoidable. *Under extenuating circumstances, the responsible anesthesiologist may waive the requirements marked with an asterisk (*); it is recommended that when this is done, it should be so stated (including the reasons) in a note in the patient's medical record.* These standards are not intended for application to the care of the obstetrical patient in labor or in the conduct of pain management.

†Note the "continual" is defined as "repeated regularly and frequently in steady succession" whereas "continuous" means "prolonged without any interruption at any time."

STANDARD I

Qualified anesthesia personnel shall be present in the room throughout the conduct of all general anesthetics, regional anesthetics and monitored anesthesia care.

OBJECTIVE

Because of the rapid changes in patient status during anesthesia, qualified anesthesia personnel shall be continuously present to monitor the patient and provide anesthesia care. In the event there is a direct known hazard, e.g., radiation, to the anesthesia personnel which might require intermittent remote observation of the patient, some provision for monitoring the patient must be made. In the event that an emergency requires the temporary absence of the person primarily responsible for the anesthetic, the best judgment of the anesthesiologist will be exercised in comparing the emergency with the anesthetized patient's condition and in the selection of the person left responsible for the anesthetic during the temporary absence.

STANDARD II

During all anesthetics, the patient's oxygenation, ventilation, circulation, and temperature shall be continually evaluated.

OXYGENATION

OBJECTIVE

To ensure adequate oxygen concentration in the inspired gas and the blood during all anesthetics.

METHODS

1) Inspired gas: During every administration of general anesthesia using an anesthesia machine, the concentration of oxygen in the patient breathing system shall be measured by an oxygen analyzer with a low oxygen concentration limit alarm in use.*
2) Blood oxygenation: During all anesthetics, adequate illumination and exposure of the patient is necessary to assess color. While this and other qualitative clinical signs may be

Table 15-4 continued

adequate, there are quantitative methods, such as pulse oximetry, which are encouraged.

VENTILATION

OBJECTIVE

To ensure adequate ventilation of the patient during all anesthetics.

METHODS

1) Every patient receiving general anesthesia shall have the adequacy of ventilation continually evaluated. While qualitative clinical signs such as chest excursion, observation of the reservoir breathing bag and auscultation of breath sounds may be adequate, quantitative monitoring of the CO_2 content and/or volume of expired gas is encouraged.
2) When an endotracheal tube is inserted, its correct positioning in the trachea must be verified. Clinical assessment is essential and end-tidal CO_2 analysis, in use from the time of endotracheal tube placement, is encouraged.
3) When ventilation is controlled by a mechanical ventilator, there shall be in continuous use a device that is capable of detecting disconnection of components of the breathing system. The device must give an audible signal when its alarm threshold is exceeded.
4) During regional anesthesia and monitored anesthesia care, the adequacy of ventilation shall be evaluated, at least, by continual observation of qualitative clinical signs.

CIRCULATION

OBJECTIVE

To ensure the adequacy of the patient's circulatory function during all anesthetics.

METHODS

1) Every patient receiving anesthesia shall have the electrocardiogram continuously displayed from the beginning of anesthesia until preparing to leave the anesthetizing location.*
2) Every patient receiving anesthesia shall have arterial blood pressure and heart rate determined and evaluated at least every five minutes.*
3) Every patient receiving general anesthesia shall have, in addition to the above, circulatory function continually evaluated by at least one of the following: palpation of a pulse, auscultation of heart sounds, monitoring of a tracing of intra-arterial pressure, ultrasound peripheral pulse monitoring, or pulse plethysmography or oximetry.

BODY TEMPERATURE

OBJECTIVE

To aid in the maintenance of appropriate body temperature during all anesthetics.

METHODS

There shall be readily available a means to continuously measure the patient's temperature. When changes in body temperature are intended, anticipated or suspected, the temperature shall be measured.

Source: Department of Anesthesiology, Harvard Medical School.

The use of end-tidal carbon dioxide measurements indicate whether the endotracheal tube is, in fact, in the trachea. It is an index of the adequacy of ventilation whether spontaneous or controlled.

The mass spectrometer monitors all the respiratory and anesthetic gases being used for both the inspired and end-tidal concentrations and allows for a more adequate assessment of what the patient is actually receiving, rather than what the anesthesiologist assumes the patient is receiving.

The geriatric population in particular contains a large number of patients with significant concurrent disease. Invasive monitoring has become a useful tool in reducing morbidity and mortality in this area.

The use of intra-arterial pressure monitoring is indicated when dealing with patients whose medical conditions include significant coronary artery disease and/or valvular dysfunction with prior ventricular compliance and minimal cardiovascular reserve. It should be considered in patients with significant hypertension, cerebrovascular disease, or significant pulmonary pathology, or when frequent arterial blood gas sampling is required.[11]

A Swan-Ganz pulmonary artery catheter is indicated for patients undergoing non–cardiac surgery; in patients with significant cardiac disease, pulmonary diseases interfering with oxygenation, shock secondary to hemorrhage or sepsis; in complicated surgery in high-risk patients and when assessments of intravascular volume are critical.[12]

TEMPERATURE CONTROL

Progressive deterioration of thermoregulation occurs with aging.[13] The common occurrence of hypothermia during operation and anesthesia has been noted, and occurs with greater frequency in the geriatric patient (Figure 15-2).[14]

It behooves us to take all necessary measures to reduce the incidence and degree of intraoperative and postoperative hypothermia in all patients, particularly the elderly, in whom homeostatic mechanisms are impaired.

A number of conditions encountered in the modern operating room tend to cause hypothermia: generally cold ambient temperature; loss of shivering caused by the use of muscle relaxants; vasodilation caused by anesthestic agents; the administration of cold blood and fluid; the use of cold, dry gases; and evaporation of fluid from exposed serous surfaces.

The effect of ambient temperature in the operating room on mean body temperature was studied by Morris.[15] He found that all anesthetized patients became hypothermic when the operating room temperature was below 21°C (70°F), regardless of other preventive measures.

Vaughan and others[16] demonstrated that the magnitude of the temperature drop during surgery was greater in the elderly patient.[3] Although the remaining rate was similar in both the elderly and the younger patient, the absolute temperatures in the

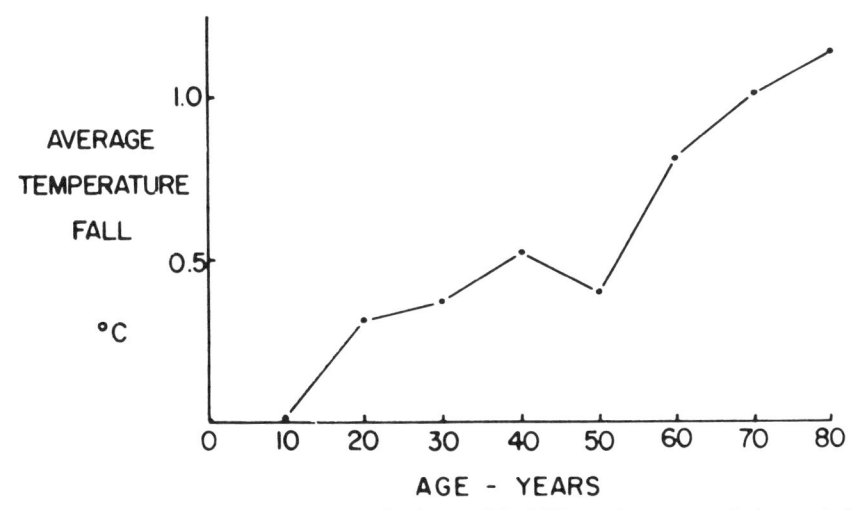

Figure 15-2 Relationship between the age of patients and the fall in rectal temperature during surgical operation. *Source:* Reprinted with permission from *Archives of Surgery* (1966;93:365–369), Copyright © 1966, American Medical Association.

older patients was significantly less on discharge from the recovery room. (See Figure 15-3.)

Some of the effects of hypothermia in the recovery room that are of concern to the anesthesiologist are related to the increased oxygen demand caused by shivering and the increased metabolic rate, and the shift of the oxyhemoglobin dissociation curve to the left, which might lead to hypoxia, as well as the increased solubility of anesthetic agents, which may delay awakening.

The maintenance of normal body temperature in the operating room oftentimes becomes a serious challenge, particularly in longer procedures. Body heat is lost through the evaporation of water from exposed body cavities; by convection into the operating room environment, which is kept at comfortable levels for the operating team; and through the administration of cold fluids (relative to body temperature).

Measures that may be taken to reduce heat loss in the operating room are summarized in Table 15-5.

Maintenance of body temperature at normal levels tends to decrease postoperative shivering, with its attendant marked increase in oxygen consumption, which may increase 400% to 500%.[18] This is of particular importance in elderly or sick patients who have difficulty increasing their oxygen supply.[19,20]

PREOPERATIVE MEDICATION

The use of preoperative medications, a required ritual for many years, has recently changed dramatically. Much of the change has been brought about by

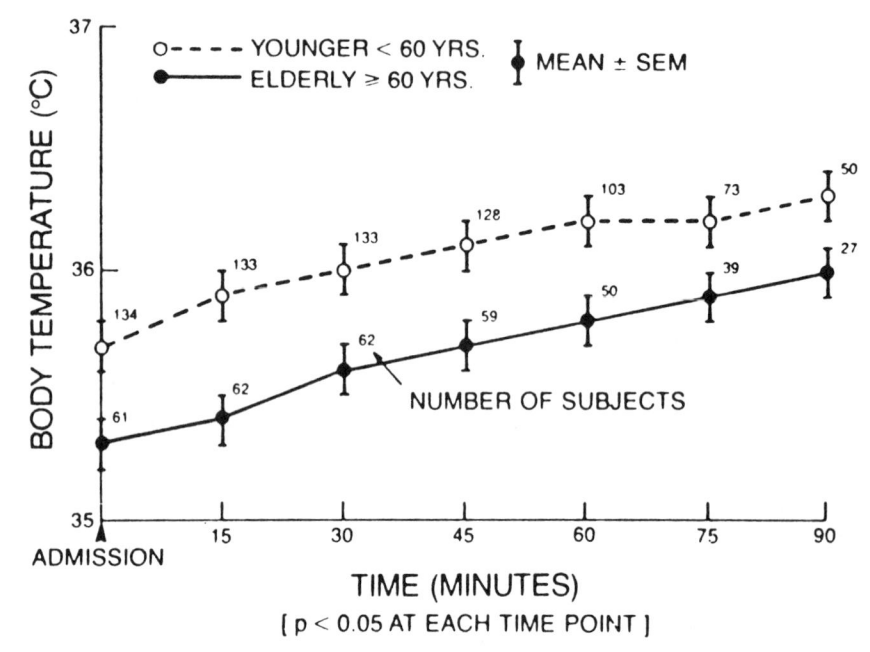

Figure 15-3 Tympanic membrane body temperatures (mean ± SEM) at time of admission to recovery room and at 15-minute intervals to 90 minutes for younger and elderly age groups. Differences in mean temperatures between groups were statistically significant both at time of admission to recovery room and at each time interval thereafter. *Source:* Reprinted with permission from *Anesthesia and Analgesia* (1981;60:746–751), Copyright © 1981, International Anesthesia Research Society.

altering patterns of care, resulting in a shift to same-day admission and ambulatory surgery, as well as the development of newer, more potent anesthetic agents.

In 1963 Egbert and associates,[21] demonstrated that the preoperative interview by an anesthesiologist exerts a calming effect on the patient apart from or in addition to that produced by barbiturate preoperative medication.

Table 15-5 Measures to Control Heat Loss in the Operating Room

- Ambient temperature in OR above 21°C (70°F)
- Use of warming blankets
- Use of blood and fluid warmers
- Use of heated solutions of crystalloids[17]
- Use of warm irrigating solutions by surgeon
- Humidification and heating of anesthetic gases
- Reduction in length of surgery

The virtual elimination of preoperative sedation in our ambulatory surgery patients in the past 4 years reinforces the fact that routine administration of preoperative sedation is no longer valid. There remain, however, many instances in which preoperative pharmacologic preparation is necessary and helpful.

Many anesthesiologists refrain from medicating elderly patients preoperatively. When necessary, preoperative medications should be tailored to the patient's requirements, which may be influenced by age, weight, physical status, duration and type of surgery, degree of anxiety, history of reactions to sedation during prior surgery, and presence or absence of pain.

It is best to medicate most inpatients preoperatively, particularly those having cancer surgery or regional anesthesia. The experience associated with being transferred and transported from the bed to the operating table is best dealt with by a patient who has received some pharmacologic assistance that provides amnesia and sedation. If pain is present or is brought on by movement, narcotics should be considered.

Patients with severe chronic lung disease or hypovolemia are generally better off without preoperative medication.

Although we are constantly barraged with literature, advertisements, and salespeople extolling the virtues of new analgesics and sedatives, the old standby medications that have been used for years serve very well and contribute to cost containment. Analgesics such as morphine and meperidine have been used extensively and are my personal preference.

Benzodiazepines are useful for the reduction of anxiety. Diazepam is both painful and unreliably absorbed when administered intramuscularly, but may be given by mouth with a sip of water. Midazolam is absorbed well after intramuscular injection and exerts its peak effect between 30 and 60 minutes after injection. The diazepams do produce some degree of anterograde amnesia.

Hydoxyzine, an antihistamine, is a mild tranquilizer with minimal cardiovascular side effects that is useful in the poor-risk or elderly patient.

The risk of aspiration must always be considered when general anesthesia is contemplated. Aspiration pneumonitis is produced if the gastric pH is below 2.5. Patients for emergency surgery, in particular, may be considered candidates to receive therapy directed at reducing gastric volume and raising the pH of gastric contents.

There are several agents that one might consider in such patients. If time before surgery is short, a clear antacid, such as 0.3 M sodium citrate (Bi citra) or two tablets of Alka-Seltzer in 30 mL of water, will raise the gastric pH.

$Histamine_2$ antagonists, such as cimetidine and ranitidine, will reduce acid production by the gastric mucosa. They are most effective in reducing gastric pH and volume when given the evening before surgery, as well as one hour before surgery. Although in some patients it will reduce the volume of gastric contents as well, it cannot be relied on to do so. There is some rationale, if an hour or more is available before surgery, to administer an H_2-antagonist in order to decrease the production of hydrochloric acid.

Regarding the volume of gastric contents, metoclopramide may have value in stimulating gastric emptying and increasing lower esophageal sphincter pressure. Its use may be considered for patients undergoing emergency surgery.

RECOVERY ROOM

A brief discussion of complications seen in the recovery room in elderly patients is certainly in order. Although the complications may be interrelated, an attempt to discuss them by major system involvement has been made.

The major respiratory complications seen in the recovery room are airway obstruction, hypoxemia, hypercapnia, and aspiration. All may be life-threatening and should be dealt with promptly.

Postoperative patients, particularly if they have received general anesthesia, should all receive oxygen by nasal prongs or face mask if they have been extubated, or through the endotracheal tube if it is still in place. The gas should always be humidified to prevent drying of secretions.

The most common cause of airway obstruction is blockage of the pharynx by the tongue. Frequently snoring sounds will be heard, but these may be absent if the patient is completely obstructed.

Extending the head while pulling the mandible forward will usually relieve the obstruction. If, however, the obstruction is not completely relieved, the insertion of a well-lubricated nasal airway or an oropharyngeal airway is indicated. A nasal airway is better tolerated by the patient during emergence from general anesthesia. If the obstruction is not relieved by the suggested maneuvers, or if laryngospasm develops, ventilation by bag and mask by a competent person is mandatory.

Hypoxemia may be caused by many factors, but generally it is due to hypoventilation, areas of low ventilation-perfusion ratios, or intrapulmonary right-to-left shunting as is seen with atelectasis from bronchial obstruction by blood or secretions.

Endobronchial intubation from endotracheal tubes that have been inserted too far and have entered the right main stem bronchus should be thought of immediately, since this complication is quickly and easily remediable. Most endotracheal tubes are calibrated.

The average distance in the adult female from the upper teeth to the carina is 24 cm. Tubes should be inserted 20 to 24 cm from the lips, aiming for the midpoint between the glottis and the carina.

Extension or flexion of the head with an endotracheal tube in place and fixed at the lips may result in an average movement of the tube of 1.9 cm. Lateral rotation of the head may result in an average movement of 0.7 cm.[22]

Auscultation of the chest to assure equal breath sounds on both sides of the upper chest, and x-rays of the chest are useful in determining the proper position of the endotracheal tube.

Hypoventilation, which results in increased arterial carbon dioxide tension ($PaCO_2$), may be caused by several factors: poor respiratory drive, inadequate respiratory muscle function, a high rate of carbon dioxide production, or preexisting chronic lung disease.

Depression of respiratory drive may be seen with any anesthetic, particularly when techniques involving intravenous narcotics and tranquilizers are used.

Neurolept anesthesia, intravenous droperidol and fentanyl combined with nitrous oxide, and muscle relaxants have been shown to produce a biphasic respiratory depression.[23]

Intraoperative respiratory depression is followed by a return to normal ventilation at the end of surgery and during the early part of the recovery room stay. This is followed by a second period of respiratory depression.

Narcotic antagonists such as naloxone, in small doses, will alleviate the respiratory depression induced by narcotics without reversing the analgesic effects. If large doses are used, the patient may exhibit signs of severe pain, nausea, hypertension, and tachycardia. Patients should be carefully observed for recurrence of narcotic-induced respiratory depression, since differences in the duration of action of the antagonist and the narcotic may require a repeat administration of antagonist.

Inadequate neuromuscular function may result from inadequately reversed neuromuscular blocking agents commonly used during surgery to provide adequate relaxation of musculature for the surgeon. Assessment of the neuromuscular block may be accomplished with the nerve stimulator, which should be part of every anesthesiologist's armamentarium, and treated if necessary with antagonists such as neostigmine, edrophonium, or pyridostigmine combined with atropine or glycopyrrolate if nondepolarizing blockade has been used.

If a depolarizing blocker such as succinylcholine chloride has been administered, intubation and controlled ventilation should be used until the block has dissipated.

A disturbing situation with respect to prolonged muscle paralysis from a single intubating dose of succinylcholine may be noted in elderly patients who have not experienced surgery or anesthesia previously or who have never received the agent during prior anesthesia. Inadequate ventilation may persist for two to four hours, requiring intubation, and controlled and assisted ventilation. This situation is caused by a genetically determined variant of the enzyme pseudocholinesterase.

The incidence of patients with homozygous atypical pseudocholinesterase is 1/3,200. Diagnosis is accomplished by measuring the level of plasma pseudocholinesterase activity as well as the dibucaine number.

The dibucaine number, which is derived from a test based on the fact that the normal enzyme is inhibited about 80% by dibucaine and the abnormal variant enzyme about 20%, is a measure of the quality of the enzyme.[24] The heterozygote will fall somewhere in between and will usually not exhibit markedly prolonged neuromuscular block.

It is important to diagnose this condition accurately so that the patient may be made aware of its existence, and a Medic-Alert ID or its equivalent should be recommended. Family members that may be so affected genetically should be notified, and testing recommended to establish their susceptibility so that this situation may be avoided in the future.

It is our policy to inform the patient and the surgeon of the findings and to follow up with a letter documenting the studies plus recommendations for testing of family members by certified mail, return receipt requested, with a copy to the surgeon.

Other factors that may result in hypoventilation include obesity, gastric dilation, tight dressings, and markedly increased carbon dioxide production from shivering, particularly if increased minute ventilation cannot be accomplished.

An arterial blood gas value is invaluable in confirming the diagnosis of hypoventilation.

Aspiration of gastric contents may occur during or after extubation. Diagnosis may be difficult to come by definitively. Tachypnea and tachycardia may be present. The chest x-ray may show diffuse infiltration, although serial roentgenograms are required, to determine the extent of pulmonary involvement. Rales and rhonchi may be present on auscultation, indicating frank pulmonary edema. A low $PaCO_2$ relative to the inspired oxygen concentration the patient is breathing is a constant finding.

Treatment should be aggressive and aimed at restoring normal pulmonary function. This will probably entail intubation and continuous positive airway pressure.[25]

Because highly acidic acid aspirate produces pulmonary damage within 12 to 18 seconds, lavage with saline or bicarbonate solution is probably of no value. Bronchoscopy may be indicated only if solid material is suspected of being aspirated.

Steroids were used for a number of years but are commonly omitted in current treatment. Prophylactic antibiotics, once commonly prescribed in this situation, are reserved for patients who demonstrate signs of infection.

Intravascular fluid shifts resulting in pulmonary edema may require the insertion of central venous pressure lines or, preferably, a pulmonary artery catheter that allows for measurements of cardiac output and the hemodynamic factors necessary for more specific therapy.

It is not uncommon for patients who have aspirated to recover in 24 to 72 hours.

HYPOTENSION

Hypotension in the recovery room is usually due to decreased ventricular preload, reduced myocardial contractility, or markedly reduced systemic vascular resistance.

Decreased ventricular preload may be due to unreplaced blood loss, third-space fluid loss, and/or unreplaced urinary fluid losses.

Pulmonary embolism may impede blood flow to the left heart.

Decreased myocardial contractility may result from the continuing effect of anesthetic agents, preexisting heart disease, or myocardial infarction. Whatever the cause, prompt diagnosis and treatment are essential, particularly in the elderly patient who is sensitive to ischemia.

HYPERTENSION

Common causes of postoperative hypertension are pain, bladder distention, hypercapnia, hypoxia, hypothermia, volume overload, and emergence delirium.

As previously discussed, the management of hypoxia and hypercapnia is related to airway management and ventilation. The hypothermic patient should be aggressively warmed. Drainage of the distended bladder is an obvious solution. Pain should be treated with carefully titrated narcotics, and sedatives may relieve emergence delirium.

Volume overload may become manifest when vasodilatory anesthetics are eliminated. Treatment consists of diuretics and vasodilators.

Sustained hypertension in the elderly may lead to myocardial infarction and, if persistent, should be aggressively treated. Mild hypertension may be successfully treated with small increments of droperidol or chlorpromazine. The use of sublingual nifedipine has recently increased. Nifedipine has a fairly rapid onset of action and two- to four-hour duration.

Carefully maintained infusions of short-acting beta blockers or nitrates may be of value.

The poorly controlled hypertensive patient is more likely to experience postoperative hypertension. This underscores the importance of adequate preoperative preparation and continued therapy of the hypertensive patient.

PAIN CONTROL

The anesthesiologist has become more active in the management of chronic pain, particularly as it relates to oncology patients. Epidural narcotics, which may be administered by way of epidural catheter, may provide long-lasting relief of chronic pain. The patient who responds well to this therapy may have the epidural catheter implanted and connected to a subcutaneously implanted continuous pump, which may be refilled by percutaneous injection of morphine at required intervals. Respiratory depression, which may be a problem in the control of postoperative pain, is seldom seen in patients with chronic cancer pain perhaps because of a tolerance resulting from the large amounts of systemic narcotics to which they have been exposed.

Administration of narcotics directly into the neuraxis was attempted at the turn of the century.[26] It was not until 1977, when opiate receptors were discovered in the neuraxis,[27] that the administration of subarachnoid and epidural narcotics was seriously investigated. Since that time much has been done regarding these techniques. The administration of subarachnoid morphine to President Ronald Reagan for postoperative pain after his colon resection in 1985 appears to have legitimated the use of these techniques.

We have been using epidural morphine more and more with great success for postoperative pain relief, particularly in major upper abdominal and thoracic surgery and for cesarean section patients. Its use has been rapidly growing.

These techniques have a place in the control of postoperative pain accompanying major abdominal procedures in the geriatric patient. The commonly encountered side effects are respiratory depression, nausea and vomiting, and itching—all of which can be controlled by intravenous naloxone, usually in a continuous drip. Surprisingly, the analgesic effect is not altered by naloxone. Urinary retention, which has been reported with an incidence of 22% in postoperative pain patients, is also reversible with naloxone.[28,29] The use of apnea monitors has made this technique more acceptable, particularly when these patients can be monitored in recovery rooms or intensive care units.

REFERENCES

1. Stephen CR, Assaf RAE (eds): *Geriatric Anesthesia: Principles and Practice.* Stoneham, Mass, Butterworth, 1986.

2. Kannel WB, Hjortland MC, McNamara PM, et al: Menopause and risk of cardiovascular disease. The Framingham Study. *Ann Intern Med* 1976;85:447–452.

3. Schneider AJL: Assessment of risk factors and surgical outcome. *Surg Clin North Am* 1983;63:1113.

4. Wilson LA, Lawson IR, Braws W: Multiple disorders in the elderly: A clinical and statistical study. *Lancet* 1962;2:841.

5. Edwards RE, Miller RD, Roizen MF, et al: Cardiovascular effects of tricyclic antidepressants in depressed patients with chronic heart disease. *N Engl J Med* 1982;306:954.

6. Kosanin R: Anesthetic considerations in patients on chronic tricyclic antidepressant therapy. *Anesthesiol Rev* 1981;8:38.

7. Glisson SN, Fajardol El-Etr AA: Amitryptyline therapy increases electrocardiographic changes during reversal of neuromuscular blockade: *Anesth Analg* 1978;57:77.

8. Hill GE, Wong KC: Lithium carbonate and neuromuscular blocking agents. *Anesthesiology* 1977;46:122.

9. Martin BA, Kramer PM: Clinical significance of the interaction between lithium and a neuromuscular blocker. *Am J Psychiatry* 1982;139:1326.

10. Eichhorn JH, Cooper JB, Cullen DJ, et al: Standards for patient monitoring during anesthesia at Harvard Medical School. *JAMA* 1986;256:1017–1020.

11. Gallo JA: Anesthesia and the geriatric patient. *Clin Anesthesiol* 1986;4(4):824W.

12. Blitt CD (ed): *Monitoring in Anesthesia and Critical Care Medicine*. New York, Churchill Livingstone, 1985.

13. Collins KJ, Exton-Smith AN: Thermal-homeostasis in old age. *Am Geriatr Soc* 1983;31:519–524.

14. Goldberg MJ, Roe LF: Temperature changes during anesthesia and operations. *Arch Surg* 1966;93:365–369.

15. Morris RH: Operating room temperature and the anesthetized paralyzed patient. *Arch Surg* 1971;102:95–97.

16. Vaughan NS, Vaughan RW, Cort RC: Postoperative hypothermia in adults: Relationship of age, anesthesia, and shivering to rewarming. *Anesth Analg* 1981;60:746–751.

17. Norman EA, Ahmad I, Zeig NJ: Delivery temperature of heated and cooled intravenous solutions. *Anesth Analg* 1986;65:693–699.

18. Bay J, Nunn JF, Prys-Roberts C: Factors influencing arterial CO_2 during recovery from anesthesia. *Br J Anaesth* 1968;40:398–406.

19. Roe CF, Goldberg MJ, Blau CS, et al: The influence of body temperature on early post operative oxygen consumption. *Surgery* 1966;60:85–92.

20. Flacke WE, Flacke JW, Ryan JF, et al: Altered temperature regulation, in Orkin FH, Cooperman LH (eds): *Complications in Anesthesiology*. Philadelphia, JB Lippincott, 1983, pp 277–313.

21. Egbert LD, Battit GE, Turndorf H, et al: The value of the preoperative visit by an anesthetist. *JAMA* 1963;185:553.

22. Conrady PA, Goodman LR, Lainge F, et al: Alteration of endotracheal tube position. Flexion and extension of the neck. *Crit Care Med* 1976;4:8.

23. Becker LD, Paulson BA, Miller RD: Biphasic respiratory depression after fentanyl-droperidol or fentanyl alone used to supplement nitrous oxide anesthesia. *Anesthesiology* 1976;44:291.

24. Kalow W, Genest K: A method for the detection of atypical forms of human serum cholinesterase. Determination of dibucaine numbers. *Can J Bio Chem* 1957;35:339.

25. Miller RD (ed): *Anesthesia*, ed 2. New York, Churchill Livingstone, 1986, vol 3, pp 2042–2045.

26. Kitagawa O: Intrathecal injection of local anesthetics. *Tokyo Ija Shinshi* 1901;1200:653. Cited in *Anesthesiology* 1963;58:290.

27. Atweh SF, Kuhar MJ: Autoradiographic localization of opiate receptors in rat brain: 1. Spinal cord and lower medulla. *Brain Res* 1977;124:53.

28. Rawal N, Molleforsk, Arelsson, et al: An experimental study of urodynamic effects of epidural morphine and naloxone reversal. *Anesth Analg* 1983;62:241.

29. Rawal N, Sjostrand UH, Dahlstrom B: Post operative pain relief by epidural morphine. *Anesth Analg* 1981;60:726.

Chapter 16

A Radiologist Looks at the Aging Patient

Alan G. Dembner

Old age is, so to speak, the sanctuary of ills: they all take refuge in it.
Antiphanes, 408 B.C., Fragment from *The Dipnosophists*.

The ills of the geriatric female patient encompass almost all current diagnostic imaging. Numerous imaging modalities, fostered by the recent technological explosion, are available to the physician for clinical problems that are, essentially, unchanged from the beginning of time. In most cases the clinician and patient have been helped; but in other instances, because of the "cascade effect,"[1] patient care has been hindered.

Conventional diagnostic imaging equipment has always been expensive. However, those costs have been small in the face of major advanced sophisticated imaging equipment, including digital angiography, computed tomography (CT),[2] and now magnetic resonance imaging (MRI) equipment. This fact, coupled with many other factors, has imposed a new hospital reimbursement system called DRGs (diagnosis-related groups), which is forcing physicians to become more efficient in the way they manage patients. Therefore, unproductive high-risk and non-cost-effective imaging procedures will have to be eliminated.[3] The logical use of present-day radiology will result in a considerable saving to the patient.[4] Unfortunately, meaningful cost benefit information of current imaging modalities is unknown.

In choosing a diagnostic imaging modality the referring physician must consider the sensitivity and specificity of the examination. Sensitivity is the likelihood of a test being positive if a patient has a disease. Specificity is the likelihood that the test is negative if the patient does not have the disease.

$$\text{sensitivity} = \frac{\text{true positives}}{\text{true positives and false negatives}}$$

$$\text{specificity} = \frac{\text{true negatives}}{\text{true negatives and false positives}}$$

Therefore, a highly sensitive test would be useful to the clinician when the disease is serious and false-positive results would not lead to undesirable consequences. A specific test is desirable when the disease is serious and false-positive results could lead to unfortunate consequences. Sensitivity identifies abnormality, whereas specificity identifies normality. This is especially true in the geriatric patient, when a medication or operation that was "unnecessary" could have serious consequences. In screening procedures false-positive studies will have checks and balances. For example, mammography uses physical examinations, follow-up mammograms, and biopsies under local anesthesia with little morbidity and mortality.

It would take a book in itself to describe the radiological workup of the geriatric patient with gynecologic problems, let alone general medical abnormalities. The strengths, weaknesses, and, even more important, limitations of present-day diagnostic imaging modalities are pertinent.

Plain film radiographic examinations are readily available and have a relatively low radiation exposure and cost. They are useful in the evaluation of chest and breast disease, trauma (iatrogenic or otherwise), and metastatic bone disease when pathological bone fractures are suspect or thought to be imminent.

Barium examinations are also relatively inexpensive and noninvasive for imaging of the gastrointestinal tract. MRI and CT will not replace those studies in the diagnosis of ulcer disease or large bowel diseases, such as pseudomembranous enterocolitis, which may develop in the gynecologic patient as a complication of her underlying disease or its treatment.

It is hoped that the newer, nonionic contrast materials will have an impact on excretory urography and angiography in the future. Currently, they are not cost effective for these imaging modalities in the general population.[5,6] Digital imaging is revolutionizing angiography and venography with its ability to use less contrast and smaller catheters in many imaging procedures that previously used conventional angiographic technique.

Technetium scanning is still the most sensitive examination for detection of metastatic bone disease. Ventilation perfusion lung scanning in nuclear medicine is the initial imaging modality after the chest x-ray for the radiographic workup of pulmonary embolism. Monoclonal antibodies scanning is a future possibility for the early diagnosis and staging of ovarian and uterine tumors.

CT has not only revolutionized neuroradiology, but changed the evaluation of disorders in the abdomen and pelvis as well. It is useful in the staging of gynecologic malignancies as well as in the diagnosis of a recurrent tumor in those patients.[7]

Diagnostic ultrasonography, a relatively low-cost procedure, is noninvasive and uses no ionizing radiation. It has the ability to differentiate solid from cystic lesions and can produce images in all planes.

MRI is in its infancy. Like diagnostic sonography, it uses nonionizing radiation, but it is extremely expensive in initial cost and maintenance. MRI has similar spatial resolution as CT, but markedly improved contrast resolution. It also has the ability for tissue characterization using hydrogen density, and specific values such as T1 and T2 relaxation times. Currently MRI is superior to CT in the imaging of many brain and spinal cord lesions. It also has tremendous promise in the evaluation of the cardiovascular system, as well as gynecologic application.

Radiation exposure must be considered in the cost benefit analysis of radiographic examinations.[8] Unlike therapeutic radiology, the possible adverse effects of radiation from diagnostic radiology are incidental to the information received from the test performed. These side effects may be divided into genetic and somatic changes, the latter being of more importance in the geriatric population.

An acute effect of radiation is changes in blood cell counts. For example, a reduction of the lymphocyte count will occur when the whole body is exposed to 25 or more rad. Evans and associates[9] estimate that 1% of all cases of leukemia that occur annually in the United States may be attributable to lifetime exposure to diagnostic radiation. The authors also suggested that 0.7% of all cases of breast cancer that occur annually in the United States can be attributed to diagnostic radiography, but this is considered high by others depending on the analysis used.[10] Modern equipment and film screen combinations have markedly reduced the radiation dose in radiographic examinations. A maximum skin dose in a posteroanterior and lateral chest is 0.05 rad, and a dose to the red bone marrow on a CT of the abdomen is approximately 0.5 rad. It must be remembered that every person receives an annual dose of approximately 0.2 rad from background radiation in our environment. We must, therefore, try to avoid clinically unproductive examinations.

The referring clinician will find the modern-day radiologist not only an interpreter of imaging examinations, but also a consultant for the effective use of diagnostic imaging examinations.[11] The clinician should feel free to call on the radiologist in formulating the appropriate diagnostic examinations and their sequence for the patient's medical problems.

REFERENCES

1. Mold JW, Stein AF: The cascade effect in the clinical care of patients. *N Engl J Med* 1986; 314:512–514.

2. Enlow RA, Hodak JA, Pullen KW, et al: The effect of the computed tomographic scanner on utilization and charges for alternative diagnostic procedures. *Radiology* 1980;136:413–417.

3. Doubilet P, Weinstein MC, McNeil BJ: Use and misuse of the term "cost effective" in medicine. *N Engl J Med* 1986;314:253–256.

4. Palmer PE, Cockshott WP: The appropriate use of diagnostic imaging. *JAMA* 1984;252:2753–2754.

5. Wolf G: Safer, more expensive iodinated contrast agents: How do we decide? *Radiology* 1986;159:557–558.

6. White RI, Halden WJ: Liquid gold: Low-osmolarity contrast media. *Radiology* 1986;159:559–560.

7. Mamtora H, Isherwood I: Computed tomography in ovarian carcinoma: Patterns of disease and limitations. *Clin Radiol* 1982;33:165–171.

8. Boice JD: The danger of X-rays—real or apparent? *N Engl J Med* 1986;315:828–830.

9. Evans JD, Wennberg JE, McNeil BJ: The influence of diagnostic radiography on the incidence of breast cancer and leukemia. *N Engl J Med* 1986;315:810–815.

10. Rall JE, Beebe GW, Hoel DG, et al: Report of the National Institutes of Health ad hoc working group to develop radioepidemiological tables. Washington, DC, Government Printing Office, 1985. (DHHS publication No [NIH] 85-2748)

11. Seltzer SE, Beard JO, Adams DF: Radiologist as consultant: Direct contact between referring clinician and radiologist before CT examinations. *AJR* 1985;144:661–664.

Part IV

Other Aspects of Aging

Chapter 17

The Cost-Effectiveness of the Geriatric Patient

Richard Caruana, Alex MacDonald, and John D. Phillips

In recent years the increased intensity and technological advancements of health care services provided to the patient have resulted in an exorbitant increase in health care expenditures. The increasing cost of these services was passed on to the patient and third party reimbursers. In view of this, the hospital and physician had neither motivation nor incentive to curb costs.

The rise in health care cost is readily demonstrated by charting the yearly increase of the proportion of the national health care cost to the overall gross national product (GNP). One survey shows that in 1950 the national health care cost was $12.7 billion and represented 4.5% of the GNP. This was compared with the year 1982, in which the national health care cost was $322 billion and represented 10.5% of the GNP.[1]

The Arthur Anderson & Company survey predicts that the upward spiral of health care costs, as measured by the percentage of the GNP devoted to health care, will continue and then level off. In 1982 the figure was 10.5%. By 1990 the panelists forecast that it will rise to 12% and remain there through 1995.[2]

The federal government's implementation of the prospective payment system of reimbursement for Medicare has forced hospitals to reduce the costs of health care. The challenge for hospital management is to provide quality care while keeping costs below the set reimbursement rates. Under this system, reimbursement is defined by diagnosis-related groups (DRGs). Many DRGs are governed by age as well as by the diagnosis and procedure, and because of the rapidly increasing geriatric population, reimbursement is greatly impacted by the elderly admission.

> Between 1970 and 1979, the elderly population increased their utilization of hospitals at a much faster rate than the general population . . . and since the number of persons 65 years and over is forecasted to increase 25% between 1979 and 1990—including a 31% rise in number

of persons over 85 years—hospital expenditures are likely to continue their upward mark.[3(p6)]

There is now a task set before hospital management in providing care for the elderly. That is to identify those special needs of the geriatric patient and how they impact the health care costs of the hospital. How management uses this knowledge to treat these patients in a compassionate, professional, and cost-effective manner is the challenge that must be met in a creative and timely fashion.

Besides the variety of diagnoses and treatment plans for the elderly, there are certain common nonmedical concerns that the geriatric patient perceives as being as crucial and important as any medical problem. These concerns include depression, loneliness, lack of communication with family, financial concerns, dependence, and a general fear and anxiousness of the hospital stay itself.

Depression is one of aging's most devastating and often undertreated health problems. A recent study showed that as many as 13% of people over 65 years of age suffer from significant depression; 2.5% experience severe depression.[4]

When several gynecologists were interviewed on the treatment of the elderly patient, a common observation was that of the changing role of the gynecologist. The role has been expanded to not only that of a primary physician, but also that of a psychiatrist, counselor, and confidant. Caring for the elderly must include a "compassionate ear" for the 80-year-old woman whose chief complaint is that nobody is paying attention to her; or the anxious patient who is concerned about her hospital stay exhausting her life savings; or the elderly hospital patient who feels abandoned and fears discharge to a nursing home.

Because of these special needs of the geriatric patient in today's health care delivery system, appropriate cost-effective actions are warranted on the part of the health care administrator. Upper management must be aware of the quality of patient care, as well as the financial concerns of the patient, while managing hospital costs in the treatment of that patient. Also, the utilization of services such as preadmission testing and the expansion of outpatient testing must be evaluated owing to the limited mobility of the elderly patient.

The illnesses and impairments of older people require services that must be sustained, in contrast with the time-limited services associated with acute illness. Older adults need housing, rehabilitation therapy, outpatient medical services, and transportation—all services that could be coordinated through the hospital.[5]

Some of the types of programs that hospitals can participate in that would have considerable impact on the care for the elderly are discussed below.

EDUCATIONAL PROGRAMS FOR THE ELDERLY

In today's society the health care delivery system has the extremely difficult task of providing a continuum of health care to our aging population. The movement is currently away from treating the elderly on an episodic, acute care basis and directed toward a multi–health care approach.[6] In addition to addressing the specific needs of the elderly by means of rehabilitation, outpatient services, and counseling programs, hospitals are stressing the importance of education for the elderly community. Hospitals have realized the benefits of community education that can teach the elderly to become more aware of the problems that may occur as a result of the aging process.

Many elderly people want to learn about how to maintain their health, yet they are unable to do so because of a lack of education. As a result of this problem, hospitals have begun to offer educational programs that would teach the aged about topics such as diabetes care, osteoporosis prevention, exercise, and proper nutrition.

The health care facility can supplement these programs with screening tests, such as physical examinations, mammography, Pap tests, and glucose tests, on an outpatient basis. The tests could be provided in a convenient, low-cost fashion and would help to identify health problems for early detection or prevention of disease that could interfere with the individual's quality of life.

In the event that the elderly person who has participated in these programs should have to be hospitalized, both she and the hospital would have the advantage of a more physically and mentally prepared admission. In addition to community education, the elderly patient's educational needs could be supplemented during the hospital stay with in-house programs. Such programs might help the patient to become more self-sufficient, which could expedite an earlier discharge.

Both community and in-house education programs could directly impact on cost reduction as a result of the hospital treating a more health conscious patient. This could lead to a potentially less acute patient, therefore reducing hospital costs and length of stay.

Through the support of hospital administration, long-term cost-effective management of health care can be realized in addition to improving the quality of life for our elderly population.

TRANSPORTATION FOR THE ELDERLY

Transportation to and from the hospital can be a difficult experience for the elderly to cope with, especially with the added stress of a hospital admission. A hospital transport system could benefit the elderly patient's hospital experience in the following ways:

- Reduce the patient's anxiety about her dependence on family and friends for means of transportation to the hospital.

- Provide a means for utilization of preadmission testing that will help to reduce the patient's stay in the hospital.
- Allow the patient to be discharged earlier if final tests or procedures can be performed on an outpatient basis.

There is generally a separate charge for hospital transport services, and most third party payers have either limited or no coverage of these fees. However, the dollar savings that this service can provide may create the incentive for payers and/or hospitals to absorb these costs in the future.

DISCHARGE PLANNING AND PLACEMENT

When addressing postdischarge care for the elderly, special emphasis must be placed on the interaction of their social, psychological, medical, and financial needs. A dynamic social work service and home health care program must be available to meet these needs. In the past, most patient referrals to the social work service department came from the physicians themselves. This captured a portion of the patients in need of discharge planning. However, in view of today's growing geriatric population and rising health care costs, a more sophisticated means for discharge planning referrals is essential.

A current, successful approach to this timely identification process or "case finding" is the development and use of high-risk screening criteria. Shortly after admission, patients who meet the screening criteria are assigned to a social worker for assessment. Consultation with the physician and interviews with the patient will determine whether the patient is a candidate for a nursing home or rehabilitation center on discharge.

> Increased interest in screening hospital patients for their need for social work services stemmed in part from studies pointing to the fact that nonmedical factors contributed to prolonged hospitalization. Other work demonstrated that appropriate and timely intervention was associated with dramatic reductions in length of stay. Support for social work case finding, an integral part of screening, grew out of research showing that, compared with more traditional patterns of referral, case finding resulted in earlier interventions and the identification of a more heterogeneous patient population, with respect to both socioeconomic status and type of social work service required. Also contributing to the growth of screening is the increasing reliance on expensive medical technology that has served to accelerate the high cost of hospital care and has led to intensified pressures to reduce hospital costs, limit hospital stays to

those periods when active, curative treatment is carried out, and hold all health care personnel more accountable.[7]

Another source of referral that is also very effective is the weekly rounds for discharge planning among the primary nurse of the patient, the social worker, and the home health care coordinator. At these meetings the patient's needs are evaluated to determine which services would be best for the patient's situation. Some patients do not meet the requirements for nursing home placement, so the utilization of home health care services might be a viable alternative. By early identification of a patient as a candidate for nursing home placement, the patient's stay in the hospital can be reduced. Even in those cases where placement has been determined but the patient requires Medicaid support before the nursing home will accept her, social work services can help to expedite discharge by beginning the application process as soon as the patient has been identified. Such patients may have no other alternative for discharge and will remain in the hospital until placement procedures are completed.

Patients who will need to be transferred to a rehabilitation facility can be identified early on in their hospital stay by weekly discharge planning rounds, review of operating room schedules, and from physician referrals. Also, to expedite transfer, some rehabilitation centers provide a weekly visit by a nurse from their facility to evaluate the patient's status and thus be able to prepare for the transfer earlier.

Home health care departments in hospitals can offer to the elderly much in the way of convenience, shortened hospital stay, and cost reduction to the patient as well as to the hospital. Most of the referrals come from physicians, who often are most familiar with the family situation, the condition of the patient, and what the patient will be faced with once at home. Home health care, in some cases, offers an alternative to a lengthy hospital stay by offering such services as visiting nurse service; homemaker and home health aides; intravenous, occupational, and physical therapists; and durable medical equipment rental or purchase.

In sum, accurate, timely, and efficient discharge planning and placement for the elderly patient benefits both the patient and the hospital; that is, it provides quality and compassionate health care while utilizing cost-effective health care management.

GERIATRIC EVALUATION UNIT

To meet the numerous needs of the geriatric patient, a holistic approach to their care and management is being provided by the development of geriatric evaluation units. These units provide the elderly with specialized programs, utilizing a team approach to evaluate the patient's medical, psychosocial, and functional needs.

The team generally consists of physicians, nurses, social workers, physical and occupational therapists, nutritionists, and psychologists—all who are experienced in the treatment of the elderly.

Periodic in-service lectures from various medical specialties and support services concerning the elderly supplement the team's education on geriatric assessment and care. The lectures also provide a mechanism to further educate the house staff in the field of gerontology.

Initially patterned after models developed in the United Kingdom, such programs usually have several goals: to increase the patient's level of functioning, to improve diagnosis and treatment, to achieve appropriate placement, to reduce the use of institutional services, and to generally increase the overall quality of care delivered to elderly patients.[8]

> The benefits of the geriatric evaluation unit can be achieved at the cost of more intensive efforts at the end of the traditional hospital stay. This expenditure of additional resources to gain later benefits can be viewed as an investment strategy. Additional costs borne during the unit stay are recouped over the ensuing year. This philosophy might be more difficult to implement in a setting where Medicare and Medicaid are the predominant sources of payment, since Medicare dollars would be used to save Medicaid expenses. In the contemporary environment of diagnosis related groups, neither the hospital nor the Medicare program has an incentive to bear these costs, although the logic of improving the functioning and survival of patients and reducing overall health costs is compelling.[8(pp1669-1670)]

In summary, it has been found that geriatric evaluation units can provide substantial benefits at minimal cost for appropriate groups of elderly patients, over and above the benefits of traditional hospital approaches.[8]

ADDITIONAL OPPORTUNITIES FOR HOSPITALS TO HELP THE ELDERLY

In addition to the alternatives for cost-effective hospital management for the elderly stated above, administrators can consider the sponsoring of medical day-care centers, life care living facilities, and emergency response systems.

Medical day-care centers would allow those individuals who are looking after their older family members at home the opportunity to go about their normal workday with the assurance that these family members are being cared for. Different levels of care can be provided by the facility, ranging from observational to skilled nursing care.

The concept of life care involves providing health care for the elderly in a comfortable condominium environment. In this setting, medical and laboratory services and physical activities are made available. Thus these elderly residents enjoy the independence of living in their own home with the added security of knowing that health care services are close at hand.

The emergency response system provides the elderly with the means of receiving immediate response to an accident or other emergency occurring in the home. This is accomplished by the person simply pressing a button on a device worn around the neck. A signal is transmitted to the emergency response center, where a monitoring operator is available 24 hours a day. Immediately on receiving the signal, all the pertinent medical information about that patient is displayed on a computer screen. The operator then contacts the patient by telephone. The patient can communicate with the operator by a voice-activated telephone hookup from anywhere in the home. Depending on the emergency situation, the operator can notify the patient's predesignated family member, friend, local first aid squad, or hospital. In addition to this kind of support, the operator, having access to the patient's medical and personal history, may be able to provide assistance over the phone by helping the patient help herself if it is not an immediate emergency or until help arrives.

CONCLUSION

It is obvious that the geriatric patient is fast becoming a major component of today's health care population. It is just as obvious, judging from government regulations and hospital budget cuts, that cost containment for quality health care is necessary for hospital survival.

In view of these factors, the cost-effectiveness of providing health care to the elderly should be considered by management as an important long-term strategy that should include the following:

- Development of health care educational programs for the elderly that would help to create a more knowledgeable community and reduce overall health care costs by admitting less acute patients to the hospital.
- Implementation of hospital policies that would include provisions for updating education directed toward the special needs and treatment plans of the elderly. These educational programs would provide residents, nurses, and support staff of the hospital with the much needed insight toward geriatric care.
- Promotion of dynamic and timely discharge planning/placement and home health programs for the elderly that can reduce length of stay and the associated costs to the hospital.

- Realization of the benefits to hospitals of sponsoring their own custodial care, intermediate care, skilled nursing care, and rehabilitation facilities, owing to the impact of the prospective payment system on earlier discharges.
- Initiation of hospital-based transport systems that would provide a convenient method for elderly patients to take advantage of preadmission testing, and outpatient services that can also lead to a reduction in length of stay.
- Creation of geriatric evaluation units, supplemented with the appropriate personnel, that will meet the medical, psychosocial, and functional needs of the elderly patient, utilizing a holistic approach to health care.

Although some of these programs may incur initial cost to the health care institution, the long-term effects on reducing hospital costs would be realized.

Management should consider the marketing potential of these programs for capturing a larger portion of the geriatric population in this competitive marketplace of the current health care delivery system.

We feel that eventually third party payers will realize the advantages of covering the costs involved in some of these programs, such as home health care and patient transport, especially when the utilization of these programs may provide reductions in length of stay, intensity of care, and readmission into the hospital.

REFERENCES

1. New England Nuclear & DuPont Inc (Boston, MA): Prospective payment and nuclear medicine: Concept, impact and action. *Symposia Summary*, 1984.

2. Arthur Anderson & Co and the American College of Hospital Administrators: Health care in the 1980's: Trends and strategies. 1984, p 5.

3. Grimaldi P, Micheletti J: *Diagnosis Related Groups—A Practitioner's Guide*. Chicago, Publishers Press, 1980, p 6.

4. Weiner M: Depression: A tragic problem in the elderly. *Clin Nurs Pract* 1986/87;4:13.

5. Hospitals diversify operations to care for the elderly. *Hospitals* 1985;59:52.

6. Mistarz JE: Multihospital systems target continuum of care strategy. *Hospitals* 1985;59:52.

7. Wolock I, Schlesinger EG: Social work screening in New Jersey hospitals: Progress, problems, and implications. Presented at The National Health Conference of the National Association of Social Workers, Washington, DC, June 11, 1984.

8. Rubenstein LZ, Josephson KR, Weiland GD, et al: Effectiveness of a geriatric evaluation unit. *N Engl J Med* 1984;311:1664.

We thank the following physicians and hospital personnel at Saint Barnabas Medical Center, Livingston, New Jersey, for information and views on the subject matter of this chapter: Kenneth Dollinger, MD; Samual Fortunato, MD; Gilbert Sugarman, MD; Harold Schwartz, MD; Marven Wallen, MD; C. Gary Walker, MBA; Shirley Weil, MSW, ACSW; Theresa Singer, MPH, BS, RN; Muriel Shore, MSN, RN, CNA.

Chapter 18

Medicolegal Issues in the Care of the Aged

Albert L. Strunk

INTRODUCTION

This is a time of considerable preoccupation with and anxiety about the legal consequences of medical treatment. It would seem that there is a medicolegal dimension to every facet of professional practice and, as one might anticipate, there are some medicolegal considerations especially applicable to the care of aged patients. Despite such considerations, the care of aged persons is not, per se, fraught with increased risk of professional liability. On the contrary, there is evidence that the geriatric patient population probably presents less risk for litigation than the patient population at large. This chapter presents several medicolegal issues that one may expect to encounter with increasing frequency as one and one's patients age.

PRELIMINARY CONSIDERATIONS

The process of aging involves profound changes of mind and body. Although this chapter primarily deals with matters of the mind, a few elemental observations concerning limitations of the body ought to be made. First, a common cause of tort liability involving aged patients is the so-called slip-and-fall case, however mundane. Injury from falls during examination or while under a physician's care is one of the ten most frequent causes of liability/malpractice claims. Assisting aged patients on and off examining tables should be the rule. Likewise, a survey of railings, steps, and access ramps in and around one's office may reveal additional obstacles or hazards to patients whose sense of balance and ability to ambulate may be impaired.

Second, geriatric patients are more likely to be taking medication than younger patients. Adverse reactions to drugs and drug interactions are likewise among the ten most frequent causes of liability/malpractice claims. A careful medication history and the avoidance of polypharmacy is essential. It is not sufficient for an aged patient to have only her gynecologist to provide care. A general internist is the logical person to coordinate care, including the use of medications, in patients who very often have multiple medical problems. Care of the wound and complications of gynecologic surgery remain the responsibility of the surgeon, but if the patient's general medical condition requires the use of intensive care facilities, an appropriately qualified internist or other intensivist ought to be involved as well.

Failure to diagnose, especially failure to diagnose cancer, is also one of the ten most frequent causes of liability/malpractice claims. In the natural tendency to focus attention on the female reproductive organs, one must not overlook bladder and bowel etiologies of pelvic and lower abdominal symptoms. Diverticulosis and diverticulitis, as well as pelvic abscesses secondary to ruptured diverticuli, inter alia, are more frequent findings in an aging population. Colorectal cancer and bladder cancer often present with signs and symptoms that will bring a patient first to her gynecologist for evaluation.

COMPETENCY

The starting point for any discussion of legal issues in the care of aged patients is the matter of competency. Legal competency is defined as the presence of those characteristics (or the absence of those disabilities) that render a witness legally fit and qualified to give testimony in a court of justice. Relative to making medical decisions that affect one's person, the patient must understand the nature of her illness, the prognosis, the alternative treatments available, and the risks and benefits of treatment or lack thereof. A competent patient has the mental capacity to reason and make judgments about the integrity and well-being of her body based on such information.

Legal competency is both time-specific and subject-specific. A patient may currently be well informed and competent to make decisions relative to her medical care and treatment, but may subsequently no longer possess the mental capacity to reason and make such judgments. It follows, therefore, that the ascertainment of competency is ongoing. Although the issue is inherent in any patient contact, it becomes significantly more important in an aged population. When competency fluctuates and it is unclear whether the patient has the capacity to make a given decision, further assessment by the treating physician or qualified consultants is mandatory. Although it is generally true that a person who is competent to reason and make judgments at a given time in regard to one subject will also be considered competent to reason and make judgments during the same period of time about another subject, legal tests of competency may be more stringent in regard to decisions that result in the withholding of medical treatment or perhaps the loss of life itself.

In order to achieve what is considered a humane result, courts have occasionally blurred the distinction between competency and credibility. Whereas the former refers to mental capacity, the latter refers to the veracity or trustworthiness to be ascribed to the patient's expression of her wishes. Thus, in cases involving the withdrawal of life-support systems, the patient may be competent according to accepted neuropsychiatric criteria, but the testimony of family members or friends may challenge the patient's credibility, particularly in situations in which the patient's choice seems to ignore a significant prospect for extending life under humane and comfortable conditions.

Considerations of competency are not, however, limited to decisions about death and dying. As suggested earlier, the question of competency arises in every patient-physician contact and influences the weight accorded by the physician to a given history, the patient's ability to consent in an informed manner to the treatment recommended, and the patient's ability to comprehend the instructions given, whether pertaining to medication usage or other treatment modalities. Not infrequently family members or friends accompany the patient to her physician's office, actively participate in articulation of the history, express the ostensible will of the patient in treatment elections, and receive instructions necessary to implement medication regimens and other treatment. Fortunately the notion that the family retains a position of confidence and respect in the treatment of the sick finds ample support in judicial opinion. Less fortunately family and friends may not always accurately reflect the wishes and intent of the patient.

INFORMED CONSENT

The common law has always recognized the right of every competent adult to determine what shall be done with her own body. This basic tenet of the common law has been brought within a penumbra of constitutional protection as a right to privacy and self-determination. When an adult satisfies the test of mental capacity and has been apprised of the nature of her illness, prognosis, alternative treatments, risks and benefits, a truly informed consent may be given. The patient then allows an invasion of her bodily integrity. That is, the patient allows a "touching," whether involving a medical or surgical intervention, that would, in the absence of the patient's consent, be considered a battery under the common law.

If a patient lacks the mental capacity to participate in decision making about her own care (ie, legal incompetency) or is unable to express her wishes by reason of disability, a surrogate decision maker must be found. In most cases the surrogate decision maker will be a family member or close friend of the patient. The priority of relationships in selecting such a person is usually as follows: (a) spouse,

(b) specific designee, (c) adult son or daughter, (d) parent, or (e) adult sibling. If the court appoints a guardian of the person (as opposed to a guardian of the property of the patient), the guardian will supersede all others as surrogate decision maker. The surrogate's responsibility is to attempt to determine what the patient's wishes were or what the patient herself would have wanted were she able to decide for herself. The surrogate may accept information from significant others in determining the unexpressed wishes of the patient.

As noted earlier, the stringency of any legal test relative to informed consent will depend on the particular circumstances involved. In emergency situations in which intervention is required to preserve life or reduce morbidity and the patient is unable, by virtue of her physical or mental condition, to provide consent, the general rule is to initiate treatment. Once the patient is out of danger and is able to make her wishes known, whether directly or through a surrogate, her wishes should be respected. The rationale here is to err on the side of safety in preserving life. Having stabilized the patient, the ascertainment of the patient's wishes can proceed in a less hurried fashion.

On the other end of the spectrum are totally elective procedures. Here treatment may not be initiated or continued without the express consent of the patient or her agreed-upon surrogate decision maker. The patient's spouse or other family members may not override the wishes of the patient, whether expressed directly or through a surrogate. Written consents on forms approved by one's institution should be used to document consent for surgical and invasive diagnostic procedures, as well as other diagnostic or therapeutic modalities having significant risks. Which modalities present significant risks to the patient is a matter for definition within the community and institution involved.

NO-CODE ORDERS

No-code orders, also referred to as DNR (do not resuscitate) orders, are a direction by the attending physician that cardiopulmonary resuscitation should not be initiated in the event of cardiac or respiratory failure. Such orders do not imply or constitute authorization to lessen or withdraw other therapeutic or supportive treatment. The appropriateness of a no-code order must be constantly reevaluated. This means reevaluation not only by the attending physician, but also in dialogue with the patient about her condition and prognosis.

Again, the wishes of the patient or her surrogate are controlling. A no-code order may not be written without the knowledge and consent of the patient or the surrogate. A competent patient's right to decide that treatment be withheld is protected both by the common law and the constitutional right of privacy. An incompetent patient does not lose her right to refuse lifesaving or life-sustaining treatment. If the patient has clearly expressed her wishes, they should be honored;

if the patient has not expressed her wishes, the surrogate decision maker shall use his or her best judgment as to whether the patient would have wanted the treatment withheld. If such a decision must be made by a surrogate, the wishes of the family may be considered in assessing what the patient herself would have wanted, but the wishes of the family are not controlling.

The best evidence of a patient's medical preference would be a living will or a durable power of attorney. An increasing number of states have enacted legislation pertaining to living wills. Such statutes enhance a patient's power to maintain her right of privacy and self-determination in circumstances in which her ability to express her wishes may otherwise be lost.

WITHDRAWAL OF LIFE-SUSTAINING TREATMENT

Generally speaking, there is no meaningful distinction between the withholding and withdrawing of life-sustaining medical treatment. As in the case of no-code orders, if it is the patient's wish that medical treatment be withdrawn, these wishes must be respected. Conversely, a medical order to withdraw medical treatment may not be written without the knowledge and consent of the patient.

It is, of course, true that the patient cannot compel the physician to enter an order that is medically inappropriate or that contravenes accepted medical standards or medical ethics. But the common circumstances of removal of a feeding tube or discontinuation of intravenous fluids, not to mention the withdrawal of supported ventilation, do not contravene medical standards or ethics when death is imminent, when there is no prospect for emergence from a vegetative state, or when there is no meaningful possibility of extending life under humane and comfortable conditions. A slightly different verbal formulation finds such orders medically appropriate when the patient is terminally ill, the prognosis for recovery extremely poor, or further intervention will only prolong the process of dying.

PROGNOSIS OR ETHICS COMMITTEES

In response to suggestions made by the courts in several jurisdictions, originally by the New Jersey Supreme Court in the *Karen Quinlan* case (1976), many health care institutions have established prognosis or ethics committees to serve in a consultative capacity in assessing a patient's prognosis and the appropriateness of a withdrawal or withholding of medical treatment. Although the specific organizational framework, composition, function, and reporting, as well as activation of such committees, vary from institution to institution, the basic purpose of such committees is to make an independent assessment of the patient's prognosis. Most such committees may be activated on request of the patient, the patient's guardian or surrogate, the patient's family, or the patient's treating physician.

An independent assessment of the patient's condition and prognosis, although obviously helpful in the medicolegal context to assure compliance with accepted medical standards and to perhaps diffuse liability, is equally helpful to the treating physician in making the decision to give or withhold care and is helpful to the family in appreciating more objectively the patient's medical condition. When, for example, a competent patient has asked to be taken off a ventilator and the family has agreed, the physician may have doubts about the medical appropriateness of such an order based on his or her assessment that death is not imminent and that the patient's life may be extended under humane and comfortable conditions. A physician may feel that the instruction of the surrogate decision maker or the family is at variance with his or her sense of what the patient would have wanted under the circumstances. Conversely, a family may insist on the continuation of life-support measures when the patient or her surrogate, as well as the physician, concur in the belief that life cannot be extended under humane conditions or death is imminent. The factual settings are myriad, but in all of these circumstances an independent assessment of the patient's condition and prognosis can be of inestimable value to physician and family alike.

It must be remembered that prognosis or ethics committees function in a consultative capacity to the treating physician. It is the treating physician who must act affirmatively to write an order that authorizes and directs the withholding or withdrawing of care. It is the treating physician who bears continuing responsibility for the care of the patient as long as she lives.

THE ROLE OF THE COURTS

Despite a popular perception that a court order is a common way of effecting medical decisions when there is disagreement among the patient, the guardian or surrogate, the family or the physician, such is seldom the case. Judicial intervention is a procedure of last resort and should be reserved for such matters as the appointment of a guardian when a family member or specified close friend is not available or when the patient's interests are not being properly protected by those exercising authority on her behalf. Resort to the courts would also be required if a departure from accepted standards of practice by the patient's physician was alleged. On the whole, courts are unsatisfactory forums in which to resolve the agonizing personal problems inherent in these cases. As was said in *In re Jones* (New Jersey Supreme Court, 1987): "Our legal system cannot replace the more intimate struggle that must be borne by the patient, those caring for the patient, and those who care about the patient." Legislatures are better equipped than the judiciary to draft guidelines and procedures for the withdrawal of life-sustaining treatment, and such legislative guidelines are increasingly forthcoming.

ABUSE OF THE ELDERLY PATIENT

Within the context of this chapter, abuse of the elderly refers to any infringement of a person's right of privacy and self-determination as a consequence of age-related incapacities, physical or mental. Although such abuse can occur in any setting, hospitals generally afford a much higher level of protection to the patient than can be guaranteed in nursing homes or, indeed, family homes. It is perhaps ironic that the hospital, an institution in which patients often complain of unwarranted intrusiveness, impersonal care, and lack of privacy, should have, by reason of its very openness to public scrutiny, developed procedures, regulations, and safeguards that largely attempt to ensure that the personal dignity of the patient, including her right of self-determination and right of privacy, will be upheld. To this end most hospitals have adopted a patient's bill of rights or similar document and have integrated policies for informed consent, procedures for implementing no-code/DNR orders, guidelines for withdrawing or withholding treatment, as well as rules and regulations creating and governing prognosis or ethics committees.

A patient's right to privacy and self-determination respecting medical treatment is technically and legally not abridged by her location in a nonhospital setting. Yet it is all too true that the very factors that increase a sense of personal privacy in the nursing home or family home setting may also deprive a patient of her ability to determine the nature of her treatment or to assert her constitutionally based right of privacy. Thus it is similarly ironic that, although the family home and the nursing home hold out the promise of more individualized care and greater sensitivity to the needs and wishes of the patient, the absence of constant public scrutiny has deprived patients of protection afforded in the hospital setting. Because of the difficulty encountered not only in ascertaining the wishes of the patient with respect to management options, but also in assessing the condition and prognosis of the patient, it has been argued that even higher standards of verification be applied to such determinations in the nonhospital setting. For example, it has been suggested that two independent physicians, rather than one, should be required to verify diagnosis and prognosis in patient care settings outside of the hospital. Similarly, nursing homes have been urged to affiliate with a hospital's prognosis committee, and state authorities have been asked to develop regional prognosis committees for nursing homes.

Care in the family home may provide the very best of care for an elderly patient, particularly in a terminal illness. Yet the potential for abuse of the patient is equally great. A salutary development in this regard is the home hospice movement and visiting nurse services, which ensure for the patient a modicum of contact with the world outside. Not only do such care providers bring important medical, nursing, and social service skills to patients confined in a family home, but they are also the eyes and ears of the larger community in observing the environment in which the patient is constrained. Such home nursing, hospice, and paramedical services are important safeguards in preventing abuse of the elderly at home.

CONCLUSION

Whether one is concerned with issues of routine gynecologic care in elderly patients or more ultimate issues encountered in terminal illness, the essential focus remains on the persona of the individual patient. As the winter of life approaches, the elements of that persona at first confront gently but ultimately war savagely with one another. Body, mind, and spirit, long and harmoniously intertwined, no longer function together in joyous concert. Physicians, usually more comfortable in caring for the body, may find it difficult to focus attention on the mind, not to mention the spirit.

Although care of the aged is not, per se, fraught with increased risk of professional liability, the wise and compassionate physician recognizes that increasing time and effort must be spent on matters of the mind in the continuing treatment of the whole patient. The issue of the patient's legal competency is implicit in every patient contact. Does the patient understand the nature and prognosis of her illness? Does the patient have the mental capacity to reason and make judgments about the integrity and well-being of her body? These questions are critical not only in regard to communications in terminal illnesses, but also in regard to all communications between physicians and patients, including patients who are quite vigorous and healthy despite their advanced years.

If the patient is legally competent, she has the capacity to exercise her constitutionally protected right of privacy and right of self-determination. In short, the patient's wishes concerning her medical care and treatment must be respected. An appropriately informed consent must be obtained from the patient before diagnostic or treatment procedures are carried out. Likewise, orders directing the withholding or withdrawal of treatment may not be entered without the patient's express consent. When the patient lacks mental capacity or is unable to express her wishes, a surrogate decision maker must be found. The surrogate shall attempt to reflect the patient's wishes were she able to decide for herself or express herself.

Prognosis or ethics committees, functioning in a consultative capacity, are of tremendous value to physician and family alike. An independent assessment of the patient's condition and prognosis aids the treating physician in deciding whether to give or withhold care and helps the family to appreciate more objectively the patient's true medical status. On the other hand, resort to the courts should be avoided, as the judicial forum is generally not well suited to resolve the agonizing personal problems inherent in such cases.

When care is not taken to ascertain the wishes of the elderly patient, she may be subjected to procedures, medications, or a manner of existence that ignores her right of self-determination and right of privacy. Although much has been heard about abuse of the elderly in institutions, it must be recognized that the family home, too, can be a place of abuse rather than a warm and supportive environment where loving care is the rule.

Finally, it is the treating physician who bears continuing responsibility for the care of the patient as long as she lives. Three centuries ago Sir William Temple observed: "In all diseases of the body or mind, it is happy to have an able physician for a friend, or a discreet friend for a physician." Medical care compassionately given by a wise and trusted physician is the best medical care. It is also, not coincidentally, the best and most defensible medicolegal care. The diligent and compassionate care of the aged patient bespeaks the sovereignty of medical professionalism and the sanctity of the physician-patient relationship. When that sacred covenant has been maintained, the requirements of secular jurisprudence, too, will have been met and far surpassed.

Part V
An Overview of Gerontology

Chapter 19

Assessment of the Older Woman

Maria A. Fiatarone and Laurence Z. Rubenstein

INTRODUCTION

The dramatic expansion of the oldest segment of our population in this century compels all physicians to understand the unique aspects of medical care of the aged. Paralleling this dramatic demographic change, the practice of medicine has shifted from being primarily a source of solace for incurable diseases to being a highly technical endeavor, perceived by both patient and physician as the potent answer to many formerly lethal conditions. However, the emergence of a large population of older people with multiple chronic diseases thrusts a new class of "incurables" on doctors who may be ill equipped, both medically and psychologically, to treat them.

The medical profession that arises from a youth-oriented society will tend to err in two ways in its treatment of the elderly. First, therapeutic nihilism may predispose to inadequate evaluation of potentially reversible conditions. Second, a misunderstanding of the physician's role in the amelioration of symptoms of "incurable" diseases may result in either inappropriate attempts at heroic cures or unwarranted disinterest in rehabilitative efforts and improvements in functional status. The answer to these problems must lie in the gradual expansion of the knowledge base of geriatric medicine to the practitioners of various subspecialties, as well as in the training of geriatricians for research, primary care, and consultative work.

One area of research that has received much attention in the past decade is geriatric assessment. Geriatric assessment can be defined as a multidimensional—usually interdisciplinary—diagnostic process designed to quantify an elderly person's medical, psychosocial, and functional capabilities and problems with the intention of arriving at a comprehensive plan for therapy and long-term follow-up. Assessment has assumed a pivotal role in geriatric care because of the complexity of the frail elderly patient, because of the vast number of unmet needs facing the rapidly growing older population, and because assessment has been increasingly associated with improvements in care outcomes. The goals of this assessment process depend on the needs of the evaluators as well as the population being studied, and have been reviewed in detail by several authors.[1,2] They generally include optimization of diagnosis, treatment planning, and assurance of long-term follow-up (case management). A considerable literature now exists, reviewed later in this chapter, showing that the assessment process leads to improvements in the quality of process and outcome of care for older adults.

The concept of geriatric assessment traces its origins to the British geriatric pioneers of the 1930s, such as Drs. Marjory Warren and Sir Ferguson Anderson, who noted a disturbingly high rate of long-term institutionalization among disabled elderly patients, most of whom had never been carefully evaluated. These early geriatricians uncovered a very high prevalence of readily identifiable remediable problems among both institutionalized and noninstitutionalized patients. They also found that most of these patients could show improvement, often dramatic, when provided with appropriate therapy and rehabilitation. When the British National Health Service was founded in 1948, geriatric medicine was accorded full specialty status, largely based on the successful experiences of the earlier pioneers. In the British system geriatric specialists are in charge of geriatric services that include acute hospital care for the elderly as well as an assortment of coordinated special care programs, such as day hospitals, geriatric rehabilitation units, and home visit services. Under the British system of "progressive geriatric care," elderly patients who require admission to hospital, except those requiring intensive medical care, are usually first admitted to an acute-care geriatric assessment/evaluation unit. There each patient receives a comprehensive assessment of medical, functional, and psychosocial problems during an approximately 2- to 3-week length of stay. Several other countries (including Sweden, Australia, Norway, Israel, and the Netherlands) have built, or are building, geriatric care systems with many similarities to the British system, most with centrally located geriatric assessment units as focal points for entry into the care system.[2] Less intensive assessments are provided to elderly patients through other programs, such as consultation clinics, home visit systems, and day hospitals.

In the United States growing awareness of the unmet health care needs facing the elderly, and realization of how other countries have met similar needs are promoting the rapid growth of American geriatric assessment programs.

In clinical practice the overall components of geriatric assessment may be reasonably outlined as follows:

- Separating normal aging from pathological disease processes
- Recognizing the interacting physical, psychological, and social components of health status
- Diagnosis of diseases that present in atypical and complex ways

- Primary and secondary prevention of disease
- Tertiary disease prevention and assessment of functional status

Each of these components is considered in greater detail in the ensuing paragraphs.

COMPONENTS OF ASSESSMENT

Separating Normal Aging from Pathological Disease Processes

Although seemingly obvious, the fundamental need to distinguish normal aging from disease processes is often ignored or unappreciated in clinical practice. Part of the problem rests with an inadequate understanding of truly normal aging processes. In addition, the persistence of stereotypes or myths about old age affects both the patient and the physician, leading to a reluctance by patients to present complaints that they consider to be inevitable accompaniments of aging (eg, memory loss, incontinence), as well as to the dismissal of potentially remediable symptoms by physicians.

Most of the earlier literature on the physiology of aging relied on cross-sectional studies that attempted to compare not necessarily comparable populations, such as healthy young subjects and institutionalized elderly patients. Not unexpectedly, an inexorable and precipitous decline in almost all organ systems and physiologic functions was described. The improved methodology of more recent cross-sectional studies and the emergence of high-quality longitudinal studies have led to improved understanding of true aging. These newer studies have been able to separate out confounding factors such as nutrition, education, environmental exposures, life style differences, and cumulative diseases from changes caused by the aging process itself. This has led to a reappraisal of some of the most widely believed geriatric dogmas. For example, cardiac output, until very recently, was thought to decline with age by as much as 40% to 50% between the ages of 30 and 80, based on the results of early cross-sectional studies.[3] In 1984 Rodeheffer and colleagues[4] demonstrated the preservation of cardiac output both at rest and with maximal exercise in a group of healthy elderly subjects who had been screened and found to be free of occult coronary artery disease. On the other hand, a recent review of the existing literature indicates that the maximal heart rate does seem to decline as a true function of aging,[5] probably secondary to a decrease in responsiveness of the aging myocardium to beta-adrenergic stimulation.[6] Similarly, a rise in systolic blood pressure (within normal range), thickening of the myocardial wall, lengthening of the contraction time of myocardial fibers, and a decrease in elasticity of the arterial wall appear at this time to represent true aging phenomena.[4–6]

Glucose homeostasis is another example of a physiological function that had been felt to deteriorate uniformly with age.[7] However, recent observations in healthy ambulatory elderly subjects demonstrated relatively minor decreases in insulin action with age in the absence of obesity.[8,9] In addition, studies of physically active older men indicate that a sedentary life style as well as an increased fat mass with age may contribute significantly to the decreased insulin sensitivity and glucose intolerance often seen in older people.[10,11]

Overall, declines in physiological function, when they are observed, tend to be milder and less homogeneous in the healthy elderly than previously thought. Much of the heterogeneity may be ascribed to genetic influences (as in the case of hepatic enzyme systems)[12] or to environmental or disease forces over the course of a lifetime (for example, renal function).[13,14] The basal function of many organ systems in the absence of disease is relatively preserved with age, whereas homeostatic mechanisms and the ability to adapt to stress may be impaired. With respect to the evaluation of an elderly patient, then, it is imperative that the physician not accept marked decline in physiological function as "normal aging" without consideration of possible pathology that may respond to intervention. Table 19-1 contrasts those findings that may be considered to be part of normal aging with more pathological alterations in physical functioning.[15,16]

The ability to make this distinction between aging and disease has been a major benefit of formalized geriatric assessment, whether conducted in an outpatient clinic,[17] an inpatient consultation service,[18] or on a geriatric evaluation unit.[19] Examples of undiagnosed and untreated conditions commonly attributed to "old age" (and often found after geriatric assessment) that may benefit from intervention include nutritional deficiencies, hearing loss, visual impairment, dementia, depression, poor dentition, hypothyroidism, incontinence, tuberculosis, hyperparathyroidism, orthostatic hypotension, anemia, and prostatic hypertrophy, among others.

Recognizing the Interacting Physical, Psychological, and Social Components of Health Status

Comprehensive assessment of the older patient must draw on an understanding of the three intersecting spheres that influence health status: the physical, the psychological, and the social. Manifestations of the same disease process may be profoundly altered by different psychological reactions to illness or variable social support networks available to the patient. Seemingly vague or complex symptomatology in the elderly is also often a result of these inseparable components of disease expression. For example, in an 85-year-old woman who presents not atypically with fatigue, anorexia, insomnia, nocturnal incontinence, confusion, and falls, two scenarios may be imagined. In one, investigation may reveal

Table 19-1 Age-Related Changes in Physiology and Common Pathological Conditions

System	Structural Change	Functional Change	Pathological Conditions Common with Age
Body composition	↓ Lean body mass ↑ Fat mass ↓ Total body water ↓ Bone mass ↓ Postmitotic cells		Obesity Malnutrition Dehydration
Muscle	↓ Cell number and size ↓ Capillary density ↓ Myosin ATPase	↓ Strength	Disuse atrophy
Skeletal	↓ Disk height ↓ Vertebral height Osteophytosis Cartilage degeneration Tendon calcification	↓ Height ↓ Joint motion	Fracture Osteoarthritis Osteoporosis
Skin	↓ Water content Thinning Elastin calcification Collagen cross-linking ↓ Subcutaneous fat ↓ Sweat glands ↓ Sebaceous glands ↓ Melanocytes ↓ Hair follicles	↓ Vitamin D synthesis Slower wound healing ↑ Wrinkling ↓ Tanning ↑ Vascular fragility ↓ Temperature homeostasis	Decubitis ulceration Ischemic changes

Table 19-1 continued

System	Structural Change	Functional Change	Pathological Conditions Common with Age
Cardiovascular	Myocardial fibrosis Left ventricular hypertrophy Calcified valve leaflets Arterial intima thickening Calcification of conduction system	↓ VO$_2$ MAX ↓ Maximum heart rate ↓ Beta-adrenergic sensitivity ↓ Slowed contraction ↓ Arterial compliance ↑ Blood pressure (within normal range) No change in cardiac output	Congestive heart failure Hypertension Atherosclerosis Conduction delays
Pulmonary	↑ AP diameter Kyphosis Cartilage calcification ↓ Rib motility Flattening of diaphragm ↓ Alveolar number Bronchiolar dilatation	↓ Chest wall compliance ↑ Lung compliance ↓ Cough efficiency ↓ Mucociliary activity ↑ Dead space ↓ Vital capacity ↑ Functional residual capacity ↓ Flow rates ↓ PO$_2$	Emphysema CO$_2$ retention Pneumonia
Renal	↓ Renal mass ↓ Nephron number Atrophy of afferent arterioles	↓ Glomerular filtration rate ↓ Renal blood flow ↓ Renal plasma flow ↓ Concentrating ability ↓ Sodium conservation ↓ Acid excretion ↓ ADH sensitivity	Proteinuria Renal artery stenosis Hypertensive nephrosclerosis

Table 19-1 continued

System	Structural Change	Functional Change	Pathological Conditions Common with Age
Gastrointestinal	↓ Parietal cell number ↓ Liver mass ↓ Liver blood flow ↓ Peyer's patches ↑ Diverticulosis ↓ Taste buds	↓ Acid secretion Presbyesophagus: ↑ Non-propulsive contractions ↓ Lower esophageal sphincter pressure ↓ Calcium absorption ↓ Pancreatic enzyme secretion ↓ Serum albumin ↑ Transit time	Atrophic gastritis Pernicious anemia Reflux esophagitis Intestinal polyposis Constipation Gallstones
Neurologic	↓ Brain weight ↓ Neuron numbers ↓ Cerebral blood flow Lipofuscin accumulation Neurofibrillary tangles Neuritic plaques ↓ Dendritic connections	↓ Nerve conduction velocity ↓ Processing speed ↓ Memory retrieval ↑ Pain threshold ↑ Taste and smell thresholds	Dementia Peripheral neuropathy
Vision	Lens rigidity Lens discoloration Arcus senilus ↓ Retinal cell number	↓ Accommodation ↓ Light-dark adaptation ↓ Narrowing of visual fields ↑ Threshold of light perception ↓ Intraocular fluid resorption ↓ Pupillary responses ↓ Depth perception ↓ Color vision	Cataracts Glaucoma Retinopathy

Table 19-1 continued

System	Structural Change	Functional Change	Pathological Conditions Common with Age
Hearing	↓ Cochlear cell number Angiosclerosis	↓ Auditory reaction time ↓ High-frequency hearing ↓ Speech discrimination	Profound hearing loss Cerumen impaction Paget's disease Environmental ototoxicity Drug-induced ototoxicity
Endocrine	Fibrosis of thyroid and pancreas ↓ Pituitary cell number Ovarian involution	↓ Insulin sensitivity ↓ Glucose tolerance ↓ PTH, FSH, LH, catecholamines ↓ Testosterone, estrogen, progestins, T_3, TSH response to TRH, renin	Diabetes Hypothyroidism Hyperparathyroidism
Immune	Thymic involution	↓ T cell proliferation ↓ IL-1 and IL-2 production and response ↓ Fever response ↓ Antibody response to immunization ↓ Delayed hypersensitivity reaction	Significant T cell dysfunction secondary to malnutrition
Psychological		↓ REM sleep Bereavement	Depression

Sources: Essentials of Clinical Geriatrics (p 7) by RL Kane, JG Ouslander, and IB Abrass, McGraw-Hill Book Company, © 1984; *Clinical Geriatrics* by I Rossman (Ed), JB Lippincott Company, © 1979.

congestive heart failure, for which she has been prescribed digitalis and diuretics, as well as degenerative arthritis, for which she has been taking increasing dosages of self-prescribed over-the-counter ibuprofen. Further analysis may disclose an exacerbation of her heart failure and decreased renal function secondary to the nonsteroidal anti-inflammatory drug use, with resultant digoxin toxicity. In the elderly, anorexia, confusion, and falls, or decreased functional status alone may be prominent manifestations of such toxicity.[20] In the second scenario, physical examination and exhaustive laboratory and radiologic studies may reveal no obvious process responsible for her complaints. When a more extensive history is later obtained, it may be found that she has no family, and has been despondent over the recent death of a friend with whom she had relied on for meals. Home evaluation and functional assessment may disclose a hazardous home environment, predisposing to falls, unhygienic conditions, and an inability to take medications, shop, or prepare meals independently. Thus identical symptom complexes may be attributed to wholly different problems (iatrogenesis versus depression and social isolation in the above scenarios), underlining the necessity of thorough exploration of physical, psychological, and social factors in each person.

Diagnosis of Diseases Presenting in Atypical and Complex Ways

One of the hallmarks of disease in old age has been said to be the frequent absence of "classic" signs and symptoms that the physician has been trained to interpret. Examples of this phenomenon would include infection in the absence of fever or leukocytosis[21]; myocardial infarction without chest pain[22]; hyperthyroidism without lid lag, hyperphagia, or tachycardia[23]; pneumonia without cough or fever[24]; or peripheral vascular disease without claudication.[25] In addition, many diverse diseases seem to converge down a final common pathway with altered mentation and reduced level of functional status as their only manifestations. Examples of such nonspecific presentations include urinary tract infection, hypothyroidism, malnutrition, depression, malignancy, and electrolyte and fluid imbalances. A listing of some of the more common conditions and their potentially altered presentation in the elderly is found in Table 19-2.

In addition, the identification of polypharmacy and iatrogenic illness as the cause of physical decline is critical,[26] as the elderly consume approximately 25% to 30% of the medications in this country, while constituting less than 12% of the population.[27] Drug–drug interactions, drug–nutrient interactions, noncompliance, and excessive medical expenditures are often the results of polypharmacy.[28] Such polypharmacy may be ascribed to the over-zealous treatment of multiple somatic complaints, inattention to the pharmacokinetic and pharmacodynamic changes of aging, lack of periodic medication review, inadequate

Table 19-2 Atypical Presentation of Disease in the Elderly Patient

Disease	Classic Signs Frequently Absent	Possibly Altered Presentation
Cardiovascular		
Angina	Substernal chest pain	Jaw pain, abdominal pain, nausea, shortness of breath
Myocardial infarction	Chest pain	Confusion, nausea, vomiting, fatigue, syncope
Congestive heart failure	Dyspnea on exertion, edema, rales	Weight loss, anorexia, insomnia, incontinence, confusion
Transient cerebral ischemia	Paralysis, sensory loss, dysarthria, amaurosis fugax	Confusion
Peripheral vascular disease	Claudication	Poor wound healing
Endocrine		
Hyperthyroidism	Tachycardia, tremors, lid lag exophthalmos, heat intolerance	Confusion, paranoia, atrial fibrillation, anorexia, weight loss, angina, congestive heart failure
Hypothyroidism	Weight gain, depressed reflexes, cold intolerance, myxedema	Depression, weight loss, confusion, fatigue
Hyperparathyroidism	Constipation, dehydration, renal stones, bone pain	Confusion, psychosis
Diabetes mellitus	Polydipsia, polyuria, polyphagia, weight loss	Anorexia, fatigue, confusion
Infections		
Urinary tract infection	Dysuria, frequency, urgency	Confusion, abdominal pain, anorexia
Endocarditis	Heart murmur, fever, peripheral emboli	Weight loss, anorexia, fatigue, confusion
Meningitis	Meningismus, fever	Confusion
Pneumonia	Fever, cough, sputum, pleuritic chest pain, tachypnea	Anorexia, abdominal pain, confusion
Surgical		
Appendicitis	RLQ pain, fever	Vomiting, diffuse abdominal pain, no pain
Peptic ulcer	Epigastric pain relieved by food	Painless hematochezia, perforation

Table 19-2 continued

Disease	Classic Signs Frequently Absent	Possibly Altered Presentation
Miscellaneous		
Dehydration	Tachycardia, increased thirst, poor skin turgor	Lethargy, confusion, falls, syncope
Pulmonary embolism	Tachycardia, tachypnea, hemoptysis, pleuritic chest pain, shortness of breath	Confusion secondary to hypoxemia, right-sided heart failure
Hip fracture	Pain, shortening of leg	Abnormal gait, falls
Depression	Dysphoric mood, suicidality, guilt, loss of libido, insomnia, anhedonia	Confusion, weight loss, fatigue, hypersomnia, psychosis

patient education regarding medication usage, and "doctor-shopping" by the patient. A reduction in medication usage as well as adverse drug reactions in the elderly population has been demonstrated after programs of drug utilization review have been instituted in nursing homes.[29] Similar benefits may be expected from physician or pharmacist review in elderly outpatients on multiple medications.[30]

Primary and Secondary Prevention of Disease

Both primary and secondary prevention are valuable and appropriate goals of geriatric assessment. Primary prevention is intended to prevent the onset of disease and may take the form of education (eg, home safety evaluation), immunization (eg, influenza, pneumococcal, or tetanus), or risk factor reduction (eg, smoking, obesity). Secondary prevention, or screening, is the early detection of conditions that are already present but remediable and may take the form of blood glucose determinations, mammography, prostate palpation, or fecal occult blood testing. These measures are intended to avert or delay the extension of the disease process while it is still in limited form. For secondary prevention to be beneficial in the elderly, at least three criteria must be satisfied:

1. The disease must have a sufficient prevalence in the population to make mass screening programs logical (eg, colon cancer).[31]
2. A screening tool that is sensitive, specific, low in risk, and acceptable to the potential screenees is available (eg, sphygmomanometer blood pressure recording).
3. Early detection of the disease will allow subsequent therapeutic intervention that can increase the quality or quantity of life remaining for the person (eg, antihypertensive medications for diastolic blood pressure elevations greater than 95 mm Hg).[32]

There is currently no consensus of opinion as to the most appropriate use of available screening tools in the elderly. In many cases efficacy data must be extrapolated from clinical trials involving only younger people. A brief review of practices in the screening for occult malignancy will highlight some of the controversy.

More than 50% of all cancer in the United States occurs in those over 65 years of age, and the probability of developing cancer in one's remaining lifetime at age 65 is between 22% and 36%, depending on race and sex.[31] The most common malignancies in those over 65 are breast, colon, and lung in women, and prostate, lung, and colon in men.[31] In the case of breast cancer, there is evidence from two randomized controlled trials that annual mammography and breast examination by a physician in women aged 50 to 65,[33] or mammography alone every 3 years in women aged 50 to 74,[34] can result in a 30% to 40% reduction in breast cancer mortality. However, only 15% to 20% of American women over age 50 have ever had mammography, and a much smaller proportion are being examined with any regularity.[35] This pattern of usage is difficult to explain, especially since in the Breast Cancer Demonstration Project[36] both the cancer detection rate and the ratio of malignant to benign disease rose significantly with the age of the screenee. In the case of mammographic screening it appears that proof of benefit alone is not sufficient to overcome deterrents to usage, such as fears of radiation, unnecessary biopsies, or overdiagnosis, financial costs, and attitudinal bias on the part of physician and patient.[35] In the case of breast self-examination, a comprehensive review by O'Malley and Fletcher[37] indicates that this modality has a low sensitivity, which diminishes with advancing age, and as yet no demonstrated impact on breast cancer mortality.

One might expect that colon cancer would similarly be an appropriate target for screening in the elderly, since 95% of cases occur in those over the age of 50.[31] There is evidence from one randomized controlled trial conducted by the Kaiser-Permanente Health Plan that those enrollees who were offered a yearly screening package that included rigid proctosigmoidoscopy and digital rectal exam had a slightly decreased mortality from colon cancer compared with nonscreened enrollees.[38] On the other hand, fecal occult blood testing, although widely recommended in this country and capable of detecting lesions at a premalignant stage, has not yet been shown to impact on the incidence or mortality of colorectal cancer in three ongoing controlled trials.[39-41] Other problems with this method of screening include high rates of false negativity (30% to 50%),[42] indirect and hidden costs (endoscopy, radiology, education and retrieval programs), and low rates of acceptability and compliance among the elderly who would be most likely to benefit.

The remainder of the screening recommendations for occult malignancy (pelvic examination, endometrial biopsy, Pap test) are directed toward detection of disease of the uterus, ovaries, and cervix. Although no randomized trial of Pap tests has been conducted, epidemiologic studies consistently demonstrate lower mortality from cervical cancer as well as a lower incidence of invasive cervical cancer in those who have been regularly screened.[43] Twenty-seven percent of all cases of cervical cancer and 41% of all cervical cancer deaths occur in those over the age of 65.[31] Several studies that have looked specifically at women over 65 indicate that the incidence of abnormal cytology or invasive cervical cancer is highest in the postmenopausal woman, who is least likely to be screened.[44-49] The conversion rate appears to be low in older women who have been previously appropriately screened (8% in women aged 70 to 79, 0% in women over 80 in a British Columbia study),[50] but it should be remembered that many older women in this country have never been screened.[49] Recognition of a long phase of carcinoma in situ (8 to 30 years in various studies)[43] has led to various recommendations for interval screening in asymptomatic low-risk women. Although the exact protocol remains a matter of debate, it seems prudent at this time to continue periodic screening by way of Pap tests in women past the age of 65, especially in those who do not have adequate screening histories.

Finally, the usefulness of routine pelvic examination in the absence of postmenopausal bleeding or risk factors for uterine or ovarian cancer has not been demonstrated.

In summary, although malignant disease is of obvious importance in the geriatric population, the efficacy of current screening recommendations is controversial in many respects. Tables 19-3 and 19-4 contrast the opinions of several consensus panels.[51-55] The evidence for benefit at this time appears strongest for mammography, breast exam, sigmoidoscopy and digital rectal exam, and Pap tests in previously unscreened women.

Secondary prevention may also be useful for nonneoplastic diseases, such as diabetes, hypertension, atherosclerosis, osteoporosis, or malnutrition. In this domain there are also many unanswered questions regarding the efficacy of preventive measures. For example, the risk of cardiovascular disease attributable to established risk factors such as glucose intolerance, obesity, hypertension, hyperlipidemia, and smoking is age-dependent, according to data from the longitudinal Framingham study.[56] The percentage of probability of developing cardiovascular disease within 8 years is increased by 50- to 100-fold in a 35-year-old person with all of these risk factors compared with a person with none of these conditions. In the 70-year-old with the same risk factor profile, cardiovascular disease is still accelerated, but by sevenfold to eightfold only compared to a low-risk person. Therefore, the risk-benefit ratio of treating these conditions is considerably altered as a person ages. In addition, the isolated effect of elevated total cholesterol levels on the occurrence of coronary disease loses statistical significance in men over the age of 65, although a positive correlation is still observed in women. As no studies have been conducted in the elderly that demonstrate that cardiovascular disease can be averted by lowering cholesterol levels, as it can in middle-aged men,[57] the dilemma of how to counsel an elderly patient with mild or moderate hyperlipidemia detected on routine screening is obvious.

One of the most common conditions noted during health screening in the geriatric population is hypertension.[58] (Blood pressure screening, incidentally, may be considered primary prevention of stroke or secondary prevention of hypertension itself.) Many misconceptions exist regarding the efficacy of treatment of hypertension in this age group. In the case of diastolic hypertension (greater than 95 mmHg), both the Hypertension Detection and Follow-up Program[59] and the Australian National Heart Foundation Study[60] have demonstrated that intervention in those who were 60 to 69 years of age at the time of diagnosis resulted in significant reductions in mortality at the end of 5 years, particularly in

Table 19-3 Recommendations for Cancer Screening in Asymptomatic Elderly People

Site	Modality	ACS	CTF	F&C	B&S	Authors	Strength of Data Behind Recommendations
Uterus and Ovaries	Pelvic exam	1	NR	NR	2 (65–74)	1	C
	Endometrial biopsy	*	NR	NR	NR	NR	C
Cervix	Pap test	NR†	5	NR	2	1–2	B
Breast	Mammography	1	NR	NR	1	2	A
	Breast exam	1	NR	NR	1	1	A
	Self-breast exam	Monthly	NR	NR	NR	Monthly	C
Colorectal	Digital rectal	1	NR	NR	2 (65–74) 1 (75+)	1	B
	Fecal occult blood	1	1	NR	1	1	B
	Sigmoidoscopy	3–5†	NR	NR	NR	NR	B
Oral	Oral exam	NR	1	NR	NR	1	C

Numbers refer to the years between testing.
*Recommended in high-risk women at menopause (obesity, infertility, estrogen therapy, polycystic ovaries).
†After two negative exams 1 year apart.

ACS = American Cancer Society, 1980[51]; CTF = Canadian Task Force, 1979, 1984[52]; F&C = Frame and Carlson, 1975[53]; B&S = Breslow and Somers, 1977[54]; NR = not recommended for routine testing; A = good support from experimental trials; B = some evidence in favor but not conclusive; C = judgment only, no hard data showing benefit.

Table 19-4 Recommendations for General Health Screening in Asymptomatic Elderly People

Category	Modality	CTF	F&C	B&S	APHA	Authors	Strength of Data Behind Recommendations
General	History and physical exam	NR	NR	2 (65–74) 1 (75+)	NR	1	C
	Nutrition evaluation (ht, **wt**, hx)	2 (65–74) 1 (75+)	NR	1	1	1	B
	Blood pressure	2	2 (65–70) NR (70+)	1	1	1	A
	Vision testing	NR	NR	2 (65–74) NR (75+)	1	1–2	C
	Tonometry	NR	NR	NR	1	NR	C
	Hearing testing	Periodic	NR	2 (65–74) NR (75+)	NR	2	C
	Dental exam	1	NR	1 (65–74) Periodic (75+)	NR	1	C
	Life style counseling†	NR	NR	1	NR	1	C
	Functional status	2 (65–74) 1 (75+)	NR	1	NR	1–2	C
Infectious Diseases							
	Tetanus vaccine	10	NR	NR	NR	10	B
	Influenza A vaccine	1	NR	1	1	1	A
	Pneumococcal vaccine	NR	NR	NR	NR	Once	B
	TB skin testing	*	NR	*	NR	*	B
	VDRL	NR	NR	*	NR	*	C

Table 19-4 continued

Category	Modality	CTF	F&C	B&S	APHA	Authors	Strength of Data Behind Recommendations
Lab Tests	Hematocrit	NR	NR	2 (65–74) NR (75+)	1	2	C
	Glucose	NR	NR	2 (65–74) NR (75+)	NR	NR	C
	Cholesterol	NR	NR	2 (65–74) NR (75+)	1	NR	C
	Thyroid function testing	2	NR	NR	NR	5	B
	ECG	NR	NR	2 (65–74) NR (75+)	NR	NR	C
	Stress testing	NR	NR	NR	NR	NR	C
	Chest x-ray	NR	NR	*	NR	NR	C

Numbers refer to the years between testing.
*In high-risk individuals only.
†Includes information on alcohol, tobacco, exercise, diet, stress reduction, marital problems, housing, and financial matters.

CTF = Canadian Task Force, 1979, 1984[52]; F&C = Frame and Carlson, 1975[53]; B&S = Breslow and Somers, 1977[54]; APHA = American Public Health Association, 1974[55]; NR = not recommended for asymptomatic individuals; A = good support from experimental trials; B = some evidence in favor but not conclusive; C = judgment only, no hard data showing benefit.

Assessment of the Older Woman 375

mortality from stroke. Conversely, although isolated systolic hypertension has been shown in numerous studies to be associated with increased mortality from cardiovascular disease in all age groups,[61] the benefits of intervention await the results of the Systolic Hypertension in the Elderly Program, which is in progress at the time of this writing.[62] Until then, treatment of isolated systolic hypertension in the elderly cannot be definitively claimed to be beneficial.

Another example of a common disease of concern in the older woman is osteoporosis. Unfortunately there are problems with both detection and treatment of this disorder. The available screening modalities for bone density measurements or estimation suffer from insensitivity (plain radiographs), lack of correlation with clinical outcome (radius densitometry), high cost, and radiation exposure (spinal computerized tomography), and are not currently recommended as screening tools in all postmenopausal women.[63] In addition, most treatment trials have focused on women within a few years of surgical or natural menopause, and there is little information regarding the efficacy of treatment in the 75- or 85-year-old woman who may have already lost 30% or 40% of her bone mass at the time of presentation.

In summary, then, much more information is needed in the area of screening in the elderly population before general recommendations can be established in all domains. Until that time, extrapolation from existing data must be made with caution and sensitivity to the adverse consequences of any diagnostic or therapeutic intervention undertaken. Current recommendations for primary and secondary prevention of nonmalignant diseases are presented in Table 19-4.[52-55] Benefit appears most established in the cases of hypertension,[32] hearing loss,[64] immunizations,[65-68] dementia,[69,70] and depression.[71]

Tertiary Disease Prevention and Assessment of Functional Status

One of the major goals of geriatric assessment is to identify medical problems and the impact they have on a patient's life—in essence, to determine how pathology translates into recognizable functional disability. When cure is no longer a realistic expectation on the part of patient or physician, efforts must be directed toward caring for the patient despite often immense life style limitations. This is the concept of tertiary prevention, or efforts to ameliorate disability from existing, noncurable conditions. The value of even minimal improvements in functional status must not be underestimated, as they may allow continued independent living rather than institutionalization, thus contributing importantly to the person's quality of life. Many tools are available today for the formalized assessment of the older person's physical, psychological, and social functioning. Their purpose is to standardize the gathering of information by various practitioners so that a clear picture of the patient's capabilities and limitations emerges.

This task is important for the planning of therapeutic and rehabilitative strategies as well as for the monitoring of change over time. Many of these assessment tools have been reviewed in terms of their reliability, validity, applicability, and general usefulness in the elderly in an excellent text by Kane and Kane.[1] Although many of these instruments are too long and cumbersome for daily use by the practicing physician, several are short, easy to administer, and of immense value. Those of most practical significance for the assessment of the older woman are reviewed below.

A basic scale of the activities of daily living (such as the Katz scale)[72] identifies the person's ability to perform tasks of self-care independently: maintaining continence of bowel and bladder, transferring, eating, bathing, dressing, and toileting. The inability to perform these tasks, for whatever reason, has been correlated with overall prognosis of geriatric patients. In addition, the ability to perform activities of daily living (ADLs) is vital for the determination of caregivers and services needed by the patient. It should be noted that even wheelchair-dependent patients may be perfectly capable of performing these ADLs, and not in need of constant supervision therefore. Many geriatric assessment programs have used improvements in functional status as measured by the Katz scale or others as markers for the effectiveness of their intervention.

More advanced tasks, the so-called instrumental activities of daily living (IADLs), may also be conveniently cataloged by use of a scale such as the Lawton scale.[73] These activities, such as shopping, cooking, handling finances, arranging transportation, and using the telephone, identify those capabilities necessary for independent living without the assistance of family or professional services. Again, there may be a variety of physical, psychological, and environmental forces at work that contribute to the maintenance of these IADLs. For the woman over age 75 in particular, who lives alone 50% of the time because of widowhood or divorce,[74] the ability to handle these tasks may be the primary determinant of continued living in the community.

Items on the Katz and Lawton functional status scales are reproduced in Table 19-5.

PRINCIPLES OF HISTORY TAKING

Standard medical textbooks and physical diagnosis courses do not offer substantial commentary on techniques of history taking particularly suited to the older adult. It is clear to anyone who has dealt with frail elderly patients with multiple medical conditions that history taking is often difficult, time-consuming, and frustratingly incomplete. In patients with sensory and cognitive deficits, substantial modifications are necessary to obtain and convey information effectively.

Table 19-5 Tasks on Functional Assessment Scales

Katz Activities of Daily Living
　Bathing
　Dressing
　Toileting
　Transfer
　Continence
　Feeding

Lawton Instrumental Activities of Daily Living
　Ability to use telephone
　Shopping
　Food preparation
　Housekeeping
　Laundry
　Mode of transportation
　Responsibility for own medications
　Ability to handle finances

Sources: *Journal of the American Medical Association* (1963;185:914), Copyright © 1963, American Medical Association; *Gerontologist* (1969;9:179–186), Copyright © 1969, Gerontological Society of America.

Specific problems and suggestions for approaching them are discussed in this section.

The Physical Environment

The physical design of an office or examining room is often inconvenient or hazardous for the frail elderly patient. Low, soft chairs without arms are difficult to get into and out of for patients with myopathy, neurologic impairments, or weakness from any cause. Thick rugs, loose carpeting, and unmarked steps may lead to falls in patients with gait disorders, peripheral neuropathy, or visual impairment. Examining tables are often too high and difficult to climb onto for older frail patients or those with arthritis or amputations. Attention to these simple details can make interaction with the older person safer and more pleasant.

Some offices are too dimly lighted for the patient with cataracts, and this interferes with effective communication. The physician should be wary of sitting in front of a bright examining light or a sunny window, as this may cast the examiner's face in a dark shadow that is both disturbing to the patient and disruptive to conversation when hearing loss makes visual cueing and lip reading essential. For similar reasons, the patient and physician should be positioned close together, so that conversation is possible at normal or only slightly increased volume. Among hearing impaired persons it is best when talking louder than normal to use a low pitch, since most hearing disorders selectively impair high pitch more than low pitch. If necessary, the patient can use a portable amplifier or even the physician's stethoscope as an earpiece for amplification. For patients with profound hearing loss, written communication may be necessary as a last resort.

Seating should be available for family members or other caregivers when the patient is not able to give an adequate history because of illness or cognitive dysfunction. However, routine inclusion of such people in the examining room during the initial history and physical is not necessary and may be embarrassing or demeaning to an elderly patient who is obviously able to communicate with the physician without such assistance.

Timing

It is often impossible to complete a detailed history and physical assessment in the time usually allotted for this process. Thus alternative strategies must be used. One approach is to instruct the patient before the visit to bring a written history or to fill out a medical questionnaire that has been provided by the office staff. Alternatively, the patient may be prescreened by allied health professionals (eg, nurse, nurse practitioner, physician's assistant, social worker) before the physician visit, at which time major medical history components can be gathered. When neither of these options is feasible, the physician must adopt history-taking techniques that provide the most important facts in the most efficient manner, without compromising the quality of the physician-patient relationship. In some cases, breaking the assessment process into two or more visits may be the best way to obtain all the desired information without overtaxing the patience of either party. In addition, the ordering of the medical history (chief complaint, history of present illness, past medical history, etc.) may have to be changed in patients with short attention spans, multiple current complaints, or tangential thought processes in order to complete the interview in a reasonable amount of time.

Components of the Medical History

Before discussing each of the components of the medical history, it should be mentioned that care must be taken that the physician's terminology is not misinterpreted by the older patient. Cultural, ethnic, generational, and educational differences in language usage abound and may lead to confusion and inappropriate workup on the part of the physician, or failure to recognize an important symptom the patient is trying to describe. For example, "dizziness" may imply dysequilibrium, anxiety, vertigo, headache, confusion, blurred vision, hypoglycemia, or hypotension to an elderly patient. "Fatigue" may be used as a description for pain, shortness of breath, depression, muscle weakness, or mental confusion. Asking patients to explain the symptom in their own words in several ways can usually clear up such differences in language usage.

Attention to the patient's conversation is also important for the assessment of mental status, which should, in reality, be ongoing throughout the interview, not simply during the administration of a mental status questionnaire. Casual history taking may not expose profound deficits in cognitive functioning, especially in the patient who confabulates or has relatively good preservation of language skills but deterioration in other spheres, such as abstraction, visuospatial orientation, calculating ability, or recent memory. The physician should be aware of speech that is "empty"—filled with repetitive phrases and clichés, continually paraphrasing the examiner's questions, lacking in abstract or meaningful words, and replete with substitutions of vague phrases such as "that place" or "those people" for more specific names of people and places.

The standard approach to the medical history begins with the elicitation of a chief complaint (usually presumed to be singular), followed by a recitation of past illnesses, numerous symptoms organized into specific organ systems, as well as details of family illnesses and social and occupational history. It is interesting to note that after obtaining such a classic "complete" history, one may have a little insight into how patients actually live, what level of emotional and physical health they enjoy, or what their expectations of the medical encounter might be. Ways in which these important pieces of information can be obtained in the setting of the medical interview are discussed below.

It is prudent to begin the interview by determining the primary concerns of the patient, even if they do not precisely fit into the definition of the "chief complaint" that the physician is used to evaluating. This establishes the rapport that will facilitate the exchange with the patient during the remainder of the interview. In addition, the insight this provides into the major disabilities and limitations as perceived by the patient illustrates how functional assessment is as crucial as the establishment of correct medical diagnoses in the elderly.

Changes in usual health status, or the "history of present illness," may be difficult to obtain because of the insidious onset of many chronic conditions in the elderly patient that defy precise localization in time. Often a history analogous to infants who "fail to thrive" is obtained, marked by lethargy, poor nutritional intake, withdrawal, and decreased functional abilities. Detecting such a trend in its early stages is essential in the frail elderly, and social and psychological correlates to such a decline should be sought during the initial evaluation so that intervention is not unduly delayed.

A detailed recitation of all past medical illnesses and their exact dates of onset is often difficult or impossible for the older patient. Certainly the details of childhood illnesses and self-limited diseases bear little relevance to the health status of a very elderly patient, and may be deferred. Focusing instead on chronic conditions, which are likely to forecast future events in the life of the patient, such as atherosclerotic disease or prior malignancy, is likely to be more profitable.

The review of systems as it is categorically taught is problematic for several reasons. For example, symptoms such as confusion or weight loss may be manifestations of disease in almost any organ system in the elderly patient. An abbreviated review of systems should focus on those areas likely to be impaired in the geriatric patient: weight loss, depression, memory loss, falls, incontinence, weakness, pain, sensory impairment, and neurologic symptomatology.

The family history is usually not helpful to the physician in this setting, as compared with the predictive role it assumes in the evaluation of a younger person in some instances. A notable exception may be a family history of affective illness, alcholism, or suicide, since major depression may present de novo in old age,[42] and a high index of suspicion in such people may avoid unnecessary delays in diagnosis if they later present with vague symptoms attributable to depression. One other use of the family history is to identify diseases with which the patient is emotionally linked (eg, from which a loved one has died), which may explain "irrational" fear of a diagnostic procedure or the sudden noncompliance with a treatment regimen.

Compared with most other aspects of medical history taking, the social history assumes a much more prominent role in the assessment of the elderly patient than it may in a younger person. The usual information obtained pertaining to occupation, smoking, and alcohol consumption is inadequate for an understanding of the health status of a geriatric patient with multiple medical problems. Other details that should ideally be obtained are listed in Table 19-6.

The final component of the medical history should include a thorough inquiry into the medication profile of the patient, including all over-the-counter medications, prescriptions, vitamins, and supplements, as well as any problems with noncompliance, cost, dosing intervals, or side effects that the patient perceives. Over-the-counter medications to be particularly aware of include those with anticholinergic side effects, those containing significant amounts of alcohol, and the nonsteroidal anti-inflammatory agents.[26]

In conclusion, medical history taking in the elderly patient often requires a departure from the traditional format in order to obtain the necessary information in a way that is tolerable to both patient and physician. Attention to environmental details as mentioned, as well as to the key role of psychosocial events as they relate to a person's health status, will facilitate the gathering of a medical history in the elderly patient.

PHYSICAL EXAMINATION

Physical examination of the older woman should be performed in a way that is expedient, sensitive to current disabilities and complaints, and respectful of the

Table 19-6 Components of the Social History

Living Arrangements	Type of dwelling
	Stairs
	Safety hazards
	Cohabitants
	Means of payment
Financial Status	Income
	Sources
	Medical insurance
	Who handles finances
Social Support Network	Family members
	Friends, neighbors
	Volunteer services
	Paid services from community
Nutrition	Source of meals
	Setting of meals, with whom
	Frequency of meals
	Alcohol intake
Transportation	Means of transportation
	Person providing transportation
	Eligibility for community services
Daily habits	Occupational history, exposures
	Smoking history
	Current daily activities
	Sleep patterns
	Exercise habits

modesty of the person. Undressing for the examination and changing positions may take longer for the older patient, and time should be allotted for this. This may be an uncomfortable time for the patient with significant functional disability or a problem such as stress incontinence. The person should always be re-covered as quickly as possible after examination, to minimize psychological and physical discomfort.

As in the history taking, the general physical examination should be directed toward the evaluation of conditions of special concern to the elderly, such as sensory deficits, malnutrition, musculoskeletal dysfunction, incontinence, gait problems, cardiovascular disease, and mental status abnormalities. Most of these problems are not assessed during the physical examination of a young person, so that the approach to the elderly patient must be altered somewhat to gather the necessary information. A brief review of those aspects of physical diagnosis that are of particular relevance in the older woman are reviewed below.

General Appearance and Vital Signs

The general appearance may provide extremely important information about the physical, psychological, and functional condition of the patient. Note should be made, for example, of cachexia, lethargy, or problems with body hygiene. These findings may provide clues to common geriatric problems, such as malnutrition, incontinence, depression, memory loss, or social isolation and neglect.

Palpation of the pulse for an extended period is important to detect atrial or ventricular dysrhythmias, to monitor drug efficacy (eg, digoxin, propranolol) or toxicity (eg, theophylline, thyroid), to suggest autonomic dysfunction (eg, lack of respiratory variation in heart rate),[75] or to assess control of disease states (eg, congestive heart failure, hyperthyroidism).

Respiratory rate should be observed at rest as well as during ambulation and change of positions. In addition to low cardiac output or obstructive pulmonary disease, tachypnea may indicate valvular heart disease, pneumonia, chronic pulmonary emboli, pleural effusion, restrictive lung disease secondary to osteoporotic kyphosis or morbid obesity, or simply deconditioning in the elderly patient.[76]

Temperature elevation cannot be relied on as an indication of infection in the older person.[21] In addition, homeostatic mechanisms of temperature regulation may also be impaired,[77] leading to hyperthermia or hypothermia during extremes of ambient temperature.

Blood pressure recording is one of the more important parts of the geriatric physical examination, and it should be obtained during every physician-patient encounter, according to some authors.[52] The blood pressure cuff should be rapidly inflated to 30 mm Hg above the level of extinction of the radial pulse to exclude the possibility of an auscultatory gap, which is more common in older people than in younger patients.[78] If the brachial or radial artery can still be palpated when the cuff is inflated above systolic pressure (Osler's maneuver),[79] this may be a sign of pseudohypertension, a falsely elevated cuff reading secondary to arteriosclerosis that may not require treatment. In all older patients the blood pressure should be recorded both supine or sitting as well as after two minutes of standing because of the high prevalence of postural hypotension in the elderly secondary to drugs, disease, or the baroreceptor changes of aging.[80]

Height and weight should always be recorded so that the percentage of ideal body weight may be calculated according to age-adjusted scales, such as those of Master and associates.[81] Unintentional loss of more than 10 pounds over the preceding 2-month period is an important sign of underlying disease or an indicator of malnutrition. Rapid weight gains in the elderly usually indicate fluid retention from congestive heart failure or medications such as nonsteroidal anti-inflammatory drugs or vasodilators.

Skin

Examination of the skin can provide clues to many disorders in the older patient. Malnutrition may be suggested by xerosis, cheilosis, or glossitis. Ecchymoses raises the suspicion of vitamin deficiency, drug effects, liver disease, multiple falls, alcoholism, or elder abuse, although some degree of increased capillary fragility with age may produce bruising after very minor trauma. Poor skin hygiene and grooming can indicate depression, dementia, social isolation, or family neglect. The high prevalence of polypharmacy in the geriatric patient raises the specter of cutaneous drug reactions in the case of unexplained rashes or excoriation secondary to generalized pruritus. Sun-exposed areas, including the scalp, should be searched for malignant lesions (basal and squamous cell carcinoma, melanoma) as well as premalignant lesions (actinic keratoses). Skin tags normally proliferate with age and are usually of no pathological significance, although they may be associated with colonic polyposis. It should be noted that the natural history of a benign nevus is to pale and become more papular with age; patterns contrary to this should provoke closer investigation.[82] Normal changes in collagen elasticity and water content of the skin, as well as loss of subcutaneous fat, make the evaluation of dehydration by way of assessment of skin turgor relatively inaccurate in the elderly as compared with the younger person. The skin over the chest or abdomen will be more informative than that of the extremities in this regard.

Head, Eyes, Ears, Nose, and Throat

Visual and auditory impairment is common in the elderly and is a major contributor to social isolation and functional decline. Because these deficits are often partially correctable, they should be aggressively sought during examination. Presbycusis (selective high-frequency sensorineural hearing loss) is the most common finding, but conduction deficit secondary to cerumen impaction may complicate the problem, and should be evaluated as well.[83] Visual acuity should be tested, as well as visual fields, which may be reduced because of glaucoma (tunnel vision), macular degeneration (loss of central vision), or cerebral infarcts (hemianopsia). Cataracts and retinal vessel abnormalities, especially in the patient with diabetes mellitus, hypertension, or atherosclerotic disease, are common findings.[84]

The oral cavity should be examined (with dental prostheses removed) for signs of leukoplakia or carcinoma, periodontal disease, candidiasis, or trauma secondary to malfitting dentures.

Thorax and Cardiovascular System

In the older woman, osteoporosis, degenerative arthritis, metastatic carcinoma, or multiple myeloma may present as vertebrae that are tender to palpation. In cases of severe osteoporosis, even minor trauma such as coughing may result in rib fracture, which should be suspected if there is pleuritic pain accompanied by discrete areas of tenderness over the ribs. Chest deformity secondary to dorsal kyphosis should be observed, as this may contribute to respiratory distress by limiting vital capacity.

Loss of glandular tissue of the breast with aging may make palpation of abnormal masses easier in the older woman. Fibrocystic disease is less common in the postmenopausal female than in her younger counterpart. (Self examination of the breast is covered elsewhere in this book.)

Rales present at the bases of the lungs may indicate atelectasis or fibrosis rather than congestive heart failure in the older patient. Emphysematous changes in the lungs may, on the other hand, obscure typical lung findings of congestive failure in some patients. If suspicion of neuromuscular impairment leading to aspiration is present, observing the patient for cough while drinking a small quantity of water may be helpful in making this diagnosis.

Cephalic, subclavian, aortic, renal, and femoral arteries should be auscultated for the presence of bruits suggestive of atherosclerotic disease. Abnormal widening (greater than 3 cm in transverse diameter) or tenderness of the abdominal aorta should be sought. In some healthy older people the aorta is easily palpable but of normal caliber, which is not a pathological finding. Distal pulses in all extremities should be palpated, and if diminished, adnexal changes consistent with peripheral vascular disease (atrophy of skin, decreased hair growth, dystrophic nails, poor capillary refill, dependent rubor, and pallor on elevation) should be noted if present.

A left-sided S_4 and soft systolic ejection murmur are present in many older people and may not be indicative of organic heart disease, representing decreased ventricular compliance and mild aortic cusp calcification with age, respectively.[85] Regurgitant murmurs, however, are always abnormal, and may indicate calcification of the mitral annulus or mitral valve prolapse, both of which are being diagnosed with increasing frequency in the older woman.[86]

Abdomen and Pelvis

Palpation may reveal fecal impaction or an enlarged uterus. The liver may be displaced caudally secondary to emphysematous changes of the lungs, and thus appear enlarged unless its size is also measured by percussion. Rectal examination should include a search for hemorrhoids, rectal mass or polyp, rectocele, and occult blood.

Gynecologic examination, which is covered in detail in other chapters, will focus on the findings of atrophic vaginitis, uterine or ovarian carcinoma, uterine prolapse, cystocele, and urinary incontinence.

Extremities

Arthritic deformities should be noted, especially those that limit the range of motion necessary for the adequate performance of the functional activities of daily living. The lower extremities should be assessed for the presence of edema, venous stasis disease, or ischemia. Podiatric problems are extremely prevalent in the older patient, especially in the older woman whose footwear (high heels and pointed toes) may have accelerated degenerative changes at the metatarsophalangeal joints. Other findings include ingrown toenails, fungal infection, calluses, ulceration, and signs of neglect.

Neurologic System

Contrary to the cursory attention it is often given in the younger person, the neurologic examination occupies a place of primary importance in the geriatric physical examination. Although some loss of lean muscle tissue is apparently normal with age, selective atrophy, severe wasting, or demonstrable weakness during specific muscle testing is not normal. Functional actions should be examined as well as the ability to resist the examiner's muscle in isometric contraction. For example, the ability to rise from a chair, climb onto the examining table, or lift the arms over the head can be quickly demonstrated during the course of the examination. Specific patterns of muscle weakness should be noted: generalized, as in malnutrition, hyperthyroidism, or hypothyroidism; peripheral nerve distribution, as in peroneal or ulnar nerve trauma or diabetic mononeuropathy; proximal, as in polymyalgia rheumatica or steroid myopathy; or hemiparesis, as from stroke. Involuntary movements may also be observed, including their variability during the examination. Essential (familial) tremors, as well as tremors secondary to muscle weakness, will be accentuated during sustained use of the involved muscle groups, whereas parkinsonian tremors or buccolingual dyskinesia can usually be interrupted by voluntary movement of the muscles involved.

Sensory examination of the lower extremities may reveal decreased vibratory sensation, widened two-point discrimination, diminished proprioception, and loss of deep tendon reflexes at the ankle in many elderly people in the absence of nervous system disease, and may reflect the mild decrease in nerve conduction velocity (approximately 10%) that occurs across the age span.[87] Severe sensory loss, or loss of pain and temperature sensation, should not be considered within the range of normality, however.

Problems with gait and balance are commonplace, and may be secondary to a variety of factors, including motor weakness, cerebellar dysfunction, sensory loss, visual impairment, orthostatic hypotension, abnormal mental status, environmental hazards, or drug toxicity.[88] Use of rating scales such as that of

Tinetti and colleagues[89] allows the examiner to quickly assess the major components of ambulation (eg, symmetry, step length, step height, ability to maintain balance while turning or bending) without the use of any equipment or tool other than observation. The results can be quantified to provide an overall score that has been found to correlate with the subsequent risk of falls in geriatric patients.

The formal assessment of mental status is one of the most important contributions of geriatric assessment because of the high prevalence of depression and cognitive dysfunction in this population. Casual history taking and conversation may not disclose even moderately severe memory deficits in some cases. The most widely validated tool for this purpose is the 30-point Folstein Mini-Mental State Exam.[90] Changes in score over time may be used in a patient to assess disease progression or response to therapy. Depression may likewise be difficult to diagnose in the elderly, as it may present without prominent dysphoria or guilt ("masked depression"),[91] or its symptoms may be ascribed to "old age." Lethargy, decreased appetite, insomnia, withdrawal, and anhedonia are not part of normal aging, however, and should point to the need for evaluation of affective disorder. The use of a geriatric depression screening scale such as that of Yesavage and associates[92] in such cases may be very informative.

In summary, then, examination of the older person must incorporate a knowledge of normal physiological changes of aging as well as a heightened awareness of common pathological conditions of the elderly. Emphasis should be placed on functional disability as well as anatomical abnormality in order to provide a complete picture of the mental and physical health of the older patient.

SPECIALIZED GERIATRIC ASSESSMENT PROGRAMS AND THEIR EFFECTIVENESS

An enlarging body of evidence indicates that the most striking unmet health care needs of the elderly population—inappropriate institutionalization, incomplete medical diagnosis, lack of coordination of community support services, overprescription of medications, and underutilization of rehabilitation[93,94]—can be ameliorated through the use of geriatric assessment programs.[2] Geared to specific local needs and conditions, these programs vary in many of their structural and functional components as well as in their stated purposes.

The major types of geriatric assessment programs, both in the United States and abroad, are listed in Table 19-7. For example, some are located within inpatient hospital wards, whereas others are outpatient or home visit programs. Some are carefully targeted to the most frail elderly populations, whereas others are open to virtually anyone over a certain age of eligibility. Nevertheless, they share many characteristics. Virtually all programs provide multidimensional assessment, using one or more sets of measurement instruments to quantify functional,

Table 19-7 Principal Types of Assessment Programs

Acute hospital inpatient units
  Geriatric assessment/evaluation units
  Geropsychiatric assessment units
  Geriatric rehabilitation units
Chronic hospital inpatient assessment units
Inpatient geriatric consultation services
Hospital outpatient departments
Home visit assessment teams
Office settings or freestanding units

---

psychological, and social parameters. Most use interdisciplinary teams to pool expertise and enthusiasm in working toward common goals. Many programs, both outpatient and inpatient, provide at least limited treatment and are sites for geriatric education and research. As a rule, only inpatient units are able to provide extensive treatment and rehabilitation. On the other hand, outpatient programs are better able to provide longitudinal primary care and case management. Costs are greater for inpatient programs, but so are the variety of services able to be offered.

A considerable literature now exists documenting the benefits from geriatric assessment programs. Table 19-8 lists the several positive outcomes various studies have shown to derive from geriatric assessment programs with the types of study evidence available (experimental, quasi-experimental, or descriptive) and the specific study references. Some kinds of benefits can be readily identified by descriptive studies. These are primarily process of care benefits, such as improved diagnosis and reduced prescribed medications. Other benefits, including the most important outcomes (eg, improved use of services and survival), require documentation by more sophisticated studies that involve equivalent control group designs with longitudinal follow-up.

Although admittedly the table cannot do justice to the individual papers in what is now a sizable literature, one can appreciate the growing body of data supporting the idea that the frail elderly population can derive great benefit from assessment programs. Of the 32 studies included, 12 used control groups,[19,95–105] and 8 of these used random allocation.[19,95,96,98,103–105] All 20 of the papers describing noncontrolled studies report positive results. Of the 12 studies using control groups, all but 2 report at least some major positive benefits of the program when compared with the controls.

A consistent area of demonstrated impact from these assessment programs has been improvement in diagnostic accuracy, usually indicated by the diagnosis of new, treatable problems. Many found substantial numbers of previously undiagnosed problems among patients undergoing geriatric assessment. Depending on each study's criteria for considering newly documented problems as new diagnoses (some included all new diagnostic labels, whereas others counted only

Assessment of the Older Woman

Table 19-8 Improvements in Patient Outcomes Derived from Geriatric Assessment Programs

Outcome	Program Type	Study Type (References)
Improved diagnostic accuracy	GAU/	
	GARU	D (106, 109, 112, 114), RCT (115)
	ICS	D (18, 110), RCT (95)
	OAS	D (107, 108, 113), RCT (103, 105)
	HVT	D (111, 116)
Improved placement location	GAU/	
	GARU	D (112, 114, 119, 120), MC (100, 101), RCT (19)
	ICS	D (110, 118)
	OAS	D (107, 108, 117)
	HVT	RCT (99)
Improved functional status	GAU/	
	GARU	D (106, 112, 114, 121, 122), MC (100), RCT (19)
	OAS	D (113), RCT (103)
	HVT	D (111)
Improved affect or cognition	GAU/	
	GARU	D (106, 112, 114, 121, 123), RCT (19, 96)
	OAS	D (113)
	HVT	RCT (104)
Reduced prescribed medications	GAU/	
	GARU	D (106, 114), MC (101)
	ICS	RCT (95)
Decreased nursing home use	GAU/	
	GARU	D (112, 114, 119, 120), MC (100, 101), RCT (19)
	ICS	D (110)
	OAS	D (117)
	HVT	RCT (99)
Increased use of home health services	GAU/	
	GARU	MC (101)
	ICS	MC (97)
	OAS	RCT (105)
	HVT	RCT (99, 104)
Reduced use of acute hospitals	GAU/	
	GARU	D (119), MC (101), RCT (19, 98)
	ICS	D (118, 124)
	OAS	RCT (103, 105)
	HVT	RCT (99)
Reduced medical care costs	GAU/	
	GARU	RCT (19, 98)
	OAS	RCT (105)
	HVT	RCT (99)
Prolonged survival	GAU/	
	GARU	RCT (19, 98)
	HVT	RCT (99, 104)

GAU = inpatient geriatric or geropsychiatric assessment unit; GARU = inpatient geriatric assessment and rehabilitation unit; ICS = inpatient consultation service; OAS = outpatient assessment service; HVT = home visit team; D = descriptive (before-after) study; MC = matched control study; RCT = randomized controlled trial.

major problems that were treatable), new diagnoses were found in frequencies varying from just under one per patient to more than four per patient. Discovery of these new diagnoses stemmed from several factors, including the geriatric assessment process itself (which includes a careful search for treatable problems), a longer period to evaluate the patient, as well as from a probable lack of diagnostic thoroughness in the referring services.[18,95,103,105–116] Although virtually impossible to prove cause and effect, it is likely that this improved diagnostic accuracy helped to produce many of the other reported benefits.

The first report that an assessment program could improve placement location and decrease use of nursing homes was published in 1973 on data from T. Franklin Williams' pioneering outpatient assessment program in Monroe County, New York.[117] This program assessed all patients referred for nursing home placement in the county and found that only 38% of patients referred for nursing home placement actually needed such skilled nursing care, whereas 23% of the patients were able to return to their homes and 39% were able to go to board-and-care facilities or retirement homes after careful assessment and recommendations for specific therapy. Expert judgments made by an independent team of observers indicated that major improvements in placement decisions were being made by the program. Several subsequent reports, including two from controlled studies,[19,99] have shown similar assessment-related improvements in placement locations.[19,99–101,107,108,110,112,114,118–120]

Several reports have examined patient functional status before and after treatment on geriatric units, particularly on units providing rehabilitation. These reports have usually used a validated measure of functional status to document change over time. They show that the majority of patients improve during their stays on the units. The absence of control groups in most of the reports prevents one from differentiating the effect of time from that arising from the geriatric program itself. However, two controlled studies clearly showed that patients in geriatric programs were more likely to improve, and to retain their improvement, than controls.[19,103]

Impacts on psychological parameters, such as cognitive status and affect, have also been examined. Although both cognitive function and affect have been shown to improve over time in noncontrolled studies,[106,112,113,121–123] only impacts on affect have been documented in controlled trials.[19,96,104]

Improvement in quality of treatment is difficult to quantify. One measurable parameter, use of prescription drugs, has been reported. In those reports, drug prescribing was made generally more appropriate, usually resulting in a decreased quantity of prescribed drugs, despite concurrent increases in the number of treatable diagnoses identified.[95,101,106,114,115]

Use of hospital services has been examined in several studies, involving inpatient units, inpatient consult services, and outpatient assessment services. All studies that included long-term follow-up of at least a year report reduced use of acute hospital services and reduced total health care costs over time.[19,99,103,115] When only the initial hospitalization period is compared, the results are mixed—some show a prolonged length of stay (LOS) associated with the assessment,[19,97,114] whereas others show a shortened LOS.[98,101,118,119,124] Whether the initial LOS is shortened or prolonged is a function of the intensity of the intervention as well as of the speed and thoroughness of the hospital services used by control patients among other things. The reduction in acute hospital use and total health care costs over time from assessment services primarily reflects a reduction in rehospitalization rates, which stems both from the initial assessment itself and from the often improved quality of follow-up services.

The only reliable way for measuring program impact on survival is to use a control group, preferably one randomly assigned, and to follow subjects for a substantial period of time. The Sepulveda randomized controlled trial showed a 50% reduction in 1-year mortality as compared with the control group.[19] The Danish randomized trial showed a 25% reduction in 3-year mortality from a group of home-living elderly receiving periodic inhome assessments.[99] A similar impact was reported in the Welsh trial of home assessment.[104] On the other hand, Mark Williams' study of an outpatient assessment program failed to show impact on survival—although, as the author discusses, the control group received additional diagnostic care from well-trained internists.[105]

Targeting programs to the most appropriate patients is a key issue. Although geriatric assessment programs can clearly be effective, it is important to identify accurately which subgroups of patients can be expected to benefit most in order to make maximal use of scarce resources. Although it might be argued that the majority of elderly probably could benefit from careful assessment, the bulk of older people generally are healthy, and the relative yield of assessment tends to be lower for healthy than for frail or ill elderly. In general, people most likely to benefit from assessment are those who are on the verge of needing institutionalization, who are in the lower socioeconomic groups, who have inadequate primary medical care, and who have poor social support networks. On the other hand, patients in the end stages of a terminal illness or irreversible dementia would be less likely to derive much benefit. The proportion of at-risk elderly who can derive especially great benefits from assessment programs appear to constitute between 5% and 10% of hospitalized elderly and a currently undetermined proportion (perhaps 2% to 5%) of nonhospitalized elderly. In systems of care in which the average level of health of the elderly population is lower, the proportions who would benefit would probably be much higher.

CONCLUSIONS

This chapter has described a clinical approach to the unique aspects of caring for the elderly patient—comprehensive geriatric assessment. The approach can be used in individual offices or as part of comprehensive assessment programs. The data reviewed here suggest that geriatric assessment programs are effective, practical, and vitally important. They can lead to better diagnosis, treatment outcomes, functional status, and living location and lower use of long-term institutional care services. It is hoped that the concepts presented here will be helpful in approaching the older woman in the clinical office setting.

REFERENCES

1. Kane RA, Kane RL: *Assessing the Elderly: A Practical Guide to Measurement.* Lexington, Mass, Lexington Books, 1981.

2. Rubenstein LZ, Campbell LJ, Kane RL: *Geriatric Assessment.* Philadelphia, WB Saunders, 1987.

3. Brandfonbrener M, Lardowne M, Shock NW: Changes in output with age. *Circulation* 1955;12:577.

4. Rodeheffer RJ, Gerstenblith G, Becker LC, et al: Exercise cardiac output is maintained with advancing age in healthy human subjects: Cardiac dilation and increased stroke volume compensate for a diminished heart rate. *Circulation* 1984;69(2):203–213.

5. Lakatta EG: Alterations in the cardiovascular system that occur in advanced age. *Fed Proc* 1979;38:163.

6. Fleg JL: Alterations in cardiovascular structure and function with advancing age. *Am J Cardiol* 1986;57:33c–44c.

7. Davidson MB: The effect of aging on carbohydrate metabolism: A review of the English literature and a practical approach to the diagnosis of diabetes mellitus in the elderly. *Metabolism* 1979;28(6):688–705.

8. Rosenthal M, Doberne L, Greenfield M, et al: Effect of age on glucose tolerance, insulin secretion, and in vivo insulin action. *J Am Geriatr Soc* 1982;30(9):562–567.

9. Zavaroni I, Dall'Aglio E, Bruschi F, et al: Effect of age and environmental factors on glucose tolerance and insulin secretion in a worker population. *J Am Geriatr Soc* 1986;34:271–275.

10. Seals DR, Hagberg JM, Allen WK, et al: Glucose tolerance in young and older athletes and sedentary men. *J Appl Physiol* 1984;56(6):1521.

11. Hollenbeck CB, Haskell W, Rosenthal M, et al: Effect of habitual physical activity on regulation of insulin-stimulated glucose disposal in older males. *J Am Geriatr Soc* 1984;33:273–277.

12. Kitani K: Hepatic drug metabolism in the elderly. *Hepatology* 1986;6(2):316.

13. Davies DF, Shock NW: Age changes in glomerular filtration rate, effective renal plasma flow, and tubular excretory capacity in adult males. *J Clin Invest* 1950;29:496–507.

14. Lindeman RD, Tobin J, Shock NW: Longitudinal studies on the rate of decline in renal function with age. *J Am Geriatr Soc* 1985;33:278–285.

15. Kane RL, Ouslander JG, Abrass IB: *Essentials of Clinical Geriatrics.* New York, McGraw-Hill, 1984, p 7.

16. Rossman I (ed): *Clinical Geriatrics.* Philadelphia, JB Lippincott, 1979.

17. Rubenstein LZ, Josephson KR, Nichol-Seamons M, et al: Comprehensive health screening of well elderly adults: An analysis of a community program. *J Gerontol* 1986;41(3):342–352.

18. Katz DR, Dube DH, Calkins E: Use of a structured functional assessment format in a geriatric consultative service. *J Am Geriatr Soc* 1985;33:681–686.

19. Rubenstein LZ, Josephson KR, Wieland GD, et al: Effectiveness of a geriatric evaluation unit. A randomized clinical trial. *N Engl J Med* 1984;311:664.

20. Portnoi VA: Digitalis delirium in elderly patients. *J Clin Pharm* 1979;11–12:747–750.

21. Norman DC, Grahn D, Yoshikawa TT: Fever and aging. *J Am Geriatr Soc* 1985;33:859–863.

22. Bayer AJ, Chadna JS, Farag RR, et al: Changing presentation of myocardial infarction with increasing old age. *J Am Geriatr Soc* 1986;34:263–266.

23. Tibaldi JM, Barzel US, Albin J, et al: Thyrotoxicosis in the very old. *Am J Med* 1986;81:619–622.

24. McFadden JP, Price RC, Eastwood HD, et al: Raised respiratory rate in elderly patients: A valuable physical sign. *Br Med J* 1982;284:626–627.

25. Lombardi G, Polotti R, Polizzi N, et al: Prevalence of asymptomatic peripheral vascular disease in a group of patients older than 50. *J Am Geriatr Soc* 1986;34(7):551–552.

26. Lamy PP: The elderly and drug interactions. *J Am Geriatr Soc* 1986;34:586–592.

27. Vestal RF: Pharmacology and aging. *J Am Geriatr Soc* 1982;30(3):191.

28. Moore SR, Ted TW (eds): *Geriatric Drug Use—Clinical and Social Perspectives.* New York, Pergamon Press, 1985.

29. Dyer CC, Oles KS, Davies SW: The role of the pharmacist in a geriatric nursing home: A literature review. *Drug Intell Clin Pharm* 1984;18:428–433.

30. Hammarlund ER, Ostrom JR, Kethley AJ: The effects of drug counseling and other educational strategies on drug utilization of the elderly. *Med Care* 1985;23:165–170.

31. Siedman H, Mushinski MH, Gelb SK, et al: Probability of eventually developing or dying of cancer—United States, 1985. *CA* 1985;35(1):36.

32. Amery A, Lijnen P, Mibuyamba-Kabangu JR, et al: Influence of hypotensive drug treatment on morbidity and mortality in elderly hypertensives—review of the published trials. *Acta Med Scand* [suppl] 1983;676:64–85.

33. Shapiro S: Evidence on screening for breast cancer from a randomized trial. *CA* 1977;39(suppl):2772.

34. Tasar L, Fagerberg CJG, GAD A, et al: Reduction in mortality from breast cancer after mass screening with mammography. Randomized trial from the breast cancer screening working group of the Swedish National Board of Health and Welfare. *Lancet* 1985;1:829–832.

35. Howard J: Using mammography for cancer control: An unrealized potential. *CA* 1987;37(1):33–48.

36. Baker LH: Breast cancer detection demonstration project: Five year summary report. *CA* 1982;32(4):194.

37. O'Malley MS, Fletcher SW: Screening for breast cancer with breast self-examination: A critical review. *JAMA* 1987;257:2196–2203.

38. Dales LG, Friedman GD, Ramcharan S, et al: Multi-physic check-up evaluation study: 3. Outpatient clinic utilization hospitalization and mortality experience after seven years. *Prev Med* 1973;2:221.

39. Hardcastle JD, Farrands PA, Balfour TW, et al: Controlled trial of fecal occult blood testing in the detection of colorectal cancer. *Lancet* 1983;2:1–4.

40. Gilbertson VA, McHugh RB, Schuman L, et al: The earlier detection of colorectal cancers. A preliminary report of the results of the occult blood study. *CA* 1980;45:2899–2901.

41. Winawer SJ, Fleisher M, Baldwin M, et al: Current status of fecal occult blood testing in screening for colorectal cancer. *CA* 1982;32:100.

42. Simon JB: Occult blood screening for colorectal carcinoma: A critical review. *Gastroenterology* 1985;88:820–837.

43. Guzick DS: Efficacy of screening for cervical cancer: A review. *Am J Public Health* 1978; 68:125.

44. Siegler EE: Cervical carcinoma in the aged. *Am J Obstet Gynecol* 1969;103(8):1093–1097.

45. Massachusetts Department of Public Health: Papanicolaou testing—are we screening the wrong women? (letter). *N Engl J Med* 1975;294(4):223.

46. Neighbor RM, Newman RL: Incidence of cervical cancer in perimenopausal and postmenopausal women detected by Papanicolaou smears. *Am J Obstet Gynecol* 1975; 124(4):348–351.

47. Oster S: Cervical vaginal screening in the over 65 female. *Mt Sinai J Med (NY)* 1980; 47(2):192–193.

48. Stenkvist B, Bergstrom R, Eklund G, et al: Papanicolaou smear screening and cervical cancer. What can you expect? *JAMA* 1984;252:1423–1426.

49. Mandelblatt J, Gopaul I, Wistreich M: Gynecological care of elderly women. Another look at Papanicolaou smear testing. *JAMA* 1986;256:367–371.

50. Fidler AK, Boyes DA, Worth AJ: Cervical cancer detection in British Columbia. *Br J Obstet Gynaecol* 1968;75:392–404.

51. Eddy D: Guidelines for the cancer-related check-up: Recommendations and rationale. *CA* 1980;30:194.

52. Canadian Task Force on the Periodic Health Examination: The Periodic Health Examination. *Can Med Assoc J* 1979;121:1193–1254 and 1984;130:1278–1292.

53. Frame PS, Carlson SJ: A critical review of periodic health screening using specific screening criteria. *J Fam Pract* 1975;2:29–36.

54. Breslow L, Somers AR: The lifetime health-monitoring program. A practical approach to preventive medicine. *N Engl J Med* 1977;296(11):601–608.

55. American College of Preventive Medicine Task Force: *Preventive Medicine USA: Theory, Practice and Application of Prevention in Personal Health Services*. New York, Fogarty International Center, Prodist, 1976, pp 27–101.

56. Kannel WB, Garrison RG, Wilson DWF: Obesity and nutrition in elderly diabetic patients. *Am J Med* 1986;80(suppl 5A):22.

57. Lipid Research Clinics Program: The Lipid Research Clinics coronary primary prevention trial results. *JAMA* 1984;251:351–364.

58. Borhani NO: Prevalence and prognostic significance of hypertension in the elderly. *J Am Geriatr Soc* 1986;34:112–114.

59. Hypertension Detection and Follow-up Program Cooperative Research Group: Five year findings of the HDFP; reduction in stroke incidence among persons with high blood pressure. *JAMA* 1982;247:633.

60. National Heart Foundation of Australia: Treatment of mild hypertension in the elderly: Report by the management committee. *Med J Aust* 1981;2:398.

61. Gifford RW: Management of isolated systolic hypertension in the elderly. *J Am Geriatr Soc* 1986;34:106–111.

62. Hulley SB, Furberg CD, Gurland B, et al: Systolic hypertension in the elderly program (SHEP): Antihypertensive efficacy of chlorthalidone. *Am J Cardiol* 1985;56:913–920.

63. Cummings SR, Black D: Should perimenopausal women be screened for osteoporosis? *Ann Intern Med* 1986;104:817–823.

64. Poposhin L, Fradis M, Ben-David J, et al: What is normal aging? 7. Hearing and old age. *Geriatr Med Today* 1984;3(11):22–29.

65. Barker WH, Mulholy JP: Influenza vaccination of elderly persons. Reduction in pneumonia and influenza hospitalizations and deaths. *JAMA* 1980;244:2547–2549.

66. Le Mintagne JR, Noble GR, Quinnan GV, et al: Summary of clinical trials of inactivated influenza vaccine—1978. *Rev Infect Dis* 1983;5:723–736.

67. Patriarca PA, Weber JA, Parker RA, et al: Efficacy of influenza vaccine in nursing homes. *JAMA* 1985;253:1136–1139.

68. Immunization Practices Advisory Committee, Centers for Disease Control: Recommendations for prevention and control of influenza. *Ann Intern Med* 1986;105:319–404.

69. Larson EB, Reifler BV, Featherstone HJ, et al: Dementia in elderly outpatients: A prospective study. *Ann Intern Med* 1984;100:417–423.

70. Erkinjuntti T, Wikstrom J, Palo J, et al: Dementia among medical inpatients. Evaluation of 2000 consecutive admissions. *Arch Intern Med* 1986;146:1923–1926.

71. Finlayson RE, Martin LM: Recognition and management of depression in the elderly. *Mayo Clin Proc* 1982;506:115–120.

72. Katz S, Ford AB, Moskowitz RW, et al: Studies of illness in the aged. The index of ADL; A standardized measure of biological and psychosocial function. *JAMA* 1963;185:914.

73. Lawton MP, Brody EM: Assessment of older people: Self-maintaining and instrumental activities of daily living. *Gerontologist* 1969;9:179–186.

74. Allan CA, Blotmen H: Chartbook on aging in America. Washington, DC, The 1981 White House Conference on Aging, 1981.

75. Bennett T: Are cardiovascular reflexes a useful means of assessing autonomic neuropathy? *Internal Medicine for the Specialist* 1983;4:55.

76. Pierson DJ, Hudson LD: Evaluation of dyspnea. *Geriatrics* 1981;36(4):48–62.

77. Collins KJ, Dore C, Exton-Smith AN, et al: Accidental hypothermia and impaired temperature homeostasis in the elderly. *Br Med J* 1977;1:353–356.

78. Larochelle P, Bass MJ, Birkett NH, et al: Recommendations from the consensus conference on hypertension in the elderly. *Can Med J* 1986;135:741–745.

79. Messerli FH, Ventura HO, Amodeo C: Osler's maneuver and pseudohypertension. *West J Med* 1985;312(24):1548–1551.

80. Robbins AS, Rubenstein LZ: Postural hypotension in the elderly. *J Am Geriatr Soc* 1984;32(10):769–774.

81. Master AM, Lasser RD, Beckman G: Tables of average weight and height of Americans aged 65–94. *JAMA* 1960;172:658–662.

82. Proper S, Fenske N: Common skin tumors on the geriatric population. *Geriatr Med Today* 1985;4(A):17.

83. Mader S: Hearing impairment in elderly persons. *J Am Geriatr Soc* 1984;32(7):548.

84. Keeney AH, Keeney VT: A guide to examining the aging eye. *Geriatrics* 1980;36(2):81.

85. Griffiths RA, Chadwick DE: Evaluation of systolic murmurs in the elderly. *Geriatr Med Today* 1983;2(12):62–65, 69–72, 81.

86. Devereux RB, Hawkins I, Kramer-Fox R, et al: Complications of mitral valve prolapse. Disproportionate occurrence in men and older patients. *Am J Med* 1986;81(5):751–758.

87. Jenkyo L, Reeves A: Neurologic signs in uncomplicated aging. *Semin Neurol* 1981;1:21–30.

88. Sabin TD: Biologic aspects of falls and mobility limitations in the elderly. *J Am Geriatr Soc* 1982;30(1):51–58.

89. Tinetti ME, Williams TF, Mayewski R: Fall risk index for elderly patients based on number of chronic disabilities. *Am J Med* 1986;80:429–434.

90. Folstein MF, Folstein SE, McHugh PR: Mini-mental state: A practical method for grading the cognitive state of patient for the clinician. *J Psych Res* 1975;12:189–198.

91. Blazer D, Williams CD: Epidemiology of dysphoria and depression in an elderly population. *Am J Psychiatry* 1981;137:439.

92. Yesavage JA, Brink TL, Rose TL, et al: Development and validation of a geriatric screening scale: A preliminary report. *J Psychiatr Res* 1983;17(1):37–49.

93. Butler R: *Why Survive? Being Old in America*. New York, Harper & Row, 1975.

94. Kane RL, Kane RA: Care of the aged: Old problems in need of new solutions. *Science* 1978;200:913.

95. Allen CM, Becher PM, McVey LJ, et al: A randomized controlled clinical trial of a geriatric consultation team: Compliance with recommendations. *JAMA* 1986;255:2617–2621.

96. Balaban DJ: Chronic care study: A randomized longitudinal study of patients with chronic diseases treated on a special care unit. Final Report. Philadelphia, Leonard Davis School of Health Economics, 1980.

97. Berkman B, Campion E, Swagerty E, et al: Geriatric consultation team: Alternate approach to social work discharge planning. *J Gerontol Soc W* 1983;5(3):77–88.

98. Collard AF, Bachman SS, Beatrice DF: Acute care delivery for the geriatric patient: An innovative approach. *QRB* 1985;11(6):180–185.

99. Hendriksen C, Lund E, Stromgard E: Consequences of assessment and intervention among elderly people: Three year randomized controlled trial. *Br Med J* 1984;289:1522–1524.

100. Lefton E, Bonstelle S, Frengley JD: Success with an inpatient geriatric unit: A controlled study. *J Am Geriatr Soc* 1983;31:149–155.

101. Popplewell PY, Henschke PJ: What is the value of a geriatric assessment unit in a teaching hospital? A comparative study. *Aust Health Rev* 1983;6(2):23–25.

102. Teasdale TA, Schuman L, Snow E, et al: A comparison of outcomes of geriatric cohorts receiving care in a geriatric assessment unit and on general medicine floors. *J Am Geriatr Soc* 1983;31:529–534.

103. Tulloch AH, Moore V: A randomized controlled trial of geriatric screening and surveillance in general practice. *J R Coll Gen Pract* 1979;29:733–742.

104. Vetter NJ, Jones DA, Victor CR: Effects of health visitors working with elderly patients in general practice: A randomized controlled trial. *Br Med J* 1984;288:369–372.

105. Williams ME: Outpatient geriatric evaluation. *Clin Geriatr Med* 1987;3(1):175–184.

106. Applegate WB, Akins D, Vanderzwaag R, et al: A geriatric rehabilitation and assessment unit in a community hospital. *J Am Geriatr Soc* 1983;31:206–210.

107. Bayne JR, Caygill J: Identifying needs and services for the aged. *J Am Geriatr Soc* 1977;25:264–268.

108. Brocklehurst JC, Carty MH, Leeming JT, et al: Medical screening of old people accepted for residential care. *Lancet* 1978;2:141.

109. Cheah KC, Beard OW: Psychiatric findings in the population of a geriatric evaluation unit: Implications. *J Am Geriatr Soc* 1980;28:153–156.

110. Lichtenstein H, Winograd CH: Geriatric consultation: A functional approach. *J Am Geriatr Soc* 1985;33:422–428.

111. Lowther CP, MacLeod RDM, Williamson J: Evaluation of early diagnostic services for the elderly. *Br Med J* 1970;3:275–277.

112. Poliquin N, Straker M: A clinical psychogeriatric unit: Organization and function. *J Am Geriatr Soc* 1977;25:132–137.

113. Reifler BV, Eisdorfer C: A clinic for impaired elderly and their families. *Am J Psychiatry* 1980;137:1399–1403.

114. Rubenstein LZ, Abrass IB, Kane RL: Improved care for patients on a new geriatric unit. *J Am Geriatr Soc* 1981;29:531–536.

115. Rubenstein LZ, Josephson KR, Wieland GD, et al: Geriatric assessment on a subacute hospital ward. *Clin Geriatr Med* 1987;3(1):131–144.

116. Williamson J, Stokoe IH, Gray S, et al: Old people at home: Their unreported needs. *Lancet* 1964;1:1117–1120.

117. Williams TF, Hill JG, Fairbank ME, et al: Appropriate placement of the chronically ill and aged: A successful approach by evaluation. *JAMA* 1973;226:1332–1335.

118. Burley LE, Currie CT, Smith RG, et al: Contribution from geriatric medicine within acute medical wards. *Br Med J* 1979;263(2):90.

119. Schuman JE, Beattie EJ, Steed DA, et al: The impact of a new geriatric program in a hospital for the chronically ill. *Can Med Assoc J* 1978;118:639–645.

120. Sloane P: Nursing home candidates: Hospital inpatient trial to identify those appropriately assignable to less intensive care. *J Am Geriatr Soc* 1980;28:511–514.

121. Gross PF: Evaluation of a geriatric assessment unit in an acute general hospital in a rural region of Australia. Institute of Health Economics and Technology Assessment, Sydney, Australia. Long-term Care Project, Working Paper no 3, 1985.

122. Liem PH, Chernoff R, Carter WJ: Geriatric rehabilitation unit: A 3-year outcome evaluation. *J Gerontol* 1986;41:44–50.

123. Spar JE, Ford CV, Liston EH: Hospital treatment of the elderly neuropsychiatric patients: 2. *J Am Geriatr Soc* 1980;28:539–543.

124. Barker WH, Williams TF, Zimmer JG, et al: Geriatric consultation teams in acute hospitals: Impact on back up of elderly patients. *J Am Geriatr Soc* 1985;33:422–428.

Index

A

Abdomen
  pain in, 144
  in physical examination, 385
Abortion, breast cancer risk and, 57, *58*
Abuse
  alcohol, 192
  laxatives, 140-141
  patient, 170, 353-354
  privacy, 353
  self-determination, 355
  substance, 191-194
Acetaminophen, in management of rheumatic disorders, 211
Acetohydroxamic acid (AHA), for treatment of renal calculi, 264
Achalasia, as cause of dysphagia, 133
Acquired immunodeficiency syndrome (AIDS), vulvovaginal lesions in, 160-161
ACTH. *See* Adrenocorticotropic hormone (ACTH)
Actinomyces infection, 159
Actinomycosis, of pelvic organs, 159
Activities of daily living (ADLs), 377
  instrumental (IADLs), 377
Acute mesenteric ischemic bowel disease, 144

Acyclovir, for herpes simplex infections, 79
Adenocarcinoma, 84
Adenomas, colorectal, 143
Adenovirus, in genital tract, 160
Adipose tissue, androgen conversion and, 29
Adjustment disorders, 187-188
  medical illness and, 178
ADLs. *See* Activities of daily living (ADLs)
Adrenal gland
  cortex, 27-28
  medulla, 28-29
Adrenocorticotropic hormone (ACTH), 28
Adult respiratory distress syndrome (ARDS), 253
Age, as risk factor
  breast cancer, 55, *56*
  heart disease, 98
  stroke, 100
Aging
  and cognition, 171
  normal vs. pathologic disease process, 361-362, *363-366*
Agoraphobia, 190
AHA. *See* Acetohydroxamic acid (AHA)

AIDS. *See* Acquired immunodeficiency syndrome (AIDS)
Airway obstruction, as postoperative complication, 326
Alcohol
  abuse vs. dependence, 192
  hallucinosis, 194
  intoxication, 192-193
    idiosyncratic, 193
  withdrawal syndrome, 193
  withdrawal delirium, 194
Aldosterone, adrenal cortex and, 28
Allopurinol, in treatment of gout, 211
Alopecia, 90-92
Alpha-agonists
  anesthesia and, 317
  in treatment of incontinence, 234
Alprazolam, in treatment of agoraphobia, 191
Alzheimer's disease, 181, 182
Ambulatory surgery, patient care approaches, 318-319
American Society of Anesthesiologists (ASA)
  intra-operative monitoring standards and, 319, *320-321*
  physical status assessment guidelines, *315*, 315-317
Amitryptyline, 180
Amnestic syndrome, 194
Ampulla of Vater, visualization of, 136
Amyotrophy, 30
Analgesics, in management of rheumatic disorders, 211
ANBP. *See* Australian National Blood Pressure (ANBP) trial
Androgen synthesis, by adrenal cortex, 28
Ancsthesia
  in ambulatory surgery, 318
  conditions following, 329-330
  monitoring, 319, 321, 322
  and preoperative medication, 323-326
  recovery from, 326-328
  risk in older patient, 313-315
    assessment of, 315-317
  temperature control during, 322-323
  See also Surgery
Angiodysplasia
  as cause of rectal bleeding, 145
  colonic, 144-145
Angiotensin blockers, as antihypertensive therapy, 119-120
Anterior colporrhaphy, 237
Anti-inflammatory drugs. *See* Nonsteroidal anti-inflammatory drugs (NSAIDs)
Antiarrhythmic drugs, TCA interaction with, 180
Antibiotics, 161
  cephalosporins, 161-163, *162*
  imipenem-cilastatin, 163
  penicillin, 163
  quinolones, 163-164
  therapy for TOA, 154-155
Anticholinergic drugs
  TCA interaction with, 179
  in treatment of incontinence, 232-233, *233*
Anticoagulation drugs, TCA interaction with, 180
Anticonvulsants, anesthesia and, 317
Antihypertensive therapy
  anesthesia and, 317
  angiotensin blockers, 119-120
  benefits of
    Framingham study, *103*, 104
    randomized prospective trials, 104-106, *107*
  beta blockers, 120
  and blood pressure measurement, 111-113
  calcium antagonists, 118-119
  centrally active agents, 120
  compliance with, 116-117
  drug vs. placebo trials, 106, *107*, 108
  as heart disease risk factor, 99
  nonmedical or behavioral, 113-114
  orthostatic hypotension, 117
  other agents, 120-121
  thiazides, 117-118
  treatment modality trials, 108-109
  trial findings, implications for patients, 109-110

in very old, uncertain benefits, 110-111
Antipsychotic medication, 183-184
Antisocial personality disorder, 186
Antispasmodic agents, in treatment of incontinence, 232-233, *233*
Anxiety
　disorders of, 189-191
　sleep patterns and, 170
Aphasia, vs. dementia, 171
Appearance, in physical examination, 382-383
ARDS. *See* Adult respiratory distress syndrome (ARDS)
Arrhenoblastomas, 30
Arteriosclerotic disease, urinary tract infection and, 254
Arteritis, temporal, polymyalgia rheumatica and, 207
Arthritis
　degenerative. *See* Osteoarthritis
　rheumatoid. *See* Rheumatoid arthritis (RA)
ASA. *See* American Society of Anesthesiologists (ASA)
Aspiration, as postoperative complication, 328
Aspirin, in management of rheumatic disorders, 211
Assessment. *See* Geriatric evaluation
Atherosclerosis, diabetes mellitus and, 30
Atrophic vaginitis, 299
Australian National Blood Pressure (ANBP) trial, antihypertensive therapy benefits and, 106, *107*, 108
Avoidant personality disorder, 187

B

Bacteremia, 253
Bacterial vaginosis, 304-305
Bacteriuria
　catheterization and, 250-251
　defined, 251
Bacteroides sp., cephalosporins against, 162
Barbiturates, TCA interaction with, 179

Barium examinations, 334
Bartholin's gland carcinoma, 88
Basal cell carcinoma, 87-88
BCDDP. *See* Breast Cancer Detection Demonstration Projects (BCDDP)
Bed rest, in treatment of rheumatoid arthritis, 208
Bed-side manner, 169-170
Behavioral therapy
　for hypertension, *114*, 114
　　judging compliance with, 115, *116*
　in treatment of incontinence, 231
Bentyl. *See* Dicyclomine
Benzodiazepines, as preoperative medication, 325
Bereavement, uncomplicated, 188
Beta blockers
　anesthesia and, 317
　as antihypertensive therapy, 120
bid dosing, vs. *tid* or *qid* dosing, 213
Bladder
　cancer of. *See* Bladder cancer
　drainage of, postoperative, 240-241
　relaxants in treatment of incontinence, 232-234
Bladder cancer, 274
　management of, 276-277
　metastatic disease, 277
　pathology and natural history, 275-276
　risk factors, 274
　signs and symptoms, 274, *275*
　staging, 276
Bleeding
　rectal, 141-146
　uterine, TOA and, 154
　See also Hemorrhage
Blepharoptosis, 20-21
Blindness, diabetes mellitus and, 32-33
Blood pressure
　ambulatory monitoring, 113-114
　evaluation, 93-94
　high, determinants of, 94
　measurement, 111-113
　treatment in very old, 110-111
　trial findings, implications for mild hypertensives, 109-110

See also Diastolic blood pressure; Systolic blood pressure
Body temperature, in intra-operative monitoring standards, 321
Bone mass, 25-26
Bonney test, in diagnostic evaluation of incontinence, 228
Borderline hypertension, 95
Borderline personality disorder, 186
Bowel disease, acute mesenteric ischemic, 144
Bowel elimination
  constipation and, 139-141
  nutrition and, 146-149
  rectal bleeding and, 141-146
Bowel motility, 139
Breast cancer
  BCDDP and HIP studies compared, 47, 48
  cases diagnosed, 49
  detection of, physical examination vs. mammography, 42, 43
    by age and modality, 46
    See also Mammography
  epidemiology, 53
  incidence and mortality rates, 39
    age-related, 42
    worldwide, 59, 60
  natural history of, 52
  pathogenesis model, 54
  risk groups for, 53, 55-59
  survival
    factors, 39
    rates, 61
  as systemic disease, 65
  treatment for, 59-64
  tumor detection in, 39-43
Breast Cancer Detection Demonstration Projects (BCDDP), 39-42
  screening mammography, 45-50
Breasts
  cancer of. See Breast cancer
  disease of, physician visits for, 9-10
  self-examination of, 51-52
Buffering mechanisms, 94-95
Bullous pemphigoid, vulval, 289-290

C

C cells, calcitonin secretion by, 22
Calamine lotion, for herpes zoster infections, 79
Calcitonin
  secretion by C cells, 22
  treatment of osteoporosis, 26-27
  use in hypercalcemia, 24
Calcium
  antagonists, as antihypertensive therapy, 118-119
  metabolism, and renal function, 122
  osteoporosis and, 26
  recommended intake, 147, 148
Cancer. See Carcinoma
Candida sp.
  albicans, 78, 250
    in monilial vulvovaginitis, 306-307
    as suspect in vulvar dystrophy, 82
    vaginal colonization by, 152
    in vulvovaginal candidiasis, 287-288
  glabrata
    in monilial vulvovaginitis, 306-307
    in vulvovaginal candidiasis, 287-288
Candidiasis, vulvovaginal, 287-288
Carbon dioxide, end-tidal, monitoring of, 319, 322
Carcinoma, 21-22
  Bartholin's gland, 88
  basal cell, 87-88
  bladder. See Bladder cancer
  of breast. See Breast cancer
  colon, 143
  colorectal, 142-143
  depression in patients with, 177
  esophageal, 132
  incidence and death by site and sex, 40
  metastatic, 89
  mortality rate, age-related, 41
  probability at birth, 54
  recommendations for early detection, 70
  renal cell. See Kidney tumors

screening for, 371-372, *373*
in situ, vulvar, 83
squamous cell, 87
Cardiovascular disease
frequency of, 10
and hypertension, 93
Framingham (Mass) study, 96-97
risk factors for elderly women, 98-100, *103*
as stroke risk factor, 100
TCA use in, 180
Cardiovascular system, in physical examination, 384-385
Caruncle, urethral, 290-291
"Case finding," 342-343
Catheterization
bacteriuria and, 250-251
problems with, 253
treatment for urinary tract infections due to, 260
Cefazolin, 162
Cefotaxime, 163
Cefotetan, 162
Cefoxitin, 162
Ceftizoxime, 163
Ceftriaxone, 163
Cellular atypia, in vulvar dystrophies, 81-82
Cellulosodium phosphate (CSP), for treatment of renal calculi, 264
Century of the Older Woman, 7
Cephalorsporins, 161, *162*
first generation, *162*, 162
second generation, *162*, 162
third generation, *162*, 163
Cervical arthritis, as cause of dysphagia, 132
Chemical vaginitis, 308-309
Chlamydia trachomatis infection, 250, 255
Cholesterol. *See* Serum cholesterol
Cigarette smoking
as heart disease risk factor, 98
as stroke risk factor, 100
Cimetidine, as preoperative medication, 325-326
Ciprofloxacillin, 164

Circulation
changes with aging, 94-95
in intra-operative monitoring standards, *321*
Citrobacter infection, 250
Climacteric. *See* Menopause
Clinoril, in management of rheumatic disorders, 213, *214*
Clonidine, as antihypertensive therapy, 120
Clostridium welchi, sepsis from atrophied gynecologic site and, 153-154
Cognition, aging and, 171
Colchicine, in treatment of gout, 211
Colic, renal, management of, 262
Colitis, ulcerative, 146
Colon
cancer of, 143
physiology of, 140
Colonic angiodysplasia, 144-145
Colonoscopy
polypectomy and, 136
rectal bleeding and, 136
Colorectal cancer, 142-143
Colorectal polyps, 142
Comfort, of patient, attitudes toward, 12
Compassion, medical care and, 340 355
Competency, legal, 348-349
Compliance
with behaviorial therapy, measuring, 115, *116*
factors affecting, 116-117
problems with, 172
Compulsive personality disorder, 187
Computed tomography (CT), 334, 335
Connecticut Cancer Registry, 39
Consent, informed, 349-350
Constipation
defined and classified, 139
evaluation of, 141
factors affecting, 140
and laxative abuse, 140-141
management of, 140
Contact dermatitis, vulval, 285-286
Contraceptives, oral, breast cancer risk and, 57-58, *58*

Conversion disorders, 188-189
Cornyebacterium vaginalis infection, 304
Cortisol, secretory rate, 27-28
Cost-effectiveness
  of geriatric patient, 339-340
    long-term strategies, 345-346
  of radiation, 335
Courts, role of, 352-353
Credé maneuver, 228
Crohn's disease, 145-146
Cryptococcus neoformans, AIDS patients and, 160
Crystal deposition diseases, 210-211
CSP. See Cellulosodium phosphate (CSP)
Cul-de-sac of Douglas, 239-240
Cystic tumors, 86
Cystitis, 256-257
  defined, 251
  interstitial
    treatment for, 260
  with vaginitis, 158-159
  treatment for, 258-260
Cystometry, in diagnostic evaluation of incontinence, 230
Cystourethroscopy, in diagnostic evaluation of incontinence, 230-231
Cysts, 86
Cytomegalovirus, in genital tract, 160

D

Daricon. See Oxyphencyclimine
Day-care centers, medical, 344
Death rates
  age-adjusted, 5, 6
  and institutionalization, 171-172
Deaths, 4, 5
  major causes, 8
Degenerative arthritis. See Osteoarthritis
Delirium, 182-183
  alcohol withdrawal, 194
Dementia, 180-182
  aphasia vs., 171
Demerol. See Meperidine
Dependent personality disorder, 187
Depression
  after stroke, 178
  in cancer patients, 177
  as cause of hospitalization, 175-176
  differential diagnosis, 176
  features, 176
  forms, 177
  incidence, 175, 340
  presentation, 177
  treatment, 178-180
Dermatitis
  artefacta, pyoderma gangrenosum vs., 158
  atopic, 76
  chronic nonspecific, 76-77
  contact, 75-76
    allergic, 76
  vulval
    contact, 285-286
    seborrheic, 286-287
Dermatobia hominis, infestation of genital tract, 158
Dermatofibrosarcoma protuberans, 88-89
Dermatoses
  papulosquamous, 77
  pruritic. See Pruritic dermatoses
Dermopathy, diabetic, 33
Desipramine, 180
Diabetes mellitus (DM), 30-36
  as heart disease risk factor, 98
  noninsulin-dependent, 30
  as stroke risk factor, 101
  urinary tract infection and, 254
Diabetic neuropathic cachexia, 30
Diagnostic and Statistical Manual of Mental Disorders (DSM)
  adjustment disorders, 187-188
  alcohol abuse vs. alcohol dependence, 192
  alcohol hallucinosis, 194
  alcohol intoxication, 192
  alcohol withdrawal delirium, 194
  amnestic syndrome, 194
  anxiety disorders, 189-191
  delirium, 182
  dementia, 180-181
  depression, 177
  panic disorders, 190-191
  paranoid disorders, 183-184

personality disorders, 185-187
schizophrenia, 184-185
withdrawal syndromes, 193-194
Diagnostic imaging
  modality strengths and weaknesses, 334-335
  sensitivity vs. specificity, 333-334
Diagnostic-related groups (DRGs), 333
  reimbursement of, 339
Diaphanoscopy, 69
Diastolic blood pressure, lowering, benefits of, 104
Diastolic hypertension, defined, 95
Diazepams, as preoperative medication, 325
Dicyclomine, in treatment of incontinence, 232-233, *233*, 234
Dienestrol. *See* Estrogen
Diet
  and constipation, 140
  low-fat, 149
  role in colonic carcinoma, 149
  salt restricted, 149
  as stroke risk factor, 102
  as therapy for diabetes mellitus, 34-35
  See also Nutrition
Digital imaging, 334
Dilation and curettage, frequency of, 10
Dimethyl sulfoxide, in therapy for interstitial cystitis, 159
Disalcid, in management of rheumatic disorders, 213, *214*
Discharge planning and placement, 342-343
Distal colonic disease, 145
Ditropan. *See* Oxybutynin
Diuretics
  anesthesia and, 317
  as antihypertensive therapy, 117-118
  TCA interaction with, 179-180
Diverticular disease, 143
Diverticulitis, 144
Diverticulosis, 142
DNR orders. *See* Do not resuscitate (DNR) orders
Do not resuscitate (DNR) orders, 350-351

Dolobid, in management of rheumatic disorders, 213, *214*
Dosage, in management of rheumatic disorders, 214
Dosing, *bid* vs. *tid* or *qid*, 213
Double voiding, 231
Douglas, cul-de-sac of, 239-240
Doxepin, 180
DRGs. *See* Diagnostic-related groups (DRGs)
Drug interactions, in management of rheumatic disorders, 215
Drug therapy. *See individually named agents*
DSM. *See Diagnostic and Statistical Manual of Mental Disorders* (DSM)
Duct pattern, breast cancer risk and, 56-57
Duodenal ulcer disease, 137
DuPont Lo-Dose system, 66-67
Dyspareunia, secondary, prevention of, 173
Dysphagia
  causes
    mechanical, 132-133
    neurologic, 132
  esophageal role, 131-132
  evaluation, 133
Dyspnea, hyperthyroidism and, 21
Dystrophy, vulvar, 292-295
Dysuria, causes of
  infectious, 250-251
  noninfectious, 250

E

Ears, in physical examination, 384
ECT. *See* Electroconvulsive shock therapy (ECT)
Educational programs, for elderly, 340-341
Elavil. *See* Amitryptyline
Elderly
  aged aged, 7, *8*
  distribution by residence, 10-11
  population statistics for, 3, *4*
  transportation for, 341-342

Electroconvulsive shock therapy (ECT), in treatment of depression, 178, 180
Elephantiasis, genital, 156
Emergency response system, 345
Empathy, vs. sympathy, 169
Emphysematous pyelonephritis, 253-255
    treatment for, 261
Emphysematous vaginitis, 309
End-tidal carbon dioxide, monitoring of, 319, 322
Endobronchial intubation, postoperative complications from, 326
Endocrine organ senescence, 17
Endometritis, tuberculous, pre- and postmenopausal symptoms compared, 157
Endoscopy
    of biliary and pancreatic tree, 136
    of colon, 136
    in dysphagic patients, 135
    gastrointestinal, 134-136
    lower esophageal pathology and, 135-136
    in treatment of renal calculi, 265-267
    upper intestinal, 135
Enterobacter infection, 250
Enterobius vermicularis, 159
Enterovaginal fistula, 152-153
Epiurethral suprapubic vaginal suspension (ESVS), 239
Epstein-Barr virus, in genital tract, 160
Escherichia coli infection, 250-251
    sepsis from atrophied gynecologic site and, 153-154
Esophagitis
    medicinal cause of, 132
    reflux, 132
Esophagus
    carcinoma of, 132
    described, 131-132
Estrogen
    breast cancer risk and
        natural, 53, 56
        therapy, 58
    as heart disease risk factor, 98
    osteoporosis and, 26
    secretion in obese women, 29
    as stroke risk factor, 101
    vaginal infections and, 304
        susceptibility reduction, 303-304
    vaginal transudate and, 300-301
Estrogen therapy
    breast cancer risk and, 58
    for incontinence, 231-232
    to raise calcitonin levels, 22
ESVS. *See* Epiurethral suprapubic vaginal suspension (ESVS)
ESWL. *See* Extracorporeal shock wave lithotripsy (ESWL)
Ethics committees, 351-352
European Working Party on High Blood Pressure in the Elderly (EWPHE), antihypertensive therapy benefits and, 105-106, *107*
    drugs vs. placebo, 106, 108
"Euthyroid sick" syndrome, 19
Evacuation, urinary, disorders of. *See* Urinary incontinence
Evaluation. *See* Geriatric evaluation
Evaluation unit, geriatric, 343-344
EWPHE. *See* European Working Party on High Blood Pressure in the Elderly (EWPHE)
Extracorporeal shock wave lithotripsy (ESWL), 266-267
Extraocular muscle paresis, 30
Extremities, in physical examination, 386
Eyes, in physical examination, 384

F

Family history, as heart disease risk factor, 99
Fecal impaction
    incidence of, 140
    management of, 139-140
Fees, attitudes toward, 11
Female. *See* Women
Fiber, constipation management and, 140-141
Fibroepithelial papillomas, 86
Fistula
    enterovaginal, 152-153

genital, 157-158
urinary vaginal. *See* Urinary vaginal fistula
Flavoxate, in treatment of incontinence, 232-233, *233*, 234
Fluoride, in treatment of osteoporosis, 205
Folding pessary, in treatment of incontinence, 234
Follicle-stimulating hormone (FSH), 29
  increase in, 17
  ovary and, 29
Fractures, 10
  osteoporotic, risk factors for, *204*
Framingham (Mass) Study, 96-97
Freckle, melanotic, 89-90
FSH. *See* Follicle-stimulating hormone (FSH)
Functional status, assessment of, 376-377, *378*
Funding, attitudes toward, 11
Fungal disease, as differential diagnosis in pyoderma gangrenosum, 158

G

Gamma benzene hexachloride, for treatment of infestations, 80
Gangrene, Meleney's synergistic, 158
Gardnerella vaginalis infection, 152, 250, 304
Gastric ulcers
  benign vs. malignant, 137
  hemorrhage, 137
  perforation, 137
Gastrointestinal endoscopy, 134-136
Gellhorn pessary, in treatment of incontinence, 234
Genital elephantiasis, 156
Genital tract
  fistulas of, 157-158
  maggots in, 158
  virus of, 160
  warts in, 79
Geriatric assessment. *See* Geriatric evaluation
Geriatric evaluation
  components of, 360-361
  atypical and complex disease presentation, 267, *368-369*, 370
  disease prevention
    primary and secondary, 370-372, *373-375*, 376
    tertiary, and functional status assessment, 376-377, *378*
  normal aging vs. pathological disease process, 361-362, *363-366*
  physical, psychological and social, 362, 367
  defined, 359
  origins of, 360
  specialized programs, 387-388
    effectiveness of, 388, *389*, 390-391
  unit for, 343-344
Glycosuria, elimination of, 36
GNP. *See* Gross national product (GNP)
Goiters, 21-22
Gonococcus, 153
Gout, 210-211
Granulosa-theca cell tumors, 30
Grave's disease
  hyperthyroidism and, 20
  hypothyroidism and, 20
Grave's ophthalmopathy, 20
Graying of America, Social Security and, 3
Griseofulvin, in treatment of tinea cruris, 78
Gross national product (GNP), health care costs and, 339
Growth hormone, changes in production, 17
Guanabenz, as antihypertensive therapy, 120
Guanethidine, as antihypertensive therapy, caution when using, 121
Gynecologic sepsis, 153-154
Gynecologist
  changing role of, 340
  visits to, 9

H

Hashimoto's thyroiditis, hypothyroidism and, 20
HDFP. *See* High Blood Pressure Detection and Follow-Up Program (HDFP)

Head, in physical examination, 384
Health care
  attitudes toward, 11-12
  costs, GNP and, 339
  in home. See Home health care
Health Insurance Plan of Greater New York (HIP), 45-50
Health problems. See Morbidity
Health services, use of, 9-10
Health status
  interacting components in, 362, 367
  and medical history, 380-381
  screening recommendations, 371-372, *373-375*, 376
Heart disease. See Cardiovascular disease
Heberden's nodes, 200
Hemoccult blood test, 142
Hemophilus sp.
  influenza, AIDS patients and, 161
  vaginalis infection, 304
Hemorrhage, rectal, as complication in diverticulitis, 144
Herpes simplex virus, 79
  AIDS patients and, 160
  in genital tract, 160
Herpes zoster virus, 79
High Blood Pressure Detection and Follow-Up Program (HDFP), *107*, 108-109
High-risk patients, 102
  See also Risk factors
HIP. See Health Insurance Plan of Greater New York (HIP)
Hirsutism, 29
Histamine$_2$ antagonists, as preoperative medication, 325-326
Histamine$_2$-receptor antagonists, as therapy for peptic ulcer disease, 137-138
Histiocytomas, 86
History taking
  jaundice, 133
  principles of, 377-378
    medical history components, 379-381, *382*
    physical environment, 378-379
    timing, 379

Histrionic personality disorder, 186
HIV screening, conditions indicating, 161
Home health care, 342-343
  elderly patient abuse and, 353-354
Hormones
  evaluation by vaginal smear, 301-303
  osteoporosis management with, 204-205
  in treatment of osteoporosis, 204-205
  See also individually named hormones
Hospitals
  average length of stay, 10
  discharge from, 10
    planning and placement, 342-343
  effect of aging population on, 9
  elderly patient abuse and, 353
  help opportunities, 344-345
  transport services, 342
Host defense, 151-152
Hutchinson, melanotic freckle of, 89-90
Hydralazine, as antihypertensive therapy, 120-121
17-Hydroxycorticoids (17-OCHS), 27-28
Hydroxyzine, as preoperative medication, 325
Hypercalcemia
  causes of, 24
  primary hyperparathyroidism, 23-25
Hyperglycemic hyperosmolar nonketotic coma, diabetes mellitus and, 33
Hyperparathyroidism, primary, 23-24
Hyperplastic dystrophy, vulvar, 82, 293-294
Hypertension
  anesthesia and, 315
  blood pressure evaluation, 93-94
  cardiovascular disease in females with, 96-97
  complications requiring immediate treatment, 112, *112*
  definitions, 95-96
  drug therapy for, 116-121
    See also individually named agents; Antihypertensive therapy
  following surgery, 329
  nonmedical or behavioral therapy for, *114*, 114

pseudohypertension, 121
  as risk factor in stroke and coronary
    artery disease, 104
  secondary, signs of, *112*, 113
  treatment recommendations in the
    elderly, 114-116
  trial findings, implications for
    patients, 109-110
Hyperthyroidism, 20-21
  therapy for, 21
Hypochondriasis, 189
Hypomagnesemia, correction of, 118
Hyponatremia, 18
Hypotension
  following surgery, 329
  orthostatic, 117
Hypothermia, during surgery, 322-323
Hypothyroidism, 19-20
  therapy for, 20
Hypoventilation, as postoperative
  complication, 327-328
Hypoxemia, as postoperative
  complication, 326
Hysterectomy, frequency of, 10

I

IADLs. *See* Instrumental activities of
  daily living (IADLs)
ICS. *See* International Continence
  Society (ICS)
Idiopathic myxedema, hypothyroidism
  and, 20
IL-2. *See* Interleukin-2 (IL-2)
Illness, depression accompanying, 178
Imidazoles
  for treatment of monilial intertrigo,
    78-79
  in treatment of tinea cruris, 78
Imipenem-cilastatin, 163
Imipramine, 180
  in treatment of incontinence, 232-233,
    233, 234
  for use with anxiety disorders, 191
Immune response, diminished,
  explanations for, 152
Immunizations, schedule for, *44*

Impedance, blood pressure and, 94
Impetigo vulgaris, 78
Implants, in surgical treatment of
  incontinence, 238-240
In re Jones, 352
Incontinence. *See* Urinary incontinence
"Incurables," 359
Indocin. *See* Indomethacin
Indomethacin, in treatment of gout, 210,
  214
Infant mortality, reduction in, 5
Infection
  of genitocrural area, 78-79
  and nutrition relationship, 149
  See also individually named infectious
    agents
Infertility, breast cancer risk and, 57
Infestation
  of genital tract by *D. hominis*,
    158
  of genitocrural area, 79-80
Informed consent, 349-350
Institutionalization, death rates and,
  171-172
  See also Hospitals
Instrumental activities of daily living
  (IADLs), 377
Insulin
  anesthesia and, 317
  role in genesis of diabetes, 34
  as therapy for diabetes mellitus, 35
  prescriptions, 35-36
Interleukin-2 (IL-2), in treatment of
  kidney tumors, 273
International Continence Society (ICS),
  221
International Prospective Primary
  Prevention Study of Hypertension
  (IPPPSH), *107*, 108
Interstitial cystitis
  treatment for, 260
  with vaginitis, 158-159
Intertrigo, 290
Intoxication, alcohol, 192-193
  idiosyncratic, 193
Intubation, endobronchial, postoperative
  complications from, 326

IPPPSH. *See* International Prospective Primary Prevention Study of Hypertension (IPPPSH)
Isoniazid, in therapy for pelvic tuberculosis, 156
Itching
skin. *See* Pruritic dermatoses
vulvar. *See* Pruritis vulvae

J

Jakob-Creutzfeldt disease, 181
Jaundice
care and evaluation of, 134
diagnostic tests, 134
patient history and, 133
physical examination in, 134
surgical causes for, 134

K

Karyopyknotic index, in hormonal evaluation, 301-302
Keratoses, seborrheic, vulval, 291
Ketamine, anesthesia and, 317
Ketoacidosis, diabetes mellitus and, 33
Ketoconazole, for herpes zoster infections, 79
Kidney tumors, 269
clinical presentation, 270
laboratory findings, 270, *271-273*
metastatic spread, 270
staging system, 271
treatment, 271-273
Kidneys
and changes in renal function, 95
diseases of, 121-122
tumors of. *See* Kidney tumors
See also renal entries
Kimmelstiel-Wilson lesion, 32
Klebsiella infection, 250

L

"La belle indifférence", 188
Labetalol, as antihypertensive therapy, 121

Laxatives, abuse of, 140-141
Legal competency, 348-349
Legal system, role of, 352-353
Length of stay (LOS), assessment program outcome and, 391
Lentigo, 291-292
Leukemias, 89
LH. *See* Luteinizing hormone (LH)
Liability claims, 347-348
Lichen planus, 77
Lichen sclerosus
et atrophicus, 82
vulval, 292-293
Life care, concept of, 345
Life expectancy, 3-4
male vs. female, 4-7
Life-sustaining treatment, withdrawal of, 351
Lindane, for treatment of infestations, 80
Lithium
anesthesia and, 317
in treatment of depression, 180
Lithotripsy
extracorporeal shock wave, 266-267
percutaneous, 265-266
Liver function tests, jaundice and, 134
LOS. *See* Length of stay (LOS)
Loss
as concept of menopause, 175
social, depression and, 176
Loxosceles spider bite, 158
Luteinizing hormone (LH), 29
ovary and, 29
Lymph nodes, tumors in, 52-53
Lymphedema, 156
Lymphomas, 89

M

Maggots, in genital tract, 158
Magnetic resonance imaging (MRI), 334, 335
MAI. *See* Mycobacterium avium intracellular (MAI)
Malakoplakia, 155-156
Male
life expectancy of, 4-7

nursing home residential rates, 9
widowerhood rates, 172
Malignancy, 86-90
    characteristic cells, 52
    as differential diagnosis in pyoderma gangrenosum, 158
    gastric ulcers, 137
    See also individually named tumors
Malignant melanoma, 88
Malnutrition
    correction of, 147, 149
    pathways leading to, *148*
Malpractice claims, 348
Mammography, 39-74
    evolution of, 65-67
    guidelines for, 69-70
    major screening programs, 45
    misconceptions about, 51
    physician ordering frequency, 70-71
    problems associated with, 45
    public opinions about, 71
    screening, 45, 64-65
        recent investigation, 47-49
    vs. breast palpation, 42
    x-ray carcinogenesis and, 50
    See also Breast cancer
MAO. *See* Monoamine oxidase (MAO)
Marital status, breast cancer risk and, 57
Mass spectrometer, 319, 322
Mastectomy, 62-63
    radical. *See* Radical mastectomy
Maturation index, in hormonal evaluation, 302
Maturation value, in hormonal evaluation, 302
Mechanical vaginitis, 308-309
Medical day-care centers, 344
Medical examination, 9
    periodic schedule for women, *44*
Medical history, in patient history, 379-381
Medical Research Council (MRC), antihypertensive therapy benefits and, 106, *107*, 108
Medication
    and nutrition, 149
    preoperative, 323-326
    See also individually named drugs
Melanoma
    freckle of Hutchinson, 89-90
    malignant, 88
Meleney's synergistic gangrene, as differential diagnosis in pyoderma gangrenosum, 158
Menarche, breast cancer risk and, 53, 59
Menopause
    breast cancer risk and, 53, 59
    complaint etiology, 174
    early psychoanalyst views of, 173
    psychological factors involved, 174-175
    societal expectations and, 174
    socioeconomic factors involved, 175
    symptoms attributed to, 174
Meperidine
    in management of renal colic, 262
    as preoperative medication, 325
Metastases, 88
    bladder cancer, 277
    malignant melanoma prognosis and, 88
    and melanotic freckle of Hutchinson, 89-90
    renal cell carcinoma, 270
Methyldopa, as antihypertensive therapy, 120
Methylphenidate, TCA interaction with, 179-180
Metronidazole, in treatment of trichomonas vaginitis, 308
Mezlocillin, 163
Microangiopathy, 32
Mild hypertension, defined, 95-96
Minoxidil, as antihypertensive therapy, 120-121
Mixed dystrophy, vulvar, 294-295
Mixed incontinence, 222
    predisposing factors, *225*
    treatment modalities for, 242-243
Moderate hypertension, defined, 96
Molluscum contagiosum virus, 79
    AIDS patients and, 160
    in genital tract, 160
Monilial intertrigo, 78-79

Monilial vulvovaginitis, 306-307
Monitoring, intra-operative standards, 319, *320-321*
Monoamine oxidase (MAO) inhibitors
 anesthesia and, 316, *316*
 in treatment of depression, 178, 180
Morbidity, women, 7-8
Morphea, 80
Morphine, as preoperative medication, 325
Mortality
 assessment program outcome and, 391
 declining rates, 6-7
 infant, reduction in, 5
 radical mastectomy and, *63*
 See also Death rates; Deaths
Moxalactam, 163
MRC. See Medical Research Council (MRC)
Muscle wasting, 30
Musculoskeletal problems. See Rheumatic disorders
Myasthenia gravis, dysphagia in, 132
Mycobacterium avium intracellular (MAI), AIDS patients and, 160
Mycostatin. See Nystatin
Myiasis, in genital tract, 158
Mythramycin, use in hypercalcemia, 24

N

Nalidixic acid, 164
Naprosyn, in management of rheumatic disorders, 213, *214*
Narcissistic personality disorder, 186
National Cancer Institute Surveillance, Epidemiology, and End Results Program (SEER), 53
Neglect, 170
Neighborhoods, 11
Neisseria gonorrhea infection, 250, 255
Neomycin, for herpes zoster infections, 79
Nephropathy, diabetic, 32
Neurodermatitis, 76-77
Neurologic examination, in diagnostic evaluation of incontinence, 228
Neurologic system, in physical examination, 386-387

Neuropathy, in diabetes mellitus, 31
 autonomic, 30
 unusual syndromes of, 30
Nevi
 nevocytic, 85
 vulval, 291
NIDDM. See Noninsulin-dependent diabetes mellitus (NIDDM)
No-code orders, 350-351
Nocardia sp., AIDS patients and, 160
Noninsulin-dependent diabetes mellitus (NIDDM), 30
Nonsteroidal anti-inflammatory drugs (NSAIDs)
 in management of rheumatic disorders, 212, *213*
 adverse effects, 213-214
 dosage, 214
 drug interactions, 215
 generalizations, 215
 in specific conditions, *214*
 ulcers and, 137
Norfloxacillin, 164
Norpramin. See Desipramine
Nose, in physical examination, 384
NSAIDs. See Nonsteroidal anti-inflammatory drugs (NSAIDs)
Nursing homes
 effect of aging population on, 9
 marital status, 10
 residential rates, 10
 men vs. women, 9
Nutrition
 and decreased ability to eat, 147
 and gut disorders, 147
 infection susceptibility and, 149
 medication effect on, 149
 recommended daily intake in U.K., *148*
 status assessment, 147, *147*
Nystatin, for treatment of monilial intertrigo, 78-79

O

OAF. See Osteoclast activating factor (OAF)

Obesity, as heart disease risk factor, 100
Obsessive-compulsive disorder, 190
Ofloxacin, 164
OHCS. See 17-Hydroxycorticoids (17-OHCS)
Oral contraceptives, breast cancer risk and, 57-58, *58*
Orthostatic hypotension, 117
Osteoarthritis (OA), 200
  clinical course, 200-201
  common sites, *201*
  treatment program, 201-202
Osteoclast activating factor (OAF), hypercalcemia secondary to, 24
Osteoporosis, 202
  clinical picture, 203
  defined, 25
  differential diagnosis/laboratory testing, 203
  fractures, risk factors for, *204*
  management, 26-27, 203-204
    with fluoride, 205
    with hormones, 204-205
  pathogenesis, 203
  predisposing factors, 25
  syndromes of, 25-26
Ovary, 29-30
  abscess, 154-155
  tumors of, 30
Overflow incontinence, 222
  predisposing factors, *226*
  treatment modalities for, 241-243, *242*
Oxybutynin, in treatment of incontinence, 232-233, *233*, 234
Oxygenation, in intra-operative monitoring standards, *320-321*
Oxyphencyclimine, in treatment of incontinence, 232-233, *233*, 234

P

Paget's disease, 83, 205
  clinical picture, 205-206
Pain
  abdominal, 144
  evaluation of, 198-199
  following surgery, control of, 329-330

Palpation, of breasts, vs. mammography, 42
Palpitations, hyperthyroidism and, 21
Panic disorders, 190-191
Pap test, 9, 43, 371-372
Papillary carcinoma, 22
Papillary necrosis, 253-254, *254*
  treatment for, 261
Papovavirus, in genital tract, 160
Papulosquamous dermatoses, 77
Paranoid disorders, 183-184
Paranoid personality disorder, 185
Paraphrenia, 185
Parathormone, 23
Parathyroid, 23-25
  osteoporosis, 25-27
Parity, breast cancer risk and, 57
Parkinson's disease, dysphagia in, 132
Paroxysms, 28-29
Passive-aggressive personality disorder, 187
Patient history. See History taking
PDR. See *Physician's Desk Reference*
Pediculosis pubis, 80
Pelvis
  actinomycosis of organs of, 159
  examination of, in diagnostic evaluation of incontinence, 228
  in physical examination, 385
  postmenopausal tuberculosis of, 156, *157*
Pemphigus vulgaris, vulval, 288-289
Penicillin, 163
Peptic ulcer disease, 137-138
Percutaneous lithotripsy, in treatment of renal calculi, 265-266
Personality disorders, 185-187
  vs. personality traits, 185
Personality traits, personality disorders vs., 185
Pessary
  infection associated with, 155
  in treatment of incontinence, 234-235
Peutz-Jeghers syndrome, 55
Phenylpropanolamine, in treatment of incontinence, 234
Pheochromocytomas, 28-29

Phobias, 190
Phosphate therapy, in hypercalcemia, 24
Physical environment, in patient history, 378-379
Physical examination, 381-382
　abdomen and pelvis, 385
　extremities, 386
　general appearance and vital signs, 382-383
　head, eyes, ears, nose and throat, 384
　neurologic system, 386-387
　skin, 383-384
　thorax and cardiovascular system, 384-385
Physical status, ASA guidelines for assessing, *315*, 315-317
Physician visits, number of, 9
Physician's Desk Reference, dosage recommendations in, 214
Physiologic function, changes with age, 314, *314*
Pick's disease, 182
Pinworm. *See Enterobius vermicularis*
Piperacillin, 163
Pituitary, 17-18
Placebo, in antihypertensive therapy trials, 106, *107*, 108
Plasma osmolality, 18
Podiatry, need for, 30
Polymyalgia rheumatica
　clinical picture, 206
　diagnosis, 206
　prognosis, 207
　therapy, 206-207
Polyps, colorectal, 142
Postmenopausal osteoporosis, 25-26
Postmenopausal tubo-ovarian abscess, 154-155
Posttraumatic stress disorder, 190
Prazosin, as antihypertensive therapy, caution when using, 121
Prednisone, in treatment of polymyalgia rheumatica, 207
Pregnancy, first, breast cancer risk and, 57, *57*
Preoperative medication, 323-326
Pressure ulcers, 157

Primaxin. *See* Imipenem-cilastatin
Privacy, abuse of, 353
Progesterone, production after menopause, 29
Prognosis committees, 351-352
Prolactin, 17
　breast cancer risk and, 53
Propoxyphene, in management of rheumatic disorders, 211
Prostaglandins, NSAIDs effect on, 212
Proteus mirabilis infection, 250-251
Providencia stuartii infection, 250-251
Prozazan, in therapy for interstitial cystitis, 159
Pruritic dermatoses, 75
　dermatitis, 75-77
　infections and infestations, 78-80
　lichen sclerosus et atrophicus, 82
　papulosquamous, 77
Pruritis vulvae, 92
　differential diagnosis, *90*
　management, *91*
Pseudogout, 211
Pseudohypertension, 121
Pseudomonas sp.
　aeruginosa infection, 250-251
　cephalosporins against, 163
　penicillin against, 163
Pseudotumors, xanthogranulomatous, 155-156
Psoriasis, 77
　vulval, 288
Psychiatric evaluation
　assessment rules, 170-171
　components in, 170
　diagnostic categories
　　adjustment disorders, 187-188
　　anxiety disorders, 189-191
　　bereavement, uncomplicated, 188
　　delirium, 182-183
　　dementia, 180-182
　　depression, 175-180
　　paranoid disorders, 183-184
　　personality disorders, 185-187
　　schizophrenia, 184-185
　　somatoform disorders, 188-189
　　substance abuse, 191-194

diagnostic issues, 171
treatment issues, 171-172
Pulse oximeter, 319
Pyelonephritis
   acute and chronic, 251-252, *252*
   defined, 251
   emphysematous. *See* Emphysematous pyelonephritis
   findings in, 257
   treatment for, 260-261
Pyoderma gangrenosum, of genitalia, 158
Pyogenic granuloma, 86
Pyomyoma, 155
Pyuria, 253

Q

Q-Tip test, in diagnostic evaluation of incontinence, 228
Quadrantectomy, 64
Quinolones, 163-164

R

RA. *See* Rheumatoid arthritis (RA)
Race
   as heart disease risk factor, 100
   as stroke risk factor, 102
Radiation
   cost benefit of, 335
   mammography and, 50
   therapy, mastectomy and, 64
   See also X-ray carcinogenesis
Radical mastectomy, 63-64
   disease-free survival rates, *65*
   modified, 64
   mortality rates, *63*
Radioactive iodine, in hyperthyroidism therapy, 21
Radiography, 334
Radiology. *See* Diagnostic imaging
Ranitidine, as preoperative medication, 325-326
Recovery room, 326-328
   hypertension in, 329
   hypotension in, 329
   pain control in, 329-330
Rectal bleeding, 141-146
   causes of, 142
   management of, 145, *145*
Rectal temperature, during surgery, *323*
Referral, source of, 343
Reflex incontinence, 222
   drugs used to treat, *233*
   predisposing factors, *226*
   treatment modalities for, 241-243, *242*
Reflux esophagitis, 132
Regional syndromes
   clinical course, 209-210
   common sites, *209*
   management, 210
Reinfection, defined, 251
Relapse, defined, 251
Renal calculi
   current treatments, 263
      drugs, 263-264
      endoscopic procedures, 265-267
      surgery, 264-265
   and renal colic management, 262
Renal cell carcinoma. *See* Kidney tumors
Renal colic, management of, 262
Renal disease, 122-123
Renal failure, acute, 122
Renal function
   calcium metabolism and, 122
   changes with aging, 95
Reserpine, as antihypertensive therapy, caution when using, 121
Residence, of elderly
   county, 11
   neighborhoods, 11
   state, 10-11
Residuals, in diagnostic evaluation of incontinence, 228-229
Resistance, blood pressure and, 94
Respiratory depression, as postoperative complication, 327
Retinopathy, diabetic, 32
Retropubic operations, 237-238
Retzius, space of, 239
Rheumatic disorders
   anatomical sites, *199*
   case discussions, 215-217

classification, 197, *198*
crystal deposition, 210-211
degenerative arthritis/osteoarthritis, 200-202
differential diagnosis, 197-198
interview, 198-199
physical examination, 199-200
osteoporosis, 202-205
Paget's disease, 205-206
pharmacologic management, 211-215
polymyalgia rheumatica, 206-207
regional syndromes, 209-210
rheumatoid arthritis, 207-208
systemic lupus erythematosus, 208-209
Rheumatoid arthritis (RA), 207
clinical picture, 207-208
treatment, 208
Rifampin, in therapy for pelvic tuberculosis, 156
Risk factors
for breast cancer, 53, 55-59
for cardiovascular disease, 98-100, *103*
and high-risk patients defined, 102
multiple, principle of, *102*, 102-104
for stroke, 100-102

S

Salicylates, in management of rheumatic disorders, 212-213
Sarcoptes scabiei, 79-80
Scabies, 79-80
Schizoid personality disorder, 185
Schizophrenia, 184-185
Schizotypal personality disorder, 185-186
Scleroderma, dysphagia and, 133
Screening tests
cancer, 371-372, *373*
general health, *373-375*
mammography, 45
schedule for, *44*
Seborrheic dermatitis, vulval, 286-287
Seborrheic keratoses, vulval, 291
SEER. *See* National Cancer Institute Surveillance, Epidemiology, and End Results Program (SEER)

Self-determination, abuse of, 353
Self-esteem, 169
Self-examination, of breast, 51-52
Senile osteoporosis, 26
Senograph, 66
Sepsis, gynecologic, 153-154
Septic shock, 253
Serratia marcescens infection, 250-251
Serum cholesterol
as heart disease risk factor, 99-100
as stroke risk factor, 102
Severe hypertension, defined, 96
Sexual activity, genital involutional change retardation and, 173
Sexuality, 172-173
Sickle cell trait, urinary tract infection and, 254
Sigmoid volvulus, 141
Silent period, breast cancer detection during, *66*
Sinequan. *See* Doxepin
Sitophagia, 144
Skin, in physical examination, 383-384
SLE. *See* Systemic lupus erythematosus (SLE)
Sleep apnea, 113
Sleep patterns, evaluation of, 170
Smears
pap. *See* Pap test
vaginal, for hormonal evaluation, 301-303
Smith-Hodge pessary, in treatment of incontinence, 234
Social history, in patient history, *382*
Social phobias, 190
Social Security, elderly population and, 3
Social work service, 342-343
Sodium cromoglyceate, in therapy for interstitial cystitis, 159
Sodium fluoride, osteoporosis and, 27
Solid tumors, 85-86
Somatoform disorders
conversion, 188-189
hypochondriasis, 189
pain, 189
Space of Retzius, 239
Sphincterotomy, endoscopic, 136

Spider bite, *Loxosceles*, 158
Spinsterhood, breast cancer risk and, 57
Squamous cell carcinoma, 87
Staphylococcus sp., 250
  aureus
    cephalosporins against, 162
    penicillin against, 163
  epidermidis, cephalosporin resistant, 162
Steroids
  anesthesia and, 317
  in management of rheumatic disorders, 211
Stone disease. *See* Renal calculi; Urinary calculi
Storage, urinary, disorders of. *See* Urinary incontinence
Streptococcus pneumoniae infection, cephalosporins against, 162
Stress incontinence, 222
  drugs used to treat, *233*
  predisposing factors, *224*
  treatment modalities for, 241-243, *242*
Stroke
  depression following, 178
  risk factors for elderly women, 100-102
  See also Cardiovascular disease
Substance abuse, 191-194
Suprainfection, defined, 251
Surgery
  ambulatory care and, 318-319
  ASA intra-operative monitoring standards and, 319, *320-321*
  discharge planning and placement, 342-343
  hypertension following, 329
  hypotension following, 329
  pain control following, 329-330
  preoperative medication, 323-326
  recovery room and, 326-328
  temperature control during, 322-323, *324*
  for treatment of incontinence, 235
    postoperative bladder drainage, 240-241
    preliminary considerations, 235-237
    synthetic alternatives, 238-240
  technical considerations, 237-238
  for treatment of renal calculi, 264-265
Survivorship, 6
Swallowing, difficulty in. *See* Dysphagia
Sweet's disease, as differential diagnosis in pyoderma gangrenosum, 158
Systemic lupus erythematosus (SLE), 208-209
Systolic blood pressure
  evaluation, 93-94
  as heart disease risk factor, 98-99
  rise with age, 96
  as stroke risk factor, 101, *101*
  wasted cardiac work and, 96, *97*
Systolic hypertension, definitions of, 96

T

T_4. *See* Thyroxine (T_4)
TA. *See* Temporal arteritis (TA)
Target organ damage
  as heart disease risk factor, 98
  as stroke risk factor, 100
TCAs. *See* Tricyclic antidepressants (TCAs)
Technetium scanning, 334
Temperature, of body
  control, 322-323, *324*
  in intra-operative monitoring standards, *321*
Temporal arteritis (TA), polymyalgia rheumatica and, 207
Tensilon, in dysphagia treatment, 132
Thermography, 67-68
Thermoregulation. *See* Temperature, of body
Thiazide diuretics, as antihypertensive therapy, 117-118
Thorax, in physical examination, 384-385
Throat, in physical examination, 384
Thyroid, 18-22
  goiters and cancer, 21-22
  hyperthyroidism, 20-21
  hypothyroidism, 19-20
Thyroid iodine uptake, 19

Thyroid-stimulating hormone (TSH), 18-19
  in hypothyroidism, 19-20
Thyrotropin. *See* Thyroid-stimulating hormone (TSH)
Thyrotropin-releasing hormone (TRH), 19
Thyroxine (T_4), 18
  hyperthyroidism and, 21
Ticarcillin, 163
Timing, in patient history, 379
Tinea cruris, 78
TOA. *See* Tubo-ovarian abscess (TOA)
Tofranil. *See* Imipramine
Tort liability claims, 347
Touching, 169
Toxic shock syndrome (TSS), 160
Transillumination, 69
Transportation, for elderly, 341-342
Transudate, vaginal, 300-301
TRH. *See* Thyrotropin-releasing hormone (TRH)
Trichomonas vaginalis infection, 152, 250, 307-308
Trichomonas vaginitis, 307-308
Tricophyton rubrum, 78
Tricyclic antidepressants (TCAs)
  anesthesia and, 316-317, *317*
  antipsychotic medication and, 184
  in treatment of depression, 178-180
Trilisate, in management of rheumatic disorders, 213, *214*
TSH. *See* Thyroid-stimulating hormone (TSH)
TSS. *See* Toxic shock syndrome (TSS)
Tuberculosis
  AIDS patients and, 160
  postmenopausal pelvic, 156, *157*
Tubo-ovarian abscess (TOA), postmenopausal, 154-155
Tumors
  breast, 43, 52-53
    See also Breast cancer
  cystic, 86
  kidney. *See* Kidney tumors
  ovarian, 30
  pituitary, 18
  solid, 85-86
  vulvar, 83, 85-90
Tympanic membrane temperature, *324*

U

Ulcerative colitis, 146
Ulcers
  duodenal, 137
  gastric, 137
  incidence in elderly, 136-137
  peptic, 137-138
  pressure, 157
Ultrasonography, 335
  in breast cancer detection, 68-69
Uncomplicated bereavement, 188
Urethral caruncle, 290-291
Urethritis, 255
  infectious causes of, 250
  treatment for, 257-258
Urge incontinence, 222
  drugs used to treat, *233*
  predisposing factors, *225*
  treatment modalities for, 241-243, *242*
Urinary calculi, 261-262
  initial presentation, 262, *263*
Urinary frequency
  infectious causes of, 250-251
  noninfectious causes of, 250
Urinary incontinence
  acute, 222-223
  chronic, 223-226
    evacuation disorders, 225-226
    storage disorders, 223-225
  classification of, 221-222, *222-223*
  diagnostic evaluation, 226-231
  predisposing factors, 222-226
  treatment modalities, 231-243, *242*
  vs. vaginitis, 153
Urinary lithiasis. *See* Urinary calculi
Urinary tract infection, 121-122
  bacterial colonization and infection, 248-249
  clinical course and symptoms, 249-257
  complications from, 253-255
  immune function and, 249
  lower, 252-253

mechanical factors, 247-248
pathogenesis, 249
treatment, 257-261
Urinary vaginal fistula, 267
  cure rates, 269
  localization, 267-268
  symptoms and diagnosis, 267
  treatment, 268-269
Urispas. *See* Flavoxate
Urodynamic investigation, in diagnostic evaluation of incontinence, 229-231
Uroflometry, in diagnostic evaluation of incontinence, 230
Urosepsis, 253
Uteroscopy, in treatment of renal calculi, 265
Uterus
  bleeding from, TOA and, 154
  and hysterectomy frequency, 10

V

VA Cooperative trial, antihypertensive therapy benefits and, 105-106, *107*
Vagina
  anatomy, 299-300
  atrophy of, 299
  ecology, 303-304
  flora, changes with age, 152
  infections, 304-308
  noninfectious inflammation of, 308-309
  physiology, 300-303
  smears for hormonal evaluation, 301-303
Vaginal colpopexy, 238
Vaginismus, prevention of, 173
Vaginitis
  atrophic, 299
  conditions confused with, 152-153
  G. vaginalis, 152
  genitourinary infections and, 255
  interstitial cystitis with, 158-159
  noninfectious
    emphysematous, 309
    mechanical and chemical, 308-309
  T. vaginalis, 152
  treatment for, 257
  trichomonas, 307-308
Vaginosis, bacterial, 304-305

Valsalva maneuver, 228
Vasculitis, as differential diagnosis in pyoderma gangrenosum, 158
Vasodilators, as antihypertensive therapy, 120-121
Vasopressin-secreting neurons, 18
Ventilation, in intra-operative monitoring standards, *321*
Virus. *See individually named viruses*
Vital signs, in physical examination, 382-383
Vitamin D
  intoxication, 24-25
  osteoporosis and, 27
Vitiligo, 80
Voiding, frequency of, 231
Vulva
  age-associated pathology
    bullous pemphigoid, 289-290
    contact dermatitis, 285-286
    intertrigo, 290
    lentigo, 291-292
    nevi, 291
    pemphigus vulgaris, 288-289
    psoriasis, 288
    seborrheic dermatitis, 286-287
    seborrheic keratoses, 291
    urethral caruncle, 290-291
    vulvovaginal candidiasis, 287-288
  carcinoma in situ, 83
  dystrophies of, 81-82, 292
    hyperplastic, 293-294
    lichen sclerosus, 292-293
    mixed, 294-295
  normal aging process, 283-285
  normal changes, 81
  plaques, differential diagnosis of, 83, *84*
  pruritic. *See* Pruritis vulvae
  tumors of, 83, 85-90
Vulvitis, vs. vaginitis, 153
Vulvovaginal candidiasis, 287-288

W

Warts, genital, 79
Wasted cardiac work, 96, *97*

Water exercise therapy (WET), in treatment of rheumatoid arthritis, 208
WET. *See* Water exercise therapy (WET)
Whipple's disease, 155-156
Widowerhood, rates for, 172
Widowhood, rates for, 172
Withdrawal
  of life-sustaining treatment, 351
  substance abuse and, 193-194
Women
  health services use by, 9-10
  life expectancy of, 4-7
  morbidity, 7-8
  widowhood rates, 172

X

X-ray carcinogenesis, mammography and, 50
Xanthogranulomatous pseudotumors, 155-156
Xeromammography, 67

Z

Zenker's diverticulum, 132
Zoster-varicella virus, 79